Reiki in Clinical Practice
A science-based guide

Reiki in Clinical Practice
A science-based guide

Ann Baldwin PhD

Professor of Physiology, Educator Scholar Track,
University of Arizona, Arizona, USA

Forewords
James L Oschman
Gary E Schwartz

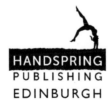

HANDSPRING
PUBLISHING
EDINBURGH

HANDSPRING PUBLISHING LIMITED
The Old Manse, Fountainhall,
Pencaitland, East Lothian
EH34 5EY, Scotland
Tel: +44 1875 341 859
Website: www.handspringpublishing.com

First published 2020 in the United Kingdom by Handspring Publishing

ISBN 978-1-912085-36-1
ISBN (Kindle eBook) 978-1-912085-37-8

British Library Cataloguing in Publication Data
A catalogue record for this book is available from the British Library
Library of Congress Cataloguing in Publication Data
A catalog record for this book is available from the Library of Congress

Commissioning Editor Mary Law
Project Manager Morven Dean
Copy-editor Kathryn Mason Pak
Designer Bruce Hogarth
Indexer Aptara, India
Typesetter Amnet, India
Printer CPI Group (UK) Ltd, Croydon, CR0 4YY

The
Publisher's
policy is to use
paper manufactured
from sustainable forests

CONTENTS

FOREWORD by James L. Oschman

Reiki in Clinical Practice: A science-based guide represents a milestone in the history of integrative medicine. Its author, Dr Ann Baldwin, is one of the most important and creative academic scientists to investigate an extremely popular and widely used healing method. Reiki has now been incorporated into clinical and hospital settings, including many of the top research hospitals around the world. This book is an invaluable resource as it shows how the science of energetics may be used to heal conditions that conventional medicine has difficulty treating.

Ann's willingness to become a practitioner of Reiki and delve into its scientific basis first-hand benefits all of us who work on the science and application of holistic therapies. Dr Baldwin is a true academic, as she places high demands on herself for scientific accuracy. Everywhere I look inside this book I see clear, scientifically correct, and very well illustrated information describing the logical basis for Ann's therapeutic successes. Everyone who prac-

tices and benefits from Reiki will find here precious information and insights.

There are literally thousands of books on Reiki, a fact that attests to the enthusiasm its practitioners have for their work. The major reasons for their enthusiasm are the remarkable benefits they see every day in their practices. Many curious patients want to know why they feel so much better or calmer after a Reiki treatment, and every practitioner wants to have good and accurate answers for them. And every delighted patient contributes to the emergence of a brighter future for our healthcare systems. Good news travels fast!

The brilliant book you are holding in your hands is destined to be the classic resource for the field.

James L. Oschman PhD
Author of *Energy Medicine: The scientific basis*

FOREWORD by Gary E. Schwartz

How many university professors of physiology and psychology exist who

1. are skilled in controlled laboratory research

2. have received substantial basic science funding from the National Institutes of Health, *and*

3. have developed strong clinical skills in practicing mind-body and energy medicine as well?

In my fifty years of having served on the faculties of Harvard University, Yale University, and the University of Arizona, I know of only one such person, and she is Dr Ann Baldwin, the author of this comprehensive and visionary book on the science and practice of Reiki.

I have had the opportunity to witness Ann's inspiring Reiki journey, from her early experiences with Reiki healing, through her emerging basic and applied Reiki research with animals and humans (as well as with other healing techniques such as Reconnective Healing), to her creating a parallel private mind-body and energy healing practice. Ann's response to Reiki has been like a duck's response to water, completely natural and seemingly effortless. Ann has a special affinity and appreciation for the science and practice of Reiki, and this historic book honors this important proclivity.

As cited in the references in Ann's Preface, I have had the privilege to collaborate with Ann on some of her basic and applied Reiki research. The truth is that if any laboratory research has convinced me that energy healing is more than just spontaneous remission or patient expectations and placebo effects, it is our controlled animal research made possible by Ann's background in physiology and biophysics.

Being an animal lover myself, I deeply appreciate Ann's sensitivities and compassion for animals' energies and feelings, regardless of whether they are laboratory rats, house cats, or stable horses. Ann's precious combination of intellectual, emotional, and intuitive qualities has resulted in this seminal book.

Reiki in Clinical Practice: A science-based guide serves skilled clinicians as well as novices, and it deserves to be celebrated.

Gary E. Schwartz PhD
Professor of Psychology, Medicine,
Neurology, Psychiatry, and Surgery,
University of Arizona; his books include
*The Energy Healing Experiments:
Science reveals our natural power to heal*

PREFACE

I am a professor of physiology at the University of Arizona and up until the late 1990s my research was focused on the mechanisms of transport of large molecules between blood and tissue. This topic is important regarding intravenous drug delivery as well as the development of disorders such as atherosclerosis (hardening of the arteries) and inflammation. To investigate the regulation of blood-tissue transport processes, I experimented on rats. So why have I written a book about Reiki in clinical practice? My interest in Reiki was actually triggered by a young woman who I hired as an assistant to help me with data analysis. She happened to be a Reiki Master. She was very enthusiastic about Reiki and it was not long before she persuaded me to try a session. I had never heard of Reiki prior to meeting her but I was open to learning more. A little later I agreed that she could train me to Reiki level one. However, even after the training I was skeptical about it and not convinced that the Reiki was actually having any significant beneficial effects on me or on other people on whom I practiced.

At this time, I discovered that my experimental rats were showing signs of stress after being moved from one animal facility to another. They were becoming more aggressive towards each other and they also exhibited signs of inflammation, including cellular damage, in the intestine. The stress response seemed to be associated with the extra noise and high levels of human activity in the new animal facility. I knew it was vital for the rats' well-being and for the integrity of the research that I find some way of reducing the stress. It was then that my assistant suggested that we apply for a grant to test whether performing Reiki on the rats would reduce the intestinal inflammation. The National Institutes of Health had recently incorporated a new institute in their research-funding center, called National Center for Complementary and Alternative Medicine (NCCAM) and so we submitted a grant proposal entitled: "Animal model in Reiki efficacy on stress-induced damage". As a result, we received funding for two years to study the effects of Reiki on rats stressed by environmental noise.

Our funded Reiki research showed that Reiki significantly reduced the stress-induced intestinal inflammation and resulted in two published peer-reviewed papers (Baldwin and Schwartz, 2006; Baldwin et al., 2008). The fact that Reiki can work on animals, even rats, to reduce their stress and to heal cellular damage, convinced me that the Reiki was working. For me, these experiments were a turning point in my career. I took the huge step of giving up my full-time tenured position at the University of Arizona so that I could devote some time to helping people reduce their stress with Reiki. I trained to Reiki Master level, started my business, Mind-Body-Science, became editor-in-chief of the Center for Reiki Research, and also continued part-time at the University of Arizona as an active researcher.

As a scientist and as a provider of Reiki to people experiencing stress-related problems, I was delighted when invited by Mary Law, Director and Co-Owner of Handspring Publishing Ltd, to write this book, *Reiki in Clinical Practice*. This book is for people who are looking for a non-invasive, inexpensive, and effective modality to use on themselves and/or their patients to reduce stress and pain and to improve well-being. This book is for people who are open-minded and who endorse treatments and techniques that are evidence-based. This book is for people who want a practical guide on how to optimize the practice of Reiki, and who want to know which populations benefit the most from Reiki. This book is for people who want advice on how to choose a Reiki practitioner; or who need a guide to help them set up their own Reiki program.

In this book I define Reiki, describe its advantages and benefits, and present a critical evaluation of the clinical research. I touch on some theories of how Reiki may work but I focus mainly on the practical aspects of Reiki. For what conditions is Reiki most likely to be beneficial? What constitutes a good Reiki session? How can you improve your Reiki practice? I address all the various physical and emotional issues that Reiki has been claimed to alleviate, and systematically evaluate the robustness of the data. I want to provide clinicians and other healthcare professionals with enough details to make choices that will most benefit their patients and themselves. In order for Reiki to become widely available to all those who need it, Reiki programs need to be set up in most hospitals. For that reason, a detailed guide on the practicalities of setting up and running Reiki programs in hospitals is included in the book.

I believe that Reiki has now earned its place in modern healthcare as an adjunct to allopathic medicine and that it should be widely available to patients and clients who are experiencing stress or pain. I hope that this book will ignite an interest in Reiki in readers who work in clinical settings and will provide them with the information and guidance

that they need to make Reiki available to their patients and clients.

Ann Baldwin
Tucson, Arizona, USA
July 2019

References

Baldwin AL, Schwartz GE. Personal interaction with a Reiki practitioner decreases noise-induced microvascular damage in an animal model. *Journal of Alternative and Complementary Medicine* 2006; 12(1): 15–22.

Baldwin AL, Wagers C, Schwartz GE. Reiki improves heart rate homeostasis in laboratory rats. *Journal of Alternative and Complementary Medicine* 2008; 14(4): 417–422.

ACKNOWLEDGMENTS

I would like to thank all the people in my town Tucson, Arizona and beyond who supported me during my switch to Reiki, and all those who believe that science and Reiki are mutually compatible.

FIGURE PERMISSIONS

Figure 1.3 From: Leadbetter CW. *The Chakras. A Monograph.* First Edition. The Theosophical Publishing House, Wheaton, Ill, USA; London, England, 1927. Plate IX.

Figure 1.4 From: http://rexresearch.com/korotkov/korotkov.htm.

Figures 2.3–2.7 From: https://hartfordhospital.org/services/integrative-medicine/patient-support/outcomes.

Figure 3.1 From: Lock and Key Theory - Chemistry@Elmhurst - Elmhurst College chemistry. elmhurst.edu/vchembook/571lockkey.html.

Figure 3.2 From: http://www.uq.edu.au/_School_Science_Lessons/UNPh29.html#29.1.1H.

Figure 3.7 From: Bentov I. Micromotion of the body as a factor in the development of the nervous system. In Sannella L. (Ed.), Kundalini: Psychosis or Transendence? Integral Publishing, Lower Lake, CA, 1976 (appendix A).

Figure 3.8 From: Becker RO. *Cross Currents: The Perils of Electric Pollution, the Promise of Electromedicine.* Jeremy P. Tarcher, Los Angeles, CA, USA, 1999. p. 80 (Figs 3-4).

Figure 3.9 From Dr. John Zimmerman.

Figure 4.5 From Rubik B, Brooks AJ, Schwartz GE. In vitro effect of Reiki treatment on bacterial cultures: Role of experimental context and practitioner well-being. *Journal of Alternative and Complementary Medicine* 2006; 12(1): 7–13.

Figure 4.6 From: Coherence and the New Science of Breath. Copyright 2006 COHERENCE L.L.C.

Figure 5.4 From: Science of the Heart. Exploring the role of the heart in human performance. An overview of research conducted by the HeartMath Institute, 2016. Figure 3.1.

Figures 5.6 & 5.7 From: HeartMath Stress Relief Program.

Figure 5.8 From: Baldwin AL, Wagers C and Schwartz GE. Reiki improves heart rate homoeostasis in laboratory rats. *Journal of Alternative and Complementary Medicine* 2008; 14(4): 417–422. Figure 4.

Figure 5.9 From: Baldwin AL and GE Schwartz. Personal interaction with a Reiki practitioner decreases noise-induced micro-vascular damage in an animal model. *Journal of Alternative and Complementary Medicine*, 12(1): 15-22, 2006. Figure 3.

Figure 6.2 From: https://opentextbc.ca/anatomyandphysiology/chapter/20-1-structure-and-function-of-blood-vessels/Figure 3.

Figure 6.3 From: Zaromytidou M, Siasos G, Coskun AU, Lucia M et al. Intravacular hemodynamics and coronary artery disease: New insights and clinical implications. *Hellenic Journal of Cardiology*, 57(6): 389-400, 2016. Figure 1.

Figure 6.5 From: Flavahan. A vascular mechanistic approach to understanding Raynaud phenomenon. *Nature Reviews Rheumatology*, 11: 146-158, 2015. Figure 4a.

Figure 6.6 Steam Artwork, steamcommunity.com

Figure 6.9 From: Baldwin A and Schwartz GE. Physiological changes in energy healers during self-practice. *Complementary Therapies in Medicine*, 20: 299-305, 2012. Figure 4.

Figure 7.1 From: Fox D. The electric cure. *Nature* 2017; 545,20–22.

Figure 7.2 From Kevin Tracey, Feinstein Institute for Medical Research.

Figure 7.3 From: How Does a GSR Sensor Work? www.tobiipro.com.

Figure 7.4 From: NIDDK Image Library.

Table 7.1 From: CDC Health Related Quality of Life article. www.cdc.gov/hrqol/wellbeing.htm#.

Figure 8.2 From: Shiflett SC, Nayak S, Bid CB, Miles P, Agostinelli S. Effect of Reiki treatments on functional recovery in patients in poststroke rehabilitation: a pilot study. *Journal of Alternative and Complementary Medicine* 2002; 8(6): 755–563. Figure 1.

Figure 8.3 From: Baldwin AL, Vitale A, Brownell E, Kryak E, Rand, W. Effects of reiki on pain, anxiety, and blood pressure in patients undergoing knee replacement surgery. *Holistic Nursing Practice* 2017; 31(2): 80–89. Figure 2.

Figure 9.1 From: Diaz-Rodríguez L, Arroyo-Morales M, Fernández-de-las-Peñas C, García-Lafuente F, García-Royo C, Tomás-Rojas I. Immediate effects of Reiki on heart rate variability, cortisol levels, and body temperature in health care professionals with burnout. *Biological Research for Nursing* 2011a; 13(4): 376–382. Figure 2.

Table 9.1 From: "2018 Survey of America's Physicians: Practice Patterns and Perspectives", The Physicians Foundation, p. 32.

Table 9.2 From: Diaz-Rodriguez et al. The application of Reiki in nurses diagnosed with Burnout Syndrome has beneficial effects on concentration of salivary IgA and blood pressure. *Revista Latino-Americana de Enfermagem* [online], 2011b; 19(5):1132–1138, Table 2.

Figure 10.1 From: American Academy of Orthopedic Surgeons.

Figure 10.2 From: Abduction and Adduction? (Biomechanics) Machine Design, 22 July 2014.

Figure 10.3 From: Manchester-Bedford Myoskeletal, "Range of Motion". http://www.mbmyoskeletal.com/learning/range-of-motion/.

Figures 10.4–10.6 From: Baldwin AL, Fullmer K and Schwartz GE. Comparison of physical therapy with energy healing for improving range of motion in subjects with restricted shoulder mobility. *Evidence-Based Complementary and Alternative Medicine* 2013; 2013: 329731. Figures 2–4.

Figures 11.1–11.3 From: Baldwin AL, Vitale A, Brownel, E, Kryak E, Rand W. Effects of reiki on pain, anxiety, and blood pressure in patients undergoing knee replacement surgery. *Holistic Nursing Practice* 2017; 31(2): 80–89.

Figures 11.4 & 11.5 From: Midilli TS, Eser I. Effects of Reiki on post-Caesarean delivery pain, anxiety, and hemodynamic parameters: a randomized, controlled clinical trial. *Pain Management Nursing*, 16(3):388-399, 2015.

Figures 11.6 & 11.7 From: Chirico A. Self-Efficacy for coping with cancer enhances the effect of Reiki treatments during the pre-surgery phase of breast cancer patients. *Anticancer Research*, 37(7): 3657-3665, 2017. Figures 1 & 2.

Table 11.1 From: Burton D, Nicholson G and Hall G. Endocrine and metabolic responses to surgery. *Continuing Education in Anaesthesia*, Critical Care & Pain, 2004; 4(5): 144-147. Table 2.

Table 11.2 From: Midilli TS, Eser I. Effects of Reiki on post-Caesarean delivery pain, anxiety, and hemodynamic parameters: a randomized, controlled clinical trial. *Pain Management Nursing*, 16(3):388-399, 2015.

Figure 12.1 From: Tsang K, Carlson L, Olson K. Pilot crossover trial of Reiki versus rest for treating cancer-related fatigue. *Integrated Cancer Therapy* 2007; 6 (1): 25–35. Figure 1.

Figure 12.2 From: NIH/Warren Grant Magnusen Clinical Center.

Tables 12.1–12.3 From: Olson K, Hanson J, Michaud M. A phase II trial of Reiki for the management of pain in advanced cancer patients. *Journal of Pain Symptom Management* 2003; 26(5): 990–997. Figures 2–4.

Table 12.4 From: Richeson NE, Spross JA, Lutz K, Peng C. Effects of Reiki on anxiety, depression, pain and physiological factors in community-dwelling older adults. *Research in Gerontological Nursing* 2010; 3(3): 187–199. Table 1.

Figure 13.1 From: Villines Z. What are the side-effects of chemotherapy? *Medical News Today*. www.medicalnewstoday.com/articles/323485.php.

Figure 13.2 From: Fleisher KA, Mackenzie ER, Frankel ES, Seluzicki C, Casarett D, Mao JJ. Integrative Reiki for cancer patients: A program evaluation. *Integrative Cancer Therapies* 2014; 13(1): 62–67. Figure 1.

Table 13.1 From: https://www.texasoncology.com/cancer-treatment/side-effects-of-cancer-treatment/common-side-effects/low-blood-counts.

Figure 14.1 From: Anderson DM, Loth AR, Stuart-Mullen LG, Thomley BS, Cutshall SM. Building a Reiki and Healing Touch volunteer program at an academic medical center. *Advances in Integrative Medicine* 2017; 4: 74–79. Figure 2.

Table 14.1 From: Johnson R, Fuerst R. Reiki at St. Charles Cancer Center. *Reiki News Magazine*, Spring 2011, 36–40. SCCC Reiki Session Data Table.

Table 14.2 From: Hahn J, Reilly PM, Buchanan TM. Development of a hospital reiki training program: training volunteers to provide reiki to patients, families, and staff in the acute care setting. *Dimensions of Critical Care Nursing* 2014; 33(1): 15–21. Figure: Reiki volunteer competency evaluation tool.

Boxes 14.1A & B From: The Leonard P Zakim Center for Integrative Therapies and Healthy Living, Dana-Faber Cancer Institute. www.dana-farber.org.

Box 14.2 From: Reiki Federation Ireland. www.reikifederation-ireland.com/Where-Reiki-is-provided-in-Ireland.pdf.

GLOSSARY

Autonomic Nervous System The part of the nervous system responsible for control of the bodily functions not consciously directed, such as breathing, the heartbeat, and digestive processes.

The autonomic nervous system is divided into sympathetic and parasympathetic fibers. Activation of sympathetic nerves increases arousal and heart rate whereas activation of parasympathetic nerves calms the mind and body for digestion, cellular maintenance, and repair.

Biofield The biofield is a complex endogenously generated sphere of energy and information that surrounds and permeates a living system and is engaged in the generation, maintenance, and regulation of physiological functions of the system.

Chakra The Sanskrit word Chakra literally translates to wheel or disk. In yoga, meditation, and Ayurveda, this term refers to wheels of energy throughout the body. There are seven main chakras, which align the spine, starting from the base of the spine through to the crown of the head.

Clinical Trial A research study in which one or more human subjects are prospectively assigned to one or more interventions (which may include placebo or other control) to evaluate the effects of those interventions on health-related biomedical or behavioral outcomes. (NIH definition)

Cortisol Cortisol is a steroid hormone that regulates a wide range of processes throughout the body, including metabolism and the immune response. It also has a very important role in helping the body respond to stress.

Heart Rate Variability Heart rate variability (HRV) is the second-by-second change in heart rate as a function of time and reflects the interaction between sympathetic and parasympathetic autonomic nervous system activity. High HRV is associated with optimal mind-body function and adaptability. Low HRV is associated with states of physical, mental, and emotional stress.

HPA Axis HPA axis is an abbreviation for a subsystem in the body called the hypothalamic–pituitary–adrenal axis. It involves a complex set of interactions between two parts of the brain (the hypothalamus and the pituitary glands) and the adrenal glands that are located at the top of each kidney. The HPA axis plays a major role in the stress response, culminating in release of cortisol from the adrenal glands.

Limbic System The limbic system is a collection of brain structures that integrate the various bodily sensations, thoughts, and memories experienced or recalled at a particular moment into a complex electrical signal.

Placebo A placebo is a substance or treatment with no active therapeutic effect (Oxford University Press). A placebo may be given to a person in order to deceive the recipient into thinking that it is an active treatment.

Skin Conductance Response The skin conductance response is a change in the electrical properties of the skin that is associated with sweat production in response to stress or anxiety.

Vagus Nerve A nerve that supplies nerve fibers to the pharynx (throat), larynx (voice box), trachea (windpipe), lungs, heart, esophagus, and intestinal tract, and interfaces with the parasympathetic control of the heart. The vagus nerve also brings sensory information back to the brain from the ear, tongue, pharynx, larynx, and heart.

Chapter 1

What Reiki is and Why it is Important

Definition and Background

According to the International Center for Reiki training, "Reiki is a Japanese technique for stress reduction that also promotes healing. It is administered by laying on hands and can be easily learned by anyone." Actually, Reiki is taught more as a lifestyle than just a technique, and all Reiki practitioners aim to follow the five Principles of Reiki that were received by founder, Mikao Usui, during his meditations:

1. Just for today I give thanks for my many blessings.

2. Just for today I will not worry.

3. Just for today I will not anger.

4. Just for today I will do my work honestly.

5. Just for today I will be kind to myself and every other living thing.

Even just following these five principles without practicing Reiki will help with the healing process. Emotions such as worry and anger produce an activation of the fight or flight response, leading to release of adrenaline into the bloodstream as well as stimulation of the sympathetic nerves that innervate all body organs. These responses cause heart rate and cardiac contractility to increase, so that blood circulation is enhanced and more oxygen and nutrients are provided to the heart, muscles and brain. In addition, the stress hormone, cortisol, is released, which helps covert carbohydrates to glucose (Robert Scaer, *Eight Keys to Brain–Body Balance* pp. 40–41). These reactions are beneficial in the short term because they provide the body with extra energy. However, they can be detrimental in the long term because chronically high concentrations of cortisol lead to sustained increases of glucose in the bloodstream and reduced release of insulin which can cause type 2 diabetes (Rosmond, 2003). Chronically high concentra-

tions of blood glucose also lead to deposition of fat around the abdominal area, muscle wasting and impaired function of the immune system (Robert Scaer, *Eight Keys to Brain–Body Balance* pp. 113–114). Elevated stimulation of sympathetic nerves (fight or flight response) for prolonged periods increases the workload of the heart and is associated with heart disease (Florea and Cohn, 2014; Holwerda et al., 2018) and impaired regulation of blood pressure (Holwerda et al., 2018). Blood circulation to the gastrointestinal tract is also restricted which may lead to digestive problems (Bonaz and Sabate, 2009). The principles, "Just for today I will not worry", "Just for today I will not anger", do not mean that one must never experience these emotions. Obviously that would be impossible and even undesirable. When these emotions arise, the object is not to be overwhelmed by them but to experience them and then let them pass. Practicing Reiki and/or receiving Reiki enables this process, partly because Reiki stimulates the parasympathetic nerves which help the body relax (Mackay et al., 2004; Baldwin et al., 2008; Diaz-Rodriguez et al., 2011).

The Reiki principles, "Just for today I give thanks for my many blessings" and "Just for today I will be kind to myself and every other living thing" also aid in the healing process because they help one focus on the positive aspects of life. Barbara Fredrickson, a psychology researcher at University of North Carolina, has performed experimental studies showing that when people experienced positive emotions, such as joy, contentment and love, they saw more possibilities in their lives. In addition, this broadened sense of possibilities enables people to build new skills and resources that they can use in other parts of their lives. Fredrickson refers to this concept as the "broaden and build" theory (Fredrickson, 2004).

The Reiki principle, "Just for today I will do my work honestly" can be interpreted as taking responsibility for one's life and for the attainment of one's goals and ambitions. Realizing that one has control over how one

Chapter 1

responds to outside events and personal interactions is a healthy, empowering experience. There is nothing more debilitating than blaming others, complaining, making excuses and waiting for others to act on one's behalf. So even just living by the Reiki principles can have profoundly beneficial effects on one's physical and psychological health. Although receiving Reiki sessions has many benefits, as will be described in later chapters, learning and practicing Reiki on oneself provides the ultimate gain.

English Oxford Living Dictionaries provides a more mechanistic definition of Reiki: Reiki is "a healing technique based on the principle that the therapist can channel energy into the patient by means of touch, to activate the natural healing processes of the patient's body and restore physical and emotional well-being". This definition leads to more questions such as: "What type of energy?" and "How does one channel the energy?"

The answer to the first question is not obvious. Some Reiki scholars, such as James Oschman, have proposed that Reiki energy is electromagnetic. This idea makes sense because the heart and brain both generate measurable electromagnetic fields (biofields) that extend away from the body. These fields are very weak and challenging to measure but, in the late 1960s, an ultrasensitive detector called a Superconducting Quantum Interference Detector (SQUID) was developed. In 1970, Cohen (1970) reported the recording of the electromagnetic field of the heart (a magnetocardiogram) using a SQUID. Two years later, Cohen (1972) described the use of a SQUID to measure the electromagnetic field of the brain (a magnetoencephalogram).

If Reiki energy were electromagnetic, then it would be able to interact with the heart and brain biofields, alter their vibration frequencies and consequently modify the electric currents producing the biofields. Since electrical conduction systems in the heart coordinate the contraction of the various heart chambers, altering these currents would influence cardiac function. Likewise, since information is passed between the brain and other parts of the body by electrical currents traveling along neural pathways, altering these currents could adjust brain function.

However, there are some major problems with this theory which will be discussed in Chapter 3.

The answer to the second question, "How does one channel Reiki?" is based on the purported existence of energy portals, called chakras, in the body. The word "chakra" is Sanskrit for "wheel" and chakras are believed to spin: pulling energy into the body from the environment and returning energy to the environment. The idea of the chakra system originates from traditional Indian religions, such as Hinduism, Buddhism and Jainism. According to Hindu and Buddhist texts (Lochtefeld, 2002; Jones and Ryan, 2006), the seven main chakras are arranged in a column along the spinal cord, from the base of the spine

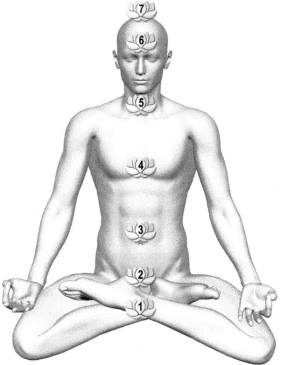

7 Crown 6 Third eye 5 Throat 4 Heart
3 Solar 2 Sacral 1 Root

Figure 1.1
Diagram of seven Chakras.

(coccyx) to the crown of the head (Figure 1.1), connected by a vertical channel. If one believes in chakras, it is easy to imagine Reiki energy entering the crown chakra, flowing through the central channel and exiting through the root chakra at the base of the spine. According to the theory, energy can also enter or exit the vertical channel through the other chakras that are not associated with the crown or coccyx. In addition, energy can flow to and from the central channel through minor chakras connected into the system. It is rather like the lymphatic circulatory system in the body, but moving energy rather than lymph (a fluid containing infection-fighting white blood cells). However, the lymphatic system connects with the blood circulation within the body whereas the chakra/channel system connects with energy in the environment. The channel concept is consistent with Reiki energy entering the chakra system from the environment and then flowing out of the minor chakras located in the hands during the healing process.

Some people have noticed that there is a correspondence between the positions of the main chakras and the locations of important glands (Roney-Dougal, 1999) (Figure 1.2). It has also been noted that the positions of the main chakras correspond to some degree with the nerve plexi or nervous networks that serve specific organs in the body (Leadbetter, 1927) (Figure 1.3) but the literature is very scant. Nevertheless, these correlations have led to the theory that chakras act as transducers, transforming environmental energies, such as Reiki, into electrical and chemical signals within the body (Wisneski and Anderson, 2009).

At present there is no convincing scientific validity for the existence of chakras. The closest evidence available for the presence of energy centers in the body arises from the use of a gas discharge visualizer (GDV), in which a small, pulsed electromagnetic field is applied to the fingertips to induce a flow of electrons in the skin and possibly deeper connective tissues (Korotkov, 2004). These free electrons accelerate towards the GDV positive electrode, gaining enough energy to cause further ionization to form an electron avalanche on the surface of the electrode. The electronic 'glow' of this discharge can be captured by an optical charge-coupled device camera system. Konstantin Korot-

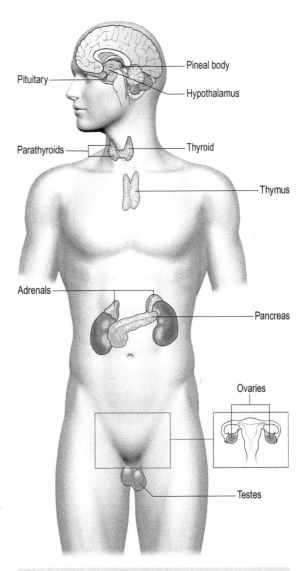

Figure 1.2
Positions of glands in body.

kov, from Saint-Petersburg Federal University of Informational Technologies, Mechanics and Optics, developed software for this device to translate the electronic responses of the fingertips to an energy profile of the whole body (Korotkov, 2009). The link between fingertip responses and functions of specific organs and organ is based on

3

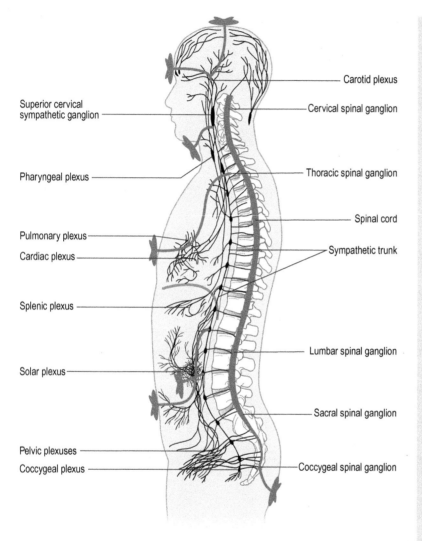

Superior cervical
sympathetic ganglion

Pharyngeal plexus

Pulmonary plexus

Cardiac plexus

Splenic plexus

Solar plexus

Pelvic plexuses

Coccygeal plexus

Carotid plexus

Cervical spinal ganglion

Thoracic spinal ganglion

Spinal cord

Sympathetic trunk

Lumbar spinal ganglion

Sacral spinal ganglion

Coccygeal spinal ganglion

Figure 1.3
Positions of nerve plexi in the body
with respect to chakras.
(From: Leadbetter CW. *The Chakras.
A Monograph.* First Edition. The Theosophical
Publishing House, Wheaton, IL, USA; London,
UK, 1927, Plate IX.)

acupuncture meridians (Mandel, 1986). When the data of the ten individual fingertips are collated and interpolated, an image of the full body energy field is created. This is illustrated in Figure 1.4. Gaps in electro-photonic emission supposedly indicate impeded transfer of electron density into the body's tissues and an abnormality in the energy supply of organs and physiological systems. Such deficiencies are seen as gaps in the image of the body's energy field that is produced by the GDV camera and software. According to Korotkov (2012), and based on the principles of Ayurvedic medicine, a specific part of every finger is also associated with a particular chakra. More information about this relationship is described in the literature (Deshpande et al., 2013) but empirical evidence is lacking. The GDV camera has been certified as a medical device by the Committee on New Medical Technique of the Russian Ministry of Health. The review of 136 exploratory studies on its use as a diagnostic instrument in medicine shows that it is comparable to other more standard devices under a wide variety of conditions (Korotkov et al., 2010).

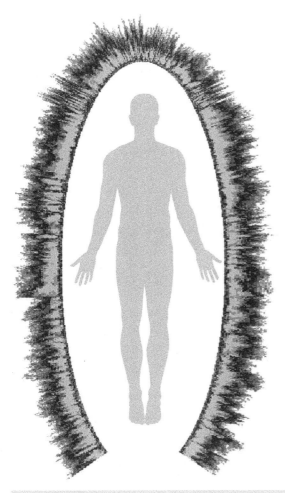

Figure 1.4
Typical image of a body biofield produced from fingertip measures using a gas charge visualizer.
(From: http://rexresearch.com/korotkov/korotkov.htm)

However, databases of results as well as methods of standardization need to be made accessible to the public and published in peer-reviewed journals to validate the GDV as a truly scientific instrument.

As a note to clinical practitioners, firstly, just because it is not possible at present to make an iron clad, evidence-based case for channeling Reiki through the body, that does not mean that it might not happen. Secondly, regardless of the mechanism by which Reiki passes from a Reiki practitioner to a client or patient, Reiki has measurable beneficial effects on physiological and emotional well-being that will be described in detail in Chapters 5–13.

Short History of Reiki

This history of Reiki is based on information from Japanese Reiki Masters, Hiroshi Doi and Tadao Yamaguchi, who are members of the original Usui Reiki association, Usui Reiki Ryoho Gakkai. More detailed information can be found in books that they have authored (Tadao Yamaguchi, *Light on the Origins of Reiki* and Hiroshi Doi, *A Modern Reiki Method for Healing*). Other information was obtained from Reiki Masters William Rand and Frank Arjava Petter, both of whom visited Japan extensively and communicated with members of Usui Reiki Ryoho Gakkai and their relatives. Their books (Frank Arjava Petter, *Reiki Fire* and Walter Lubeck, Frank Arjava Petter and William Lee Rand, *The Spirit of Reiki*) provide an accurate view of Reiki from a Westerner's context.

Reiki is related to Buddhist Qigong which is used as a means of attaining better health, higher self-awareness, and developing the higher potentials of the mind and body. Qigong is a Chinese practice of aligning breath, movement, and awareness for exercise, healing, and martial arts training, and extends back more than 4,000 years. Reiki was rediscovered by Mikao Usui (1864–1926), of Kyoto, Japan at the end of the nineteenth century. Usui chose the name "Reiki" which is usually translated as "universal life force energy". Mikao Usui was a well-educated man who had studied Christianity, Buddhism, psychology, history and medical science and had traveled to Europe and America. However, he was not always successful in his various businesses and had reached a point where he needed to seek something other than material gain. According to historical information, he used to meditate near a waterfall on Mount Kurama and one day, while on a meditation retreat, he received a sudden experience of healing energy. During this process, he realized that his purpose in life was to use this energy to heal others and to train those who wanted, to join him in the healing practice. In 1922 he founded the Reiki association Usui Reiki Ryoho Gakkai to preserve and promote the teachings of Reiki. Usui trained more than 2,000 people to practice Reiki, but only 21 people reached the highest level. Several of those were officers in the Japanese Navy, including Captain Chujiro Hayashi. Hayashi (1879–1940) was the last high level practitioner certified by Usui (in 1925). Hayashi opened a Reiki clinic in Tokyo under Usui's instructions to develop Reiki Ryoho. Usui died in 1926 after suffering a stroke.

Hayashi worked actively in his Reiki clinic with 16 healers until the outbreak of World War II. During this time, he met a woman named Hawayo Takata who was referred to his clinic because she was suffering from some serious diseases. Takata received Reiki sessions and she completely recovered. As a result, she decided to study Reiki with Hayashi for a year before returning to her home in Hawaii and starting a Reiki clinic. After further training from Hayashi, Takata taught 22 Reiki instructors before her death in 1980, and is considered to be responsible for bringing Reiki to the West. However, she simplified Hayashi's Reiki style, omitting some of its Tibetan roots and developing a simplified hand position system. Some of the instructors Takata had trained altered her teachings somewhat and formed their own groups. On the other hand, until her recent death, Takata's granddaughter, Phyllis Furumoto, continued to train Reiki practitioners while adhering closely to Takata's teachings.

After Hayashi's death in 1940, it was thought by most westerners that Reiki had more or less disappeared in Japan. However, in the 1980s it was discovered by several Western Reiki teachers that the Usui Reiki association, or Usui Reiki Ryoho Gakkai, had been perpetuated in Japan, but on a members-only basis. Since the 1990s, there have been successful efforts by several Western Reiki instructors, such as William Rand, to re-establish some of the lost Usui Reiki teachings previously dropped from Western Reiki. In addition, Japanese Reiki Masters are being encouraged to promote Reiki in Japan and, as a result, it has gained in popularity. In 2014, William Rand became aware of, and developed for teaching, a more refined Reiki

energy called "Holy Fire" which is available for Reiki Masters to learn if they choose. The use of the word holy in the name Holy Fire is not intended to have a religious meaning, but rather a meaning of being whole and complete. It is claimed that once a Reiki Master receives the Holy Fire energy, the energy continues to grow in strength and vibration, cleansing more deeply and healing more powerfully.

What Happens During a Session?

Healing Space

Reiki sessions are usually performed in a quiet room dedicated for that purpose. It is preferable that there is minimal disturbance. The room might be in a private house (Figure 1.5) or in a clinic and will contain a Reiki table, similar to a massage table, equipped with a headrest and pillow and covered with a clean sheet. In many cases, soft, ambient music will be playing to help the relaxation response, but most practitioners will ask whether or not you would like silence. Reiki is also being offered increasingly in hospitals. In this case, the Reiki practitioner will give Reiki to the patient while they rest in their hospital bed in the ward or private room. The ward will probably not be quiet, and other people will be entering and leaving the area, but Reiki can be given anywhere under most conditions.

Meeting the Client

The practitioner will greet the client and usually ask for a short history about any existing physical, emotional, mental or spiritual issues and problems. If the client is new, the practitioner will explain the process and ask them if they mind being lightly touched or whether they would prefer to receive Reiki from a distance. Placement of the hands is never intrusive or inappropriate. Most clients do not mind having the practitioner place their hands on them in the approved hand positions. However, the practitioner can just as easily hold their hands a few inches from the surface of the client's body if necessary. This is the time when clients should inform the practitioner if they have any special needs or restrictions with regard to lying on their back. The practitioner can modify the client's posi-

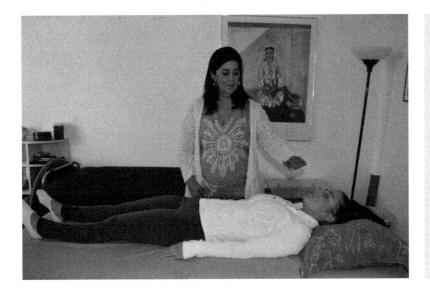

Figure 1.5
Reiki session in a private house.

tion on the table so that they are comfortable, and will also supply support cushions or blankets if needed.

Experiencing the Session

Next, the client removes their shoes and lies on the padded Reiki table, face upwards, with their arms resting by their sides. They remain fully clothed but usually remove their coat or jacket. Normally the client closes their eyes. The practitioner may scan the surface of the client's body with their palms a few inches away to locate any areas of heat or coldness, which usually indicate areas that need healing. Then they will begin the hand positions, starting at the crown of the head and working towards the feet. During this time, the practitioner will be channeling Reiki to the client. The client may feel heat, tingling, a pulsing sensation or nothing at all. If the client is not aware of sensations during the Reiki session, this does not mean that nothing is happening. Clients almost always feel refreshed, more at ease and deeply relaxed after a session and may experience other physical or psychological benefits later on, regardless of whether or not they were aware of sensations during the session. Reiki is cumulative and clients usually experience additional sensations and responses if they continue with further sessions. Sometimes, the prac-

titioner will inform the client what they are sensing while the session is in progress, but often practitioners will work in silence and wait until the end to speak with the client.

Clients with Back Problems

If the client has issues relating to their back, the practitioner will usually ask them at some time to lie prone on the Reiki table. To ensure that the client is comfortable in this position, the headrest cushion encircles a hole in which the client places their face. The cushion is draped with a clean, soft piece of fabric, which is changed for every client, and is shaped so as not to block the hole. This headrest cover may be disposable or may be made of cotton or flannel (freshly laundered). The Reiki practitioner will not manipulate the back but will apply Reiki using similar hand positions as for the front of the body.

Time Duration of Session

There is no specified time duration for Reiki sessions but they usually last for 30 or 60 minutes, agreed by the client and practitioner in advance. Sessions given in hospitals or hospices are usually shorter (15–20 minutes) because other staff in the hospital will often need to provide a variety of other services and care to the patient.

After the Session

When the session is over, the client will be invited to open their eyes, sit up and dismount from the table in their own time. They will be offered a drink of water because Reiki can cause mild dehydration. Then the practitioner will speak with the client and answer any questions that arise. The practitioner will not give a diagnosis; that is not part of Reiki. A good practitioner will just inform the client about what they felt with their hands. They may say, for example, that they felt increased or decreased sensations in their hands as they worked on certain areas of the body which could indicate that those areas require further attention. In the presence of health challenges, the practitioner may advise an additional three or four sessions over the next week or two.

Who Can Practice Reiki?

Reiki can be administered by anybody who has received training at any level. In most branches of Reiki, there are three levels. Training to level one equips a person to provide Reiki to themselves and to others, either hands-on or with their hands a few inches distant from the Reiki recipient.

When a Reiki practitioner trains to level two, they receive Reiki symbols that strengthen their practice and enable them to send Reiki to a recipient from any distance. Reiki can also be sent to issues; these may include general issues, such as depleting the Earth of its natural resources, or personal issues, such as a challenging relationship. In addition, Reiki can be sent to events in the future or to the past. Training to level three is sometimes divided into two sublevels, "Advanced" and "Master". In Advanced level training, Reiki practitioners receive one or more additional symbols, depending on the specific branch of Reiki, and they experience an even greater strengthening and increased effectiveness of their Reiki practice. At this level, Reiki has become part of the person's being and is used on a daily basis for physical healing and for mental, emotional and spiritual guidance. Practitioners who study to the Master level learn how to teach Reiki and to pass it on to others at all levels. For more detailed information on the training involved in the different Reiki levels, the following books are highly recommended: Hiroshi Doi, *A Modern Reiki Method for Healing*; Walter Lubeck, Frank Arjava Petter and William Lee Rand, *The Spirit of Reiki*; Nicolas Pearson, *Foundations of Reiki Ryoho*.

Usually, people who practice Reiki professionally have studied Reiki to the Master level and have accrued at least several years of experience offering Reiki to clients. Experience is important because it is the actual practice of Reiki that helps practitioners become more sensitive to the subtle energy and able to discern imbalances and depletions in that energy when they are treating clients. Unlike complementary therapies such as acupuncture, massage and chiropractic, there are no national board certification procedures for Reiki practitioners. For this reason, other methods must be used to select a Reiki practitioner who is likely to be effective and appropriate for one's needs.

First, it is useful to find out where, and under whom, the practitioner received their training. This information is part of the Reiki practitioner's "lineage". The full lineage starts with the practitioner's personal teacher and goes back through each preceding teacher's succession. Ultimately, all authentic lineages trace back to Mikao Usui. The main reason for requesting information about a Reiki practitioner's lineage is to ensure that they are really trained in an authentic branch of Reiki. Within the genuine Reiki "family tree", their actual lineage is unlikely to influence their ability to practice effective healing.

Second, membership of an international or national professional Reiki association is desirable because these associations require their members to adhere to listed professional and ethical standards.

Examples of professional Reiki associations include:

i. International Center for Reiki Training

ii. UK Reiki Federation

iii. Canadian Reiki Association

iv. Association of Australian Reiki Professionals

v. International Association of Reiki Professionals

These associations all have excellent websites that provide information about Reiki practitioners who they have approved and who are available in various geographical locations throughout the world. The International Center for Reiki Training (ICRT) has developed its own standardized Reiki courses that are taught by Reiki Masters who have successfully completed the ICRT training and licensing procedures. Curricula for all levels of Reiki are presented on the website. Reiki practitioners who have trained under the guidance of an ICRT instructor are most likely to practice Reiki in an effective and professional manner.

Third, plenty of excellent Reiki practitioners are not members of professional associations and so may be more challenging to locate. The internet provides contact information about Reiki practitioners in given locations. The next step is to ask the practitioners for references and testimonials and question them further to determine whether they are suitable for your needs. Sample questions are listed below:

- How long have you practiced Reiki?

- How many students have you trained to first, second and Master levels?

- What system of Reiki do you teach?

- What do the Five Principles mean to you?

- How many Reiki treatments do you provide to others, on average, per week?

- What medical issues are common in clients who come to you for Reiki?

- How many sessions do you usually recommend for people with a particular problem such as mild anxiety, chronic pain, acute pain or depression?

- Do you engage in self-treatments?

Advantages of Reiki

Complementary medicine covers a range of medical therapies that fall beyond the scope of allopathic medicine (in which disease is combated mainly by using drugs and surgery) but may be used alongside it in the treatment of disease and ill health. Examples include Reiki, massage, Qigong, biofeedback, trauma release exercises, hypnosis, homeopathy, chiropractic, osteopathy, acupuncture, Chinese or oriental medicine and herbal medicine.

Two advantages that Reiki shares with several other complementary therapies, such as clinical Qigong, biofeedback, trauma release exercises and hypnosis, is that it is non-invasive and can be used safely in conjunction with other therapies. No substances are imbibed and no part of the body is manipulated in any way. As with most complementary therapies, Reiki addresses physical, emotional and mental issues. In addition, like massage and trauma release exercises, Reiki is simple and easy to administer. Similar to massage, chiropractic and osteopathy, no special equipment is needed apart from a treatment table. In common with trauma release exercises and Qigong, Reiki can be self-administered. In fact, because Reiki is channeled through the practitioner, the practitioner will also receive Reiki every time they give it to another person. Unlike any of the other complementary therapies listed, Reiki is easy to learn and benefits can result even after a few minutes. Reiki can be performed in any environment. Most importantly, Reiki has no side effects.

Benefits of Reiki

Reiki is an integrative therapy that treats the whole person, mind and body. Usually, between one and four 30–60-minute sessions are sufficient to reduce fear and anxiety, ease chronic and acute pain, relieve side effects of chemotherapy, help cancer (and hospice) patients come to terms with their diagnosis, improve challenging relationships, speed up recovery after surgery and reduce length of hospital stay post-surgery. In addition, Reiki puts the patient in a calm state so that other medicines and treatments can work more effectively.

The most rigorous data suggest Reiki's positive effects in four areas:

- Acute and chronic pain.

- Pain and well-being during cancer treatment.

- Stress, anxiety, and depression.

- Practitioner well-being.

Scientific research supporting these effects, and others, will be discussed in detail in Chapters 5–13.

References

Baldwin AL, Wagers C, Schwartz GE. Reiki improves heart rate homeostasis in laboratory rats. *Journal of Alternative and Complementary Medicine* 2008; 14: 417–422.

Bonaz B, Sabate JM. Brain–gut axis dysfunction. *Gastroentérologie Clinique et Biologique* 2009; 33(Suppl. 1): S48–S58.

Cohen D. Magnetocardiograms taken inside a shielded room with a superconducting point-contact magnetometer. *Applied Physics Letters* 1970; 16: 278.

Cohen D. Magnetoencephalography: Detection of the brain's electrical activity with a superconducting magnetometer. *Science* 1972; 175: 664–666.

Deshpande PB, Madappa KP, Korotkov K. Can the Excellence of the Internal Be Measured? – A Preliminary Study. *Journal of Consciousness Exploration & Research* 2013; 4(9): 977–987.

Diaz-Rodríguez L, Arroyo-Morales M, Fernandez-de-las-Penas C, Garcia-Lafuente F, Garcia-Royo C, Tomas-Rojas I. Immediate effects of reiki on heart rate variability, cortisol levels, and body temperature in health care professionals with burnout. *Biological Research for Nursing* 2011; 13: 376–382.

Doi H. *A Modern Reiki Method for Healing.* Vision Publications, Southfield, MI, USA, 2014.

Florea VG, Cohn JN. The Autonomic Nervous System and Heart Failure. *Circulation Research* 2014; 114: 1815–1826.

Fredrickson BL. The broaden-and-build theory of positive emotions. *Philosophical Transactions of the Royal Society B: Biological Sciences* 2004; 359(1449): 1367–1378.

Holwerda SW, Luehrs RE, Gremaud AL, Wooldridge NA, Stroud AK, Fiedorowicz JG, Abboud FM, Pierce GL. Relative burst amplitude of muscle sympathetic nerve activity is an indicator of altered sympathetic outflow in chronic anxiety. *Journal of Neurophysiology* 2018; 20(1): 11–22.

Jones C, Ryan JD. *Encyclopedia of Hinduism.* Infobase Publishing, New York, NY, USA, 2006; p. 102.

Korotkov K, ed. *Measuring Energy Fields: State of the Art.* GDV Bioelectrography series, Vol. I. Backbone Publishing Co., Fair Lawn, NJ, USA, 2004.

Korotkov KG. *The Principles of GDV Analysis.* Marco Pietteur Editions, Embourg, Belgium, 2009.

Korotkov KG, Matravers P, Orlov DV, Williams BO. Application of electrophoton capture analysis based on gas discharge visualization technique in medicine: a systematic review. *Journal of Alternative and Complementary Medicine* 2010; 16(10): 13–25.

Korotkov KG. *Energy Fields Electrophotonic Analysis in Humans and Nature.* Amazon, 2012.

Leadbetter CW. *The Chakras: A Monograph.* First Edition. The Theosophical Publishing House, Wheaton, IL, USA; London, UK, 1927.

Lochtefeld JG. *The Illustrated Encyclopedia of Hinduism: A–M.* The Rosen Publishing Group, New York City, NY, USA, 2002; p. 137.

Lubeck W, Petter FA, Rand WL. *The Spirit of Reiki: The Complete Handbook of the Reiki System.* Lotus Light. Shangri-La, Twin Lakes, WI, USA, 2003.

Mackay N, Hansen S, McFarlane O. Autonomic nervous system changes during Reiki treatment: a preliminary study. *Journal of Alternative and Complementary Medicine* 2004; 10(6):1077–1081.

Mandel P. *Energy Emission Analysis: New Application of Kirlian Photography for Holistic Medicine.* Synthesis Publishing Co., Germany, 1986.

Petter FA. *Reiki Fire. New Information about the Origins of the Reiki Power. A Complete Manual.* Lotus Light. Shangri-La, Twin Lakes, WI, USA, 1997.

Roney-Dougal SM. On a possible psychophysiology of the yogic chakra system. *Indian Journal of Psychology* 1999; 17(2): 18–40.

Rosmond R. Stress-induced disturbances of the HPA axis: a pathway to Type 2 diabetes? *Medical Science Monitor* 2003; 9(2): RA35–39.

Scaer R. *Eight Keys to Brain–Body Balance.* W.W. Norton & Co. Inc., New York, NY, USA; London, UK, 2012.

Wisneski LA, Anderson L. *The Scientific Basis of Integrative Medicine*, Second Edition. CRC Press, Taylor and Francis Group, Boca Raton, FL, USA, 2009.

Yamaguchi T. *Light on the Origins of Reiki: A Handbook for Practicing the Original Reiki of Usui and Hayashi.* Lotus Light. Shangri-La, Twin Lakes, WI, USA, 2007.

Personal Reiki Experiences

Colonoscopy Without Anesthesia

When it was time for me to have a routine colonoscopy and I was speaking with my doctor, I soon realized that it was assumed I would have anesthesia. However, since I had just started studying Reiki I thought this would be a fine opportunity to test whether Reiki really does promote relaxation and pain relief. On the assigned day, I drove to the hospital and was soon lying on the table running Reiki energy through my body in preparation for the event. Twice I had to assure the doctor that there was no need for anesthesia. Then he started. To be honest, I was surprised how little discomfort I felt as the four-foot tube snaked through my intestine. Soon it was over and I jumped off the table and drove myself back to work. A few years later, I went to pick up a friend who had just had a routine colonoscopy and I must admit I gloated when I saw him lying in bed dressed in a hospital gown and looking somewhat drowsy. Certainly unable to drive himself home!

Painless Wisdom Teeth Extraction

During an emergency visit to the dentist, I was informed that I needed to have two wisdom teeth removed. On the day of the extraction, I gave myself a 15-minute Reiki session before leaving the house. As the dentist was preparing me for the local anesthetic he said, "The anesthetic we inject into the roof of the mouth has a very painful sting". I waited for the pain and then heard him say, "You're past the worst of it now". But I hadn't felt anything! After the extractions I drove home and then gave myself a very pleasant 45-minute Reiki session. I did not need to buy the prescribed pain relieving medicine or even apply an icepack to my face because I had no pain or swelling. The next day I taught a class at the university as planned.

Reiki and Eyelid Surgery

After studying Reiki for several years, I was convinced that Reiki was effective at reducing pain and anxiety. For that reason, when I had an elective eyelid surgery, I decided that I would just have the local anesthetic and not the Valium because I did not want to feel lightheaded or confused afterwards. During the surgery, I breathed deeply and slowly and let the Reiki energy flow up and down my body. I heard the surgeon's assistant say, "She's so calm and she didn't have Valium!" I had already been told that I would experience a lot of bruising and swelling so when I returned home I gave myself another 45 minutes of Reiki. I did notice some very slight swelling of my eyelids that day but no bruising. I know that bruising takes some time to develop and so I expected to see some the next day but there was no sign of bruising. Four days later, even the slight swelling had disappeared.

Chapter 2

Why Should Therapists Trust that Reiki is an Effective Therapy?

Introduction

Whenever a clinician or practitioner offers their client or patient a new or different therapy, one of the first questions that comes to the client's mind is: "What evidence is there that this therapy will help me with my problem?" There is no point in spending time, effort and money on a procedure that has little chance of working unless there is absolutely no alternative. General claims and testimonials about the effectiveness of a therapy are useful, but by themselves are not sufficient. For example, perhaps the person who claimed that Reiki alleviated their headache was also having acupuncture treatments and so it is not clear that it was actually the Reiki that helped them. Perhaps the patient who was sure that Reiki greatly decreased her feelings of anxiety, was in fact just being soothed by lying in a quiet room and having another person pay them compassionate attention. In either case, the Reiki itself may not have produced the beneficial effects.

Sometimes practitioners may record the experiences of their client before and after they receive one or more sessions of a particular therapy, and then write it as a case study. Case studies may be published in the peer-reviewed scientific literature. In an article entitled "Writing Case Reports for Reiki", Jane van de Velde, RN, DNP defines a case study as follows (van de Velde, 2009):

The case study is an accurate, brief and clear narrative of a clinical experience.[. . .] Most commonly, a single patient's situation is described. Included in the report are the patient's presenting symptoms, diagnosis, treatment and follow-up care. A case report often presents anecdotal evidence by telling the story of a patient's experience and describing the emotions, personal insights and impacts on the quality of life for the individual.

Practitioners who chronicle and pass on their experiences with clients in this way provide an invaluable record of the clinical practices of the profession. Editor-in-chief of *Journal of Alternative Therapies in Health and Medicine*, Dr. David Riley maintains that clearly documented individual case histories can meet the need for evidence that Reiki works not just in the laboratory, but also in "a real world medical setting" (Miles, 2002). Six Reiki case studies, published in scientific journals, are currently listed on the Center for Reiki Research (CRR) website (centerforreikiresearch.org). Although such studies are certainly useful, there are two main problems with relying on them as evidence that Reiki is an effective healing modality. Firstly, the number of published case studies for Reiki is very small and so they only cover a very limited number of different medical or psychological issues. Secondly, the client needs to know whether the average person who has their particular ailment and who receives Reiki is significantly better off than people with the same ailment who do not receive Reiki. Case studies are highly individual and cannot provide specific guidance for the management of successive patients with a particular condition. However, they are very helpful in framing questions to be answered by more rigorously designed clinical studies.

The real proof of clinical effectiveness is evident when the effects of Reiki alone are systematically compared to the effects of sham Reiki, in which a person not trained in Reiki mimics the hand positions of a Reiki practitioner, and also to the effects of no treatment other than standard care. Such investigations are known as "placebo controlled" studies, where "placebo" means the inactive treatment. By comparing Reiki with a placebo or sham treatment, other possible factors that might induce a beneficial outcome, otherwise known as "confounding variables", such as rest, lying horizontally, being in the presence of a caring person, can be separated from the effects of Reiki itself. If the patients are also randomly assigned to a given group and if they do not know whether they are receiving Reiki or sham Reiki, the study is referred to as a "randomized, blinded, controlled" study. The term "blinded" means that the patient does not know their group assignment and so will not have a preconceived notion of expected treatment outcome. It is important that the patients are randomly assigned to a treatment group to remove bias. Examples of bias would be assigning older or sicker patients to one particular group, or allowing patients to choose their own group assignment. Bias will always skew the results, making a treatment appear to be more or less effectual than it really is. The "randomized, blinded, controlled" (RBC) study removes effects of bias, expectation and confounding variables and is considered the gold standard in clinical trials.

Apart from the experimental design, the type of outcome parameter is a critical component of a clinical trial. The strongest evidence for the effectiveness of a therapy derives from objective measured outcomes, such as: lowered blood pressure; decreased concentrations of the stress hormone, cortisol, in the blood or saliva; reduced scores on anxiety or depression questionnaires; or diminished perception of pain as assessed on a visual analog scale. However, Reiki also affects a person's emotions and feelings towards others. Reiki also connects with individual spiritual qualities such as ideas about one's purpose in life or one's connection with a higher force. These qualities cannot be measured objectively. However, qualitative studies that include analysis of interviews with patients and clients after Reiki sessions may be vital to understanding the unique and personal effects of Reiki. Currently, there are both quantitative and qualitative studies in the literature that provide evidence for the effectiveness of Reiki. The relevance of these publications will be described in detail in Chapters 5–13.

Status of Clinical Research on Reiki

As of June 2019, there are 77 original Reiki research articles published in peer-reviewed scientific journals. Peer review "is the process of subjecting an author's scholarly work, research, or ideas to the scrutiny of others who are experts in the same field, before a paper describing this work is published in a journal, conference proceedings or as a book" (Wikipedia.com). If an article does not stand up to such robust criticism, it is not accepted for publication in the journal. For that reason, the number of peer-reviewed publications relating to a certain topic of research provides a good estimation of the current status of research in that area. For this book, in June 2018, in order to compare the status of Reiki research with research in other areas of complementary medicine, a search of the scientific database Medline (via Ovid) was employed. The number of articles containing the descriptive word of a particular therapy (i.e. "Reiki" or "acupuncture" or "biofeedback") in the title was determined. The results

Table 2.1 Numbers of Medline citation titles that contain the name of each specific complementary therapy		
Complementary therapy	**Number of articles 1946–June 2018**	**Number of articles 1946–1990**
Reiki	131	1
Qigong	368	22
Osteopathy	892	533
Tai Chi	922	5
Meditation	1789	384
Chiropractic	2610	515
Biofeedback	3004	1263
Massage	3848	1411
Hypnosis	4361	2720
Acupuncture	13429	2979

are shown in Table 2.1. It should be noted that these numbers do not just refer to research articles, but also include reviews, case studies and opinion articles. Although Reiki currently only appears in the titles of 131 peer-reviewed scientific articles, it is apparent from the numbers of articles published before 1990 that clinical Reiki research is at an early stage compared to most other complementary therapies. In fact, for Reiki, Qigong and Tai Chi, less than 1% of peer-reviewed articles were published before 1990, whereas the corresponding percentages for meditation, chiropractic and acupuncture were about 20% and for osteopathy and hypnosis, about 60%. Therefore, although Reiki research is in its infancy, there has been a surge of research productivity in recent decades. The robustness of this research will be discussed in the next section, focusing on the 77 peer-reviewed, published original Reiki research studies. As will be demonstrated in the next section, the higher quality research indicates that Reiki shows some promise as a noninvasive tool for healing at the physical and nonphysical levels, particularly regarding the alleviation of pain, depression, and anxiety and the maintenance of well-being.

The Touchstone Process – An Ongoing Evaluation of Reiki Research

In 2009, William Lee Rand, founder and president of the International Center for Reiki Training (ICRT), brought together a team of experts who had experience in scientific research and Reiki practice, to develop procedures to evaluate the state of Reiki research on an ongoing basis and to make those evaluations available to the public and to academic and medical communities. Another goal was to provide a framework for future investigational design including guidelines for conducting high quality Reiki research and a consultation service. The experts, selected from 5,000 possible candidates, included seven researchers with doctoral degrees and five nurses from pharmaceutical, biotechnology and healthcare settings, most of whom had contributed to the scientific literature. This team became known as The Center for Reiki Research (CRR), operating as part of ICRT. Although many of the members have changed throughout the years, all their replacements

are at least equally qualified as the original team in terms of credentials, expertise and experience in research, peer review and Reiki knowledge and practice. The CRR has been continuous in fulfilling its goals since 2009 and meets regularly every month.

Development of the Touchstone Process

Members of CRR began by developing a set of specific aims (listed on the website www.centerforreikiresearch.org) as follows:

1. Review the current status of basic and clinical Reiki research as reflected by publications only in peer-reviewed journals.

2. Evaluate existing basic, preclinical, and clinical studies for evidence (or otherwise) of Reiki's effectiveness.

3. Summarize the main goals, results, and conclusions of each peer-reviewed study.

4. Identify gaps in knowledge and recommend areas for future study.

5. Identify components critical to rigorous study design.

6. Create a consultative resource for investigators in planning clinical and/or preclinical protocols.

The immediate focus was to develop a robust review process (named the "Touchstone Process") for Reiki research articles. A diagram of the steps of the Touchstone Process used to evaluate and summarize Reiki research articles is shown in Figure 2.1. Details of the Touchstone Process can be found in the scientific literature (Baldwin et al., 2010). In order to review and score the articles, standardized forms were developed: a quantitative form for studies involving collection of objective, numerical data; and a qualitative form for the relatively small number of studies involving analysis of questionnaires and personal interviews that reveal the actual

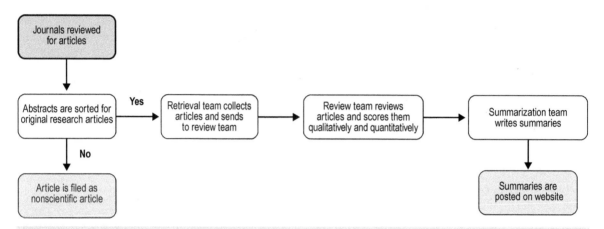

Figure 2.1

Flowchart of Reiki research literature review by the Touchstone Process.

experiences of Reiki recipients. These evaluation forms were based loosely on the CONSORT (Consolidated Standards of Reporting Trials) criteria (Olivo et al., 2008). A short list of these criteria is available at: www.consort-statement.org/ (click on CONSORT 2010 Checklist).

Not all the CONSORT criteria were included because they are designed solely for randomized, controlled clinical trials, whereas Reiki research also includes basic scientific experiments and pilot studies. A pilot study is a small scale preliminary study conducted to evaluate feasibility, time, cost, adverse events, and effect size (statistical variability) in an attempt to predict an appropriate participant sample size and improve upon the study design prior to performance of a full-scale research project.

At any stage of research, critical components of good study design include:

1. Inclusion and exclusion criteria for participants.

2. Randomization of participants between groups.

3. Comparison conditions.

4. Appropriate control groups.

5. Blinding of participants and data collectors regarding participant grouping.

6. Standardized implementation of treatment protocol.

7. Careful selection of outcomes and their measurement with reliable relevant instruments.

8. Appropriate analyses.

In the Touchstone Process, additional components pertaining to Reiki were included, such as:

1. Standardization of Reiki treatments with each participant within a study.

2. Information about training level and years of experience of Reiki practitioners partaking in the research.

3. Using Reiki practitioners trained to the same level in a given study.

A scoring system was incorporated in the quantitative and qualitative evaluation forms based on the chosen criteria and each paper is scored by at least two independent reviewers from the team. Based on the score, each reviewer

Table 2.2 Numerical score ranges for "Overall Impression".

	Qualitative (out of 15)	Quantitative (out of 34)
Weak	0–8	0–20
Satisfactory	9–11	21–25
Very good	12–13	26–29
Excellent	14–15	30–34

scientific training. Finally, the summary is read by the editor-in-chief who determines whether the summary accurately reflects the reviewers' scores and comments, and edits accordingly prior to placing it on the website: www .centerforreikiresearch.org.

Summary of Evaluations Using the Touchstone Process

rates the article for "Overall Impression" (i.e. excellent, very good, satisfactory, or weak). To ensure consistency between a reviewer's score and Overall Impression, exact numerical ranges were defined for each Overall Impression category (Table 2.2). After evaluation, each article is passed onto the Summarization Team, one of whom translates the reviews to a short summary stating the purpose or hypothesis, methods, results, conclusions, strengths and weaknesses, and impact, if any, of the study. The summaries are written for lay people who do not necessarily have

Figure 2.2 shows a histogram of the number and quality (based on evaluation scores) of the "quantitative" articles evaluated since 1996. The average number of quantitative articles published per year, and to some extent their quality, have increased greatly during the last 10 years compared to the previous decade. Articles that are rated as "Very Good" or "Excellent" by at least one reviewer and are not rated as "Weak" by any reviewer, are separated into an upper tier and further examined to determine to what degree they lend support, or not, to Reiki as a healing modality. Of the 77 current peer-reviewed, published Reiki research articles, CRR placed 33 of them (including three

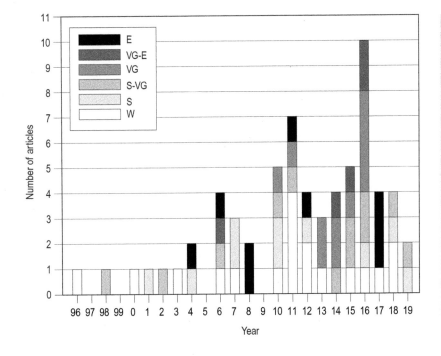

Figure 2.2
Number and quality of quantitative Reiki published papers derived by the Touchstone Process.

basic science studies) in the top tier. The three basic science studies, which will not be discussed here, addressed:

i. Physiological changes in energy healers during self-practice (Baldwin and Schwartz, 2012).

ii. Whether measurable electromagnetic fields are produced by the hands and hearts of Reiki practitioners during practice (Baldwin et al., 2013a).

iii. Whether the Reiki healing process influences the output of a random number generator in the room used for Reiki (Morse and Beem, 2011).

The other 30 papers that reported the effect of Reiki on clinical indications or conditions are categorized in Table 2.3, according to the demonstrated effectiveness of Reiki. These papers are listed as a separate group in the

Table 2.3 Papers characterized for effectiveness of Reiki

	Solid initial evidence of no effect	Suggestive initial evidence of no effect or placebo	Mixed or conditional (study design and/or execution issues)	Suggestive initial evidence of positive effect	Solid initial evidence of positive effect
CLINICAL Indication or condition	1. Pain in fibromyalgia (Assefi and Bogart, 2008)	1. Post stroke rehabilitation and recovery (Shiflett et al., 2002)	1. Well-being (Witte and Dundes, 2001)	1. Well-being in Reiki practitioners (Whelan and Wishnia, 2003)	1. Chronic pain (Dressen and Singg, 1998)
		2. Painful diabetic neuropathy (Gillespie et al., 2007)	2. Cognition in elderly (Crawford et al., 2006)	2. Well-being in nurses (Vitale, 2009)	2. Depression and stress (Shore, 2004)
		3. Well-being during chemotherapy (Catlin and Taylor-Ford, 2011; Orsak et al., 2015)	3. Pre-op anxiety & post op pain (Vitale, 2006)	3. Well-being in elderly with HIV (Mehl-Madrona et al., 2011)	3. Stress and anxiety in health workers (Diaz-Rodriguez et al., 2011)
			4. Well-being & stress (Bowden et al., 2010)	4. Well-being in students (Bowden et al., 2011)	4. Pain and shoulder movement (Baldwin et al., 2013b)
			5. Depression in adolescents (Charkhandeh et al., 2016)	5. Pain with knee surgery (Notte et al., 2016)	5. Depression in elderly (Erdogan and Cinar, 2014)
			6. Pain, stress, anxiety with HIV (Bremner et al., 2016)	6. Stress & anxiety (Kurebayashi et al., 2016)	6. Stress in mental health workers (Rosada et al., 2015)
			7. Pain and Caesarean (Midilli and Gunduzoglu, 2016)	7. Well-being with blood cancer (Alarcao and Fonseca, 2016)	7. Pain & anxiety with knee surgery (Baldwin et al., 2017)
			8. Pain and vein incision (Shaybak, 2017)	8. Well-being & anxiety pre-surgery (Chirico et al., 2017)	
PRECLINICAL Indication or condition					1. Stress response in rats (Baldwin and Schwartz, 2006; Baldwin et al., 2008)

references. As shown in Table 2.3, there was only one solidly negative result (Assefi and Bogart, 2008). This study showed no statistically significant effect of Reiki on *fibromyalgia-associated* pain levels. This observation suggests that although Reiki intervention may be useful in some settings, it is not universally effective in all clinical indications, as is also the case for more conventional drug treatments. Negative results such as these can be quite helpful in guiding the direction of future controlled studies.

The nine papers that showed solid initial evidence of a positive effect were selected on the basis of one or more of the following criteria:

- Inclusion of sham Reiki group.

- Longer-term study with multiple Reiki treatments.

- Participants blinded as to group they were assigned to.

The eight papers characterized as providing suggestive initial evidence of a positive effect were well designed and demonstrated statistically significant benefits of Reiki but were flawed by one or more of the following problems:

- Low number of participants (20 or fewer).

- Did not include a sham Reiki group.

- Did not demonstrate benefits of Reiki in all measured parameters.

The 17 papers showing solid or suggestive evidence of a positive effect of Reiki were associated with improvements in well-being and alleviation of pain, emotional stress, anxiety and depression. These studies will be discussed in detail in Chapters 5–13.

Although, at first sight, experiments involving people, rather than laboratory animals, may seem more relevant to testing the effectiveness of Reiki in clinical settings, animal experiments do have distinct advantages over human experiments with regard to scientific robustness. Mary Kearns, PhD, psychologist and Reiki Master, contributed

an article for the CRR website which addresses this viewpoint: "Conclusion. Does the Reiki Touchstone Process show support of Reiki?" (www.centerforreikiresearch.org /RRConclusion.aspx):

Perhaps the strongest evidence that Reiki has a demonstrable biological effect comes from the carefully controlled studies on rats by Baldwin and colleagues (2006, 2008; both rated 'Excellent'). In a laboratory setting, Reiki (performed at a distance from the animals) significantly reduced stress responses relative to sham Reiki. It should not be surprising that animal studies form the strongest indication of Reiki's effectiveness, as experiments in the laboratory can be designed to control for most variables that would otherwise complicate studies on human subjects. Interestingly, depression and stress were also the two clinical conditions that responded in a significant way to Reiki intervention (Shore, 2004; rated 'Excellent'), consistent with the preclinical findings of Baldwin. Further evaluation in expanded preclinical and clinical studies on stress, anxiety and depression reduction are therefore warranted.

In summary, well over half of the 30 higher-quality Reiki research studies support Reiki as a healing modality for clinical indications that are among the most common issues experienced by individuals. Evidence for the widespread incidence of problems involving pain, anxiety and depression is presented below.

According to data from the 2012 National Health Interview Survey (NHIS) (nccih.nih.gov/research/statistics/ NHIS/2012/pain/severity) published in Nahin (2015), 11.2% of American adults (25.3 million people) have experienced some form of pain every day for the past three months. Pain is one of the leading reasons Americans turn to complementary health approaches. Evidence of large-scale problems with pain is not just limited to the USA. An article in *The British Medical Journal (BMJ)* (Fayaz et al., 2016) estimates that between a third and half (43%) of the UK population, roughly 28 million adults, live with chronic pain. Based on seven studies, the prevalence of chronic pain was estimated to range from 35% to 51% of the adult population, with the prevalence of moderate to severely disabling chronic pain (based on four studies), ranging from 10% to 14%, which is equal to about eight million people. With regard to anxiety, this disorder is the most common mental illness in the USA. According to the Anxiety and Depression Association of America (ADAA), 40 million Americans over the age of 18 are affected by anxiety (18% of the population). Major Depressive Disorder affects more than 16.1 million American adults, or about 6.7% of the US population age 18 and older in a given year (adaa.org/about-adaa/press-room/facts-statistics). According to a recent report from the UK House of Commons Library (Baker, 2018), one in six people in England (17%) said they had experienced a "common mental disorder" like anxiety or depression in the last week. The same report stated that one million people (out of a population of 53 million) were in contact with mental health services as of December 2017 and the waiting time for psychological therapy ranged from 16 to 167 days. There is clearly a great need for a large number of clinical practitioners who are effective at reducing the severity of pain, anxiety and depression in their clients and patients. Based on the peer-reviewed research on the effectiveness of Reiki, which, although limited in extent, is largely positive, it seems that Reiki practitioners can fill this gap.

Reports of patient and staff outcomes from hospitals with Reiki programs

Reiki has been used in hospital operating rooms since the mid-1990s (Brown, 1995). Hospitals are incorporating it into their options for patient services, often with their own Reiki-trained volunteers, nurses, physicians and support staff.

A 2010 American Hospital Association survey (2010 Complementary and Alternative Medicine Survey of Hospitals by Sita Ananth, Samueli Institute) revealed that patient demand (85%) is by far the primary rationale in offering complementary medicine services, including Reiki. In addition, Reiki is now one of the top three complementary in-patient therapies offered in US hospitals. The survey showed that of the patients asking for complementary services, massage was requested by 37% of patients, music and art therapy by 25%, and "healing touch therapies" including Reiki and Therapeutic Touch, by 25%. According to a study published in *USA Today* (Gill, 2008), in 2007, more than 60 US hospitals offered Reiki as a hospital service, and Reiki education was offered at 800 hospitals.

One reason why hospital patients request Reiki is that hospital culture, particularly in emergency departments, emphasizes medical and technical skill and efficiency at the expense of bedside manner. As a result, patients' psychosocial and emotional needs are often neglected (Gordon et al., 2010). Patients feel vulnerable, anxious, stressed and fearful. There is a pattern of fragmentation of care, with one nurse assigned to triage, another to blood tests, a third to check the patient's temperature and so on. The patients long for the personal contact that is lacking when overworked nurses and physicians have to rush onto their next case. When a patient receives Reiki, they are treated as a whole person; their physical, emotional, and spiritual dimensions all receive attention. Anecdotal reports and patient surveys from several hospitals in the USA, along with detailed, extensive data from Hartford Hospital, Connecticut, USA are presented in the following section. A list of 64 hospitals that incorporate Reiki programs can be found at the Center for Reiki Research website:

www.centerforreikiresearch.org/HospitalList.aspx

Reiki programs have also been developed in other countries but at this stage few, if any, data are available about the effectiveness of the programs. In the UK, the **Full Circle Fund Therapies** is an award-winning charity that relies on integrative medicine in order to improve the quality of life of patients who are treated at **St. George's Hospital, London.** Their mission is to introduce, evaluate and research Reiki in clinical practice. Presently, Full Circle Fund Therapies is working at the funding and logistics level of a project, called "Connecting Reiki with Medicine", whose aim is to perform well-designed research studies to explore the benefits of Reiki.

University College London Hospitals NHS offer Reiki to patients with stress and mood disorder, and to complement the treatments of cancer and endometriosis. Wallace Cancer Care works with **Addenbrooke's Hospital-Cambridge University Hospitals NHS** to provide Reiki to complement conventional cancer treatments. More information about hospitals in the UK that offer Reiki can be found on the websites of the UK Reiki Federation and The Reiki Council. In Canada, the **Cross Cancer Institute, Edmonton**, conducted a study on the effects of Reiki with 20 oncology patients in chronic pain. A visual analog scale was used to measure pain before and after Reiki and it was concluded that Reiki greatly improved pain levels. In Spain, Reiki Master John Curtin, head of Fundación Sauce, has initiated 400 volunteer Reiki practitioners who gave more than 8,000 Reiki sessions in Madrid hospitals in 2013.

Reiki in Hospitals – Patient Outcomes

According to an International Association of Reiki Professionals (IARP) study, 60% of "America's Best Hospitals" (the top 25 ranked by *US News and World Report* in 2002) had Reiki programs in place. All hospitals using Reiki indicated that they thought Reiki was at least somewhat beneficial for patients, and 67% said they believed Reiki to be highly beneficial.

A Reiki program was introduced in 1997 at **Portsmouth (New Hampshire) Regional Hospital** by Patricia Alandydy, Reiki Master and operating room nurse manager, to address patient anxiety before surgery. This program is still in operation and Reiki volunteers cover the hospital seven days a week. If patients request Reiki, it is given the morning of surgery, and an additional 15–20-minute session is given prior to their transport to the operating room. Some patients have also received Reiki in the operating room at Portsmouth Regional Hospital. Since the start of the program, Reiki has gained wider acceptance and is not just limited to those patients who are undergoing surgery. Reiki is currently available in every department of the hospital to patients, their visitors and staff. According to Alandydy:

It has been an extremely rewarding experience to see Reiki embraced by such a diverse group of people and spread so far and wide by word of mouth, in a positive light. Patients many times request a Reiki [session] based on the positive experience of one of their friends. It has also been very revealing to see how open-minded the older patient population is to try Reiki. In the hospital setting, Reiki is presented as a technique which reduces stress and promotes relaxation, thereby enhancing the body's natural ability to heal itself.

Alandydy also offers a philosophical underpinning for establishing hospital-based Reiki programs:

The focus of offering Reiki in [our] hospital [is] to <u>bring compassion and humanity back into the patient's experience</u>. Additionally, at a time when patients can feel passive in their care, Reiki offers a <u>sense of empowerment</u>. By choosing to receive Reiki, patients can actively participate in their healing process.

A voluntary survey is given to surgical patients who receive Reiki asking them to rate their anxiety on a 10-point scale before and after their procedure. In January to March 2003, the average stress score was 4.9 points lower after Reiki and the average pain score was 3.7 points lower. Twenty-three percent of patients receiving Reiki in January to March 2003 fell asleep during treatment. Ana Drexler RN, Director of Integrative Services and Palliative Care, says that patients almost universally report a marked decrease in both stress and pain. However, Portsmouth Regional Hospital has not compared lengths of stay, pain medication use, or patient satisfaction among inpatients who have received Reiki therapy with those who have not. Nevertheless, patients who have become calmer and feel less pain are easier for the staff to care for, and likely to have a more positive hospital experience. They are also likely to have better medical outcomes.

The Reiki program at **Brigham and Women's Hospital** is staffed by over 60 volunteer Reiki practitioners, as well as nurses and other staff members certified to perform Reiki. According to the article "BWH Volunteer Reiki Program" on their website www.brighamandwomens.org/ (note to readers: to access this article enter "Reiki" in the search box:

Chapter 2

Over the past eight years, our Reiki volunteers alone have provided over 40,000 Reiki sessions to patients, family members, and hospital staff.[...] Our data, based on feedback from patients, family members, and staff members who receive Reiki sessions, as well as outside research, show that Reiki promotes relaxation, relieves stress and anxiety, reduces pain and fatigue, and improves overall quality of life.

The California Pacific Medical Center is one of the largest hospitals in northern California. Its Health and Healing Clinic provides care for both acute and chronic illness using a wide range of complementary care including Reiki. Dr. Mike Cantwell, a pediatrician specializing in infectious diseases, is also a Reiki Master. Dr. Cantwell provides 1–3-hour-long Reiki sessions, after which he assigns the patient to a Reiki II practitioner who continues with Reiki sessions outside the clinic. Patients who respond well to the Reiki treatments are referred for Reiki training so they can practice Reiki self-treatments on a continuing basis. Dr. Cantwell states:

I have found Reiki to be useful in the treatment of acute illnesses such as musculoskeletal injury/pain, headache, acute infections, and asthma. Reiki is also useful for patients with chronic illnesses, especially those associated with chronic pain.

Reiki is an ongoing clinical program offered in cardiac units at **Yale New Haven Hospital,** Connecticut, USA. The Section of Cardiology, Department of Internal Medicine at Yale University conducted a study to determine whether Reiki would improve heart rate variability in patients recovering from acute coronary syndrome. Heart rate variability (HRV) indicates how well the heart adapts to the body's needs. Acute coronary syndrome refers to a situation in which blood flow decreases in one or more coronary arteries such that the surrounding area of the heart muscle is unable to function properly. Five Reiki-trained nurses who were employed in the program were the Reiki practitioners for the study. Twelve patients received Reiki, 13 listened to music and 12 did not receive any extra treatment beyond standard of care (the control group). The increase in HRV was significantly greater in the Reiki group than in the music or control groups (Bremner et al., 2016). Low HRV is a predictor of

death after acute coronary syndrome (Balenescu et al., 2004). These data support the idea that the patients who received Reiki were given an extra boost regarding their chances of full recovery.

In 1998, **Hartford Hospital,** Connecticut, USA approved the development of a Reiki volunteer pilot program in Women's Health. Patients and staff reported statistically significant reductions in pain and anxiety, as well as improvement with sleep. As a result, the program became part of a formal Integrative Medicine Department in 1999. In 1998, 10 volunteers provided 523 Reiki sessions. In 2012, approximately 40–50 volunteers provided 3,167 Reiki sessions. The total number of Reiki sessions provided over the 15 years is 58,214. Over 84% of patients say they would be more likely to choose Hartford Hospital for future admissions because of Reiki and other complementary and alternative therapies offered by Integrative Medicine (Figure 2.3).

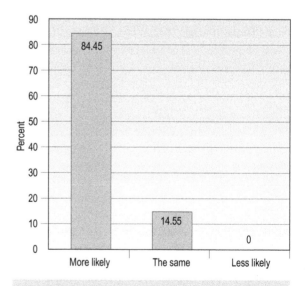

Figure 2.3

Patient Satisfaction Rating: Likelihood of choosing Hartford Hospital for future admissions because of the Integrative Medicine Program.

(From: https://hartfordhospital.org/services/integrative-medicine/patient-support/outcomes)

Some comments from patients taken from an online article, "Hartford Hospital's Reiki Volunteer Program Celebrates its 15th Year Anniversary", dated March 1st 2016, that appears on the website www.hartfordhospital.org are shown below:

I hope Reiki is always available because it helped me a lot in relaxing and healing, giving me energy to think positive and forget the bad things wrong with me. I thank you for Reiki; it really, really helped me!

I felt the Reiki program helped me to relax and deepen my breathing patterns which, in turn, reduced my pain. I am very grateful for the Reiki volunteers.

I will never go to another hospital again because of the effect Reiki has had on me. I have had eight operations and the last one at HH was the most painful. The Reiki session helped me handle it and believe I can go through it again with Reiki.

Even on pain medications, after a Reiki session was the only time I was pain free!

Data obtained from patients who obtained Reiki during the initial pilot phase (December 1999–December 2000) are presented in Figures 2.4 and 2.5. Figure 2.4 demonstrates that 570 patients felt significantly less pain and were more relaxed after a Reiki session than before. Figure 2.5 shows that a group of 44 employees felt significantly less pain, were more relaxed, and felt significantly less fatigue after their Reiki sessions than before. Data obtained from patients after the pilot study when the Reiki program had expanded (July–December 2004) are presented in Figures 2.6 and 2.7. After Reiki or massage, 97% of patients said that their sleep improved and 91% said that their nausea was reduced. Patients attending the Brownstone Ambulatory Clinic, Hartford Hospital, between August 2003 and December 2004 who received Reiki, massage or acupuncture once a week for six weeks showed significantly less anxiety and pain after their treatment. In 2008, Hartford Hospital Reiki Program was extended to the Cancer Center. Reiki is being used increasingly to comfort cancer patients and to and decrease their pain and anxiety.

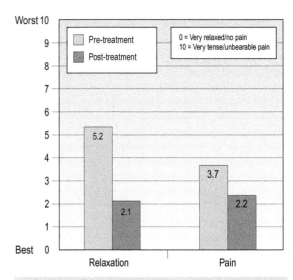

Figure 2.4

Effects of Reiki on patient relaxation and pain.

(From: https://hartfordhospital.org/services/integrative-medicine/patient-support/outcomes)

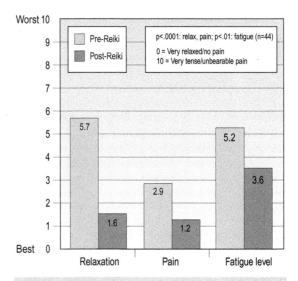

Figure 2.5

Effects of Reiki on employee relaxation, pain and fatigue.

(From: https://hartfordhospital.org/services/inte grative-medicine/patient-support/outcomes)

Chapter 2

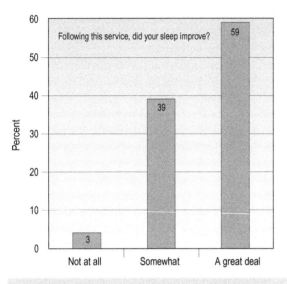

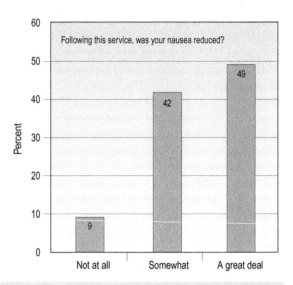

Figure 2.6

Effects of massage or Reiki on sleep and nausea in patients.

(From: https://hartfordhospital.org/services/integrative-medicine/patient-support/outcomes)

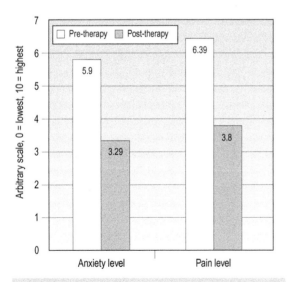

Figure 2.7

Effects of acupuncture, massage or Reiki on patient anxiety and pain levels.

(From: https://hartfordhospital.org/services/integrative-medicine/patient -support/outcomes)

Reiki in Hospitals – Cancer Patients

Three of the most prestigious cancer hospitals in the USA, as ranked by *US News*, are: (i) MD Anderson Cancer Center, Texas; (ii) Memorial Sloan Kettering Cancer Center, New York; (iii) Mayo Clinic, Minnesota. All three of these hospitals offer Reiki to their patients. MD Anderson Cancer Center is ranked No. 1 and their Integrative Medicine Center provides holistic treatments in which the mental, spiritual and emotional needs of the patient are provided. Founded in 1884 as the New York Cancer Hospital, the Memorial Sloan Kettering Cancer Center is ranked No. 2. Their Integrative Medicine Service offers acupuncture, personal training, nutrition and dietary supplement counseling, massage, and mind-body therapies (where Reiki is included). Their goal is to soothe and alleviate symptoms such as pain, muscle tension, post-operative discomfort, musculoskeletal problems, anxiety, depression, insomnia, stress, and fatigue. Mayo Clinic is ranked No. 3 in Cancer Hospitals. Mayo Clinic has also focused on a holistic approach, including the spiritual and emotional conflicts and needs that might arise during treatment. Reiki practitioners provide volunteer services to patients at both Mayo Clinic Hospital campuses and some outpatient areas.

Reiki for Hospice Care

Reiki is particularly effective for patients undergoing palliative and/or hospice care. The International Association of Reiki Practitioners states on its website (iarp.org/reiki-for-hospice-and-home-health-care/): "As a complementary treatment, Reiki is becoming more and more popular in the spheres of hospice, palliative and home care." According to the Merlene Bullock, RN BSN, Case Manager, Hospice of the Valley, Phoenix, Arizona, USA (Bullock, 1997), Reiki has been associated with improved quality of life in palliative situations:

Some general trends seen with Reiki include: periods of stabilization in which there is time to enjoy the last days of one's life; a peaceful and calm passing if death is imminent; and relief from pain, anxiety, dyspnea (shortness of breath) and edema. Reiki is a valuable complement in supporting patients in their end-of-life journey, enhancing the quality of their remaining days.

Pamela Miles, Reiki Master, educator and author, who has consulted with hospital administrators about integrating Reiki practice into clinical care, says:

Caring family members can learn Reiki as easily as the palliative patient can. Caregivers experience stress and the first thing taught in Reiki Level 1 is self-care. This ability can be used to care for the palliative patient, thereby making the family member "feel useful" (Miles, 2003).

In 2012, the Penn Wissahickon Hospice, part of the University of Pennsylvania Health System, tested a volunteer Reiki program for its effectiveness in a hospice setting. Ellen Inglesby-Deering, a volunteer coordinator, commented:

It's very exciting. I've heard nothing but positive feedback from patients, families and volunteers.

A volunteer mentioned a patient with advanced dementia who giggled after the treatment and then started having a conversation with her daughter. The daughter later commented that she had not been able to have a conversation this beneficial with her mother in over a year. The Reiki program for hospice care is still active as judged by the online requests for more Reiki volunteers.

A small study was performed at Alpert Medical School of Brown University, Providence, Rhode Island, USA (Connor and Anadarajah, 2017) to explore the experiences of hospice patients and their caregivers who received Reiki.

Three major themes emerged:

1. Trust plays an important role in both trying Reiki and experiencing benefits.

2. Sensations are felt in the body during Reiki; notable similarities in descriptions included somatic sensations (arising from skin, muscles, joints, etc.), temperature changes and visual sensations.

3. Some symptoms are relieved by Reiki, the most common being anxiety. Others include: pain, agitation, nausea, and insomnia. Participants reported no side effects. It was concluded that although symptom management in hospice patients remains a challenge, Reiki has the potential to serve as a useful adjunctive therapy in treating several symptoms, particularly anxiety.

Effects of Self-Reiki Practice on Nurses

Hospital nurses often practice Reiki on themselves because they find it to be a very effective tool for maintaining general well-being. Nurses who are taught Reiki experience immediate stress relief and relaxation after just a few minutes of self-treatment while on the job (Brathovde 2006, 2017; Cuneo et al., 2011).

Brathvode's study of Reiki as a self-care practice among nurses demonstrated that the nurses who participated increased their self-care and caring towards others after Reiki education. In Cuneo's study, 26 nurses completed a perceived stress assessment questionnaire and were then taught Reiki Level 1. After 21 days of Reiki self-practice, they repeated the questionnaire. There was a statistically significant decrease in their perceived stress. Further analysis of the results indicated that the more self-Reiki was performed, regardless of the degree of reported stress of the participant, the more effective self-Reiki was in supporting stress reduction. Common comments after Reiki self-practice were: slept better, felt relaxed/calm/peaceful, felt warm/hot.

Whelan and Wishnia (2003) studied the experiences of nurses who were already trained in Reiki and who practiced Reiki on their clients. As Reiki practitioners, these nurses also concurrently received the benefits of Reiki themselves. More than 75% reported satisfaction with the time they spent with patients, were less affected by environmental stress, experienced increased intuition and insight, and noticed a significant decrease in feelings that contribute to burnout. In addition, 75% felt they had helped clients in the healing process by bringing relaxation and calmness to the clients. However, 37.5% also reported a perceived disadvantage of practicing Reiki: decreased credibility with nursing and medical professionals despite research that demonstrated Reiki's efficacy (Whelan and Wishnia, 2003).

Vitale (2009) interviewed 11 registered nurses who were also Reiki practitioners to determine how they thought they benefited from Reiki self-practice. The nurses reported that they firstly used Reiki to relax because it promoted an immediate relaxation response. They said that they felt more energized and less tired after self-Reiki use and also mentioned that they would gain a clearer perspective on an issue, after which they would feel calm. According to the article author, Anne Vitale, herself also a nurse: "The ability to quickly restore the self to a tranquil state and awareness to shifting back into a centered state are essential for nurses working in today's healthcare environments."[...] "The nurses in this study report that the use of Reiki in self-care is useful for daily and workday stress management."

Summary

Overall, the anecdotal and clinical data obtained from Reiki programs in hospitals show that patients receiving Reiki experience enhanced relaxation and well-being, as well as reduced sensations of anxiety and pain. These responses are an essential part of the healing process and are consistent with findings from the published, peer-reviewed, scientific data. Of course, the comments and data obtained from hospital patients can be criticized because there was no systematic comparison made with patients in similar conditions who did not receive Reiki, or with patients who received frequent visitation from a friend or family member who was not a Reiki practitioner but offered them comfort. Perhaps it is not the Reiki that is improving their well-being, but just the presence of a caring person who pays them attention. This is known as the "placebo effect". The placebo effect definitely contributes to Reiki's success, but there are currently nine placebo-controlled studies that demonstrate Reiki's beneficial effects are statistically significantly greater than can be explained just by the placebo effect. Obviously, more high-quality placebo-controlled studies are needed that address the effects of Reiki on a variety of clinical conditions, but as shown by the analysis of the quality of Reiki research studies presented in the first half of this chapter (see Table 2.3), the evidence so far is heavily weighted in support of Reiki as an effective therapy. Of course, there are skeptics who carefully handpick the negative studies and ignore the positive results. For example, Stephen Barrett MD, author of *Reiki is Nonsense* (www.quackwatch.org) states:

The most comprehensive review of reiki research was done by Edzard Ernst MD PhD and his colleagues at the University of Exeter. After surveying studies published through January 2008, they concluded that most were poorly designed and "the evidence is insufficient to suggest that reiki is an effective treatment for any condition".

The entry in Wikipedia for Reiki states the following:

Reiki is a pseudoscience. Clinical research has not shown reiki to be effective as a treatment for any medical condition.

There has been no proof of the effectiveness of reiki therapy compared to placebo.

These comments are false, biased and ignore the more recently published studies, as well as the placebo-controlled experiments outlined earlier in this chapter. The main goal of the CRR is to make all of the scientific information pertaining to Reiki available to anyone who chooses to read it so that they have an informed basis from which to decide whether Reiki is likely to fulfill their needs.

References

Baker C. Mental Health Statistics for England: prevalence, services and funding. Briefing Paper 6988, 25th April, 2018.

Baldwin AL, Vitale A, Brownell E, Kearns M, Rand W. The Touchstone Process: an ongoing critical evaluation of Reiki in the scientific literature. *Holistic Nursing Practice* 2010; 24 (5): 260–276.

Baldwin AL, Schwartz GE. Physiological changes in energy healers during self-practice. *Complementary Therapies in Medicine* 2012; 20: 299–305.

Baldwin AL, Rand W, Schwartz GE. Practicing Reiki does not routinely appear to produce high intensity electromagnetic fields from the heart and hands of Reiki practitioners. *Journal of Alternative and Complementary Medicine* 2013a; 19(6): 518–526.

Balenescu S, Corian A-D, Dorobantu M, Gherasim L. Prognostic value of heart rate variability after acute myocardial infarction. *International Medical Journal of Experimental and Clinical Research* 2004; 10(7): CR307–315.

Brathovde A. A pilot study: Reiki for self-care of nurses and healthcare providers. *Holistic Nursing Practice* 2006; 20(2): 95–101.

Brathovde A. Teaching Nurses Reiki Energy Therapy for Self-Care. *International Journal for Human Caring* 2017; 21(1): 20–25.

Bremner MN, Blake BJ, Wagner VD, Pearcy SM. Effects of Reiki with music compared to music only among people living with HIV. *Journal of the Association of Nurses in AIDS Care* 2016; 27(5): 635–647.

Bullock M. Reiki: a complementary therapy for life. Hospice of the Valley, Phoenix, Arizona, USA. *American Journal of Hospice and Palliative Medicine* 1997; 14(1): 31–33.

Brown C. The Experiments of Dr. Oz. *The New York Times Magazine*, July 30, 1995, pp. 20–23.

Conner K, Anadarajah G. Reiki for hospice patients and their caregivers: an in-depth qualitative study of experiences and effects on symptoms. *Journal of Pain and Symptom Management* 2017; 53(2): 420–421.

Cuneo CL, Curtis Cooper MR, Drew CS, Naoum-Heffernan C, Sherman T, Walz K, Weinberg J. The effect of Reiki on work-related stress of the registered nurse. *Journal of Holistic* Nursing 2011; 29(1): 23–33.

Gill L. More hospitals offer alternative therapies for mind, body, spirit. *USA Today.* September 2008 http:// www.usatoday.com/news/health/2008-09-14-alternative -therapies_N.htm.

Gordon J, Sheppard LA, Anaf S. The patient experience in the emergency department: A systematic synthesis of qualitative research. *International Emergency Nursing* 2010; 18: 80–88.

Fayaz A, Croft P, Langford RM, Donaldson LJ, Jones GT. Prevalence of chronic pain in the UK: a systematic review and meta-analysis of population studies. *BMJ Open*, June 2016. DOI: 10.1136/bmjopen-2015-010364.

Miles P. The bridge to conventional medicine: a call for case reports. *Reiki Magazine International* 2002; 4(3): 32–33.

Miles P. Preliminary report on the use of Reiki for HIV-related pain and anxiety. *Alternative Therapies* 2003; 9(2): 36.

Morse ML, Beem LW. Benefits of Reiki therapy for a severely neutropenic patient with associated influences on a true random number generator. *Journal of Alternative and Complementary Medicine* 2011; 17(12): 1181–1190.

Nahin RL. Estimates of pain prevalence and severity in adults: United States, 2012. *Journal of Pain* 2015; 16(8): 769–780.

Olivo SA, Macedo LG, Gadotti IC, Fuentes J, Stanton T, Magee DJ. Scales to assess the quality of randomized controlled trials: a systematic review. *Physical Therapy* 2008; 88: 156–175.

Van de Velde J. Writing case reports for Reiki. *The Reiki News Magazine*, Summer Issue, 2009.

Touchstone papers

Alarcao Z, Fonseca JRS. The effect of Reiki therapy on quality of life of patients with blood cancer results from a randomized controlled trial. *European Journal of Integrative Medicine* 2016; 8: 239–249.

Assefi N, Bogart A, Goldberg J, Buchwald D. Reiki for the treatment of fibromyalgia: a randomized, controlled trial. *Journal of Alternative and Complementary Medicine* 2008; 14(9): 1115–1122.

Baldwin AL, Schwartz GE. Personal interaction with a Reiki practitioner decreases noise-induced microvascular damage in an animal model. *Journal of Alternative and Complementary Medicine* 2006; 12(1): 15–22.

Baldwin AL, Wagers C, Schwartz GE. Reiki improves heart rate homeostasis in laboratory rats. *Journal of Alternative and Complementary Medicine* 2008; 14(4): 417–422.

Baldwin AL, Fullmer K, Schwartz GE. Comparison of physical therapy with energy healing for improving range of motion in subjects with restricted shoulder mobility. *Evidence-Based Complementary and Alternative Medicine* 2013b; 2013: 329731.

Baldwin AL, Vitale A, Brownell E, Rand W. Effects of Reiki on pain, anxiety and blood pressure in knee replacement patients. *Holistic Nursing Practice* 2017; 31(2): 80–89.

Bowden D, Goddard L, Gruzelier J. A randomized controlled single-blind study of the effects of Reiki and positive imagery on well-being and salivary cortisol. *Brain Research Bulletin* 2010; 81: 66–67.

Bowden D, Goddard L, Gruzelier J. A randomized controlled single-blind trial of the efficacy of Reiki at benefitting mood and well-being. *Evidence-Based Complementary and Alternative Medicine* 2011: 381862.

Bremner MN, Blake BJ, Wagner VD, Pearcy SM. Effects of Reiki with music compared to music only among people living with HIV. *Journal of the Association of Nurses in AIDS Care* 2016; 27(5): 635–647.

Catlin A, Taylor-Ford RL. Investigation of standard care versus sham Reiki placebo versus actual Reiki therapy to enhance comfort and well-being in a chemotherapy infusion center. *Oncology Nursing Forum* 2011; 38(3): E212–E220.

Charkhandeh M, Talib, MA, Hunt CJ. The clinical evidence of cognitive behavior therapy and an alternative medicine approach in reducing symptoms of depression in adolescents. *Psychiatry Research* 2016; 239: 325–330.

Chirico, A, D'Aiuto G, Penon A, Mallia L, De Laurentiis M, Lucidi F, Botti G, Giordano A. Self-efficacy for coping with cancer enhances the effect of Reiki treatments during the pre-surgery phase of breast cancer patients. *Anticancer Research* 2017; 37(7): 3657–3665.

Crawford SE, Leaver VW, Mahoney SD. Using Reiki to decrease memory and behavior problems in mild cognitive impairment and mild Alzhemier's Disease. *Journal of Alternative and Complementary Medicine* 2006; 12(9): 911–913.

Diaz-Rodríguez L, Arroyo-Morales M, Fernández-de-las-Peñas C, García-Lafuente F, García-Royo C, Tomás-Rojas I. Immediate effects of Reiki on heart rate variability, cortisol levels, and body temperature in health care professionals with burnout. *Biological Research for Nursing* 2011; 13: 376.

Dressen LJ, Singg S. Effects of Reiki on pain and selected affective and personality variables of chronically ill patients. *Subtle Energies & Energy Medicine* 1998; 9(1): 53–82.

Erdogan Z, Cinar S. The effect of Reiki on depression in elderly people living in nursing home. *Indian Journal of Traditional Knowledge* 2014; 15(1): 35–40.

Gillespie E, Gillespie B, Stevens M. Painful diabetic neuropathy: impact of an alternative approach. *Diabetes Care* 2007; 30(4): 999–1001.

Kurebayashi, LFS, Turrini, RNT, Souza, TPB, Takiguchi, RS, Kuba, G, Nagumo, MT. Massage and Reiki used to reduce stress and anxiety: randomized clinical trial. *Revista Latino-Americana de Enfermagem* 2016; 24: e2834.

Mehl-Madrona L, Renfrew NM, Mainguy B. Qualitative assessment of the impact of implementing Reiki training in a supported residence for people older than 50 with HIV. *Permanente Journal* 2011; 15(3): 43-50.

Midilli TS, Gunduzoglu NC. Effects of Reiki on pain and vital signs when applied to the incision area of the body after Cesarean section surgery. *Holistic Nursing Practice* 2016; 30(6): 368–378.

Notte BB, Fazzini C, Mooney RA. Reiki's effect on patient with total knee arthroplasty: A pilot study. *Nursing* 2016; 46(2):17–23.

Orsak G, Stevens A, Brufsky A, Kajumba M, Dougall AL. The effect of Reiki therapy and companionship on quality of life, mood, and symptom distress during chemotherapy. *Evidence-Based Complementary and Alternative Medicine* 2015; 20(1): 20–27.

Rosada RM, Rubik B, Mainguy B, Plummer J, Mehl-Madrona L. Reiki reduces burnout among community mental health clinicians. *Journal of Alternative and Complementary Medicine* 2015; 21(8): 489–495.

Shaybak E. Effects of Reiki energy therapy on saphenous vein incision pain: A randomized clinical trial structure. *Der Pharmacy Lettre* 2017; 9(1): 100–109. 2017.

Shiflett SC, Nayak S, Bid C, Miles P, Agostinelli S. Effect of Reiki treatments on functional recovery in patients in post-stroke rehabilitation: a pilot study. *Journal of Alternative and Complementary Medicine* 2002; 8(6): 755–763.

Shore AG. Long-term effects of energetic healing on symptoms of psychological depression and self-perceived stress. *Alternative Therapies in Health and Medicine* 2004; 10(3): 42–48.

Whelan KM, Wishnia GS. Reiki therapy: the benefits to a nurse/Reiki practitioner. *Holistic Nursing Practice* 2003; 17(4): 209–217.

Witte D, Dundes L. Harnessing life energy or wishful thinking? Reiki, placebo Reiki, meditation and music. *Alternative & Complementary Therapies* 2001; 7(5): 304–309.

Vitale AT, O'Conner PC. The effect of Reiki on pain and anxiety in women with abdominal hysterectomies. *Holistic Nursing Practice* 2006; 20(6): 263–272.

Vitale AT. Nurses' lived experience or Reiki for self care. *Holistic Nursing Practice* 2009; 23(3): 129–145.

Chapter 3
How Does Reiki Work?

Introduction

To facilitate the acceptance, by mainstream medicine, of a therapy as a viable method of healing, it is useful to know its mechanism of action. In the case of drugs, the mechanism usually refers to the precise molecular targets, (receptors or enzymes), to which the drug binds. Receptor sites have specific affinities for drugs based on the chemical structure of the drug and the specific action that occurs there. For example, benzodiazepines, such as Librium, which are used to treat anxiety, work by binding to specific receptors located on neurons in the brain that are also sensitive to the neurotransmitter, gamma-aminobutyric acid. The binding of Librium inhibits the activity of the nerve cells, leading to decreased arousal and less anxiety. By knowing the mechanism of action of a therapy, it is easier to identify patients who will be most likely to respond to the treatment and to determine convenient and accurate methods of evaluating the correct dosage.

Non-pharmaceutical therapies, such as Reiki, Qigong, acupuncture, chiropractic, osteopathy, and hypnosis, are much less specific than most drugs in their effects on the body, and as a result their mechanisms of action are much more complicated and difficult to elicit. For example, although several theories exist regarding the ways that acupuncture might work, they do not explain the immediate suppression of pain that is usually experienced by acupuncture recipients; an alternative mechanism is required to account for this observation (Kawakita and Okata, 2014). In addition, although acupuncture points are considered the essential components of acupuncture therapy for diagnosis and treatment, no clear evidence of their existence has been established, despite numerous studies. Non-pharmaceutical therapies usually affect the whole body and exert their influence on multiple systems simultaneously, such as the nervous system, circulatory system, and hormonal system. This means that non-pharmaceutical therapies can only work through a means by which

information is communicated throughout the whole body. The "lock and key" model in which a molecule or "substrate" (the key) binds to a specific receptor or enzyme (the "lock"), which is often located in the cell membrane (Figure 3.1) is an accurate descriptor of drug interactions, but is not inclusive enough to explain the workings of complementary therapies. For this reason, the proposed mechanisms for complementary therapies, including Reiki, usually involve concepts or paradigms pertaining to the idea of a biofield. The term biofield was proposed in 1992 by an ad hoc committee of CAM practitioners and researchers convened by the newly established Office of Alternative Medicine (OAM) at the US National Institutes of Health (NIH). The committee defined "biofield" as (Rubik et al., 2015): "a massless field, not necessarily electromagnetic, that surrounds and permeates living bodies and affects the body."

Consideration of the biofield in terms of an electromagnetic field and how it relates specifically to Reiki is included later in this chapter. Unfortunately, although the concept of Reiki being mediated through an electromagnetic biofield is an attractive proposal, it cannot explain distance Reiki, mentioned previously in Chapter 1, in which a person may benefit from Reiki even if the Reiki practitioner performs the Reiki from another building, another city, or even another country. Electromagnetic force decreases with the square of the distance away from the field, and so if a Reiki practitioner is even just a kilometer away from the recipient, the chances are infinitesimal, based on classical physics, that the Reiki would influence the recipient's biofield. The scientific evidence for distance Reiki is actually very sparse and not very convincing and is briefly summarized following this introduction. However, there is more evidence for distance/distant healing in general (i.e. not just restricted to Reiki). Dr. Daniel J. Benor has published an excellent review of distant healing (Benor, 2000) focusing on randomized controlled trials in humans, animals, plants, bacteria, yeasts, cell cultures, and DNA. Due

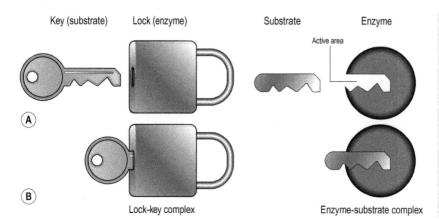

Key (substrate) Lock (enzyme) Substrate Enzyme

Active area

(A)

(B)

Lock-key complex Enzyme-substrate complex

Figure 3.1

Diagram depicting "lock and key" theory of molecular binding to receptor.

(From: Lock and Key Theory - Chemistry@Elmhurst - Elmhurst College chemistry. elmhurst.edu/ vchembook/571lockkey.html)

to the need to account for the purported far-reaching and multifaceted effects of Reiki, it is not surprising that, similar to acupuncture, there is presently no clear science-based, all-encompassing explanation of how Reiki might work.

One other purported mechanism, torsion, has been proposed as a mechanism for Reiki. The word "torsion" may be defined as a variable that describes rotation. A torsion field can be detected by an elementary particle (such as a proton or electron) with a net microscopic intrinsic spin, as predicted by the Einstein-Cartan theory. Although physicists have validated the existence of the "torsion field", the link to Reiki is tenuous at best. Russian scientist, Nikolai Kozyrev, proposed that torsion is the same as subtle energy and that right-handed torsion is beneficial to humans and left-handed torsion is deleterious. He performed experiments using macroscopic gyroscopes that apparently were detecting left- and right-handed torsion fields (Kozyrev, 1967). These experiments are not founded on fact. Physicists Stoeger and Yasskin (1979) proved that it is impossible to detect a torsion field with a macroscopic gyroscope. Torsion fields can only be detected by microscopic particles. In addition, the founding theoretical research, led by Anatoly Akimov and Gennady Shipov, was exposed as fraudulent by the Russian Academy of Sciences in 1991. For those reasons, the torsion model for Reiki will not be discussed in this chapter. However, for interested readers, more

details can be found in the references Yurth, 2000 and Swanson, 2010.

Although it is unlikely that a scientifically robust model of the mechanism of action of Reiki will be developed in the near future, this is not a reason to discard its use as a healing modality. Many drugs are used for decades before their mechanisms are discovered, for the simple reason that they work. For example, the first clinical study on the active component of aspirin, salicylic acid, was published in 1763 (Stone, 1763) but its mechanism of action as an anti-inflammatory agent was not discovered until 1971 by Robert Vane.

Distance Reiki: A Summary of Research

There are currently only four peer-reviewed published research papers that address distance Reiki. One of these papers (Shore, 2004) was ranked as "superior" using the Touchstone evaluation process. Participants were 45 adults needing treatment for mild depression or stress. They were divided into three treatment groups (hands-on Reiki, distance Reiki, and sham distance Reiki) and received a treatment once a week for six weeks. The hands-on Reiki group was told they might not receive Reiki and both distance groups were told they would receive Reiki. At the end of treatment and one year later, both Reiki groups showed significantly less depression and stress than the control group, as measured using standardized, established questionnaires. This study was a random, controlled, clinical study, and so the results are fairly convincing, even though the number of participants in each group was small. The other three papers are flawed in major ways and/or utilized only a small number of experimental participants. In the study by Demir et al. (2015), distance Reiki was sent to nine cancer patients receiving chemotherapy every day for five days. A control group of nine patients did not receive Reiki. Neither of the groups knew whether they received Reiki. Patients in the Reiki group showed significantly less pain, stress, and fatigue after treatment, as assessed using a numerical scale, whereas in the non-Reiki group, these values increased. A study by Vasudev and Shastri (2016) addressed the effect of distance Reiki on perceived stress among software professionals in Bangalore. Sixty software professionals working for a company in India were recruited. Thirty participants received distance Reiki for five minutes a day for 21 days and the other 30 participants did not. By administering a Perceived Stress Scale before and after the treatment or control period, it appeared that the distance Reiki group, but not the control group, showed significantly less stress after the treatment than before. However, there were several major flaws: first, the participants were aware of their grouping; second, one of the study authors administered the Reiki and so introduced bias; third, most of the control group was single, whereas half of the participants in the Reiki group were married; fourth, the statistical comparison between the two groups as measured after the treatment was stated as significant in the test but not in the table of data. Finally, the study by vanderVaart et al. (2011) did not show a positive effect of distance Reiki on pain in 20 women having elective Caesarian sections. This group of women received distance Reiki immediately before surgery and during the next two days. A second group received no extra treatment. The women did not know to which group they had been assigned. There was no significant difference between the groups regarding pain scores or medication use, but the Reiki group had significantly lower heart rates and blood pressures after surgery compared to the control group. Interestingly, the only information that the Reiki practitioner had concerning the patients was their hospital identity numbers. This may have hindered treatment.

Overall, the data from these four experiments are insufficient to draw any positive conclusions about the effectiveness of distance Reiki as a healing modality. A review of distance healing in general, not just Reiki, came to a similar conclusion (Crawford et al., 2002). It was stated that:

. . . methodological flaws were identified in many of these studies, including inadequacy of blinding, dropped data, poor outcome measures, lack of statistical power estimations, lack of confidence intervals, and lack of independent replication. Thus no firm conclusions could be drawn.

Despite the continuing popularity of distance healing as an alternative healing modality, when it comes to assessing clinical efficacy, high-quality experiments have so far failed to show reliable effects.

The Body Biofield and Healing

In 2015, the initial definition of biofield was extended to include its relationship to other bodily systems (Muehsam et al., 2015) as follows:

. . . an organizing principle for the dynamic information flow that regulates biological function and homeostasis. Biofield interactions can organize spatiotemporal biological processes across hierarchical levels: from the subatomic, atomic, molecular, cellular, organismic, to the interpersonal and cosmic levels. As such, biofield interactions can influence a variety of biological pathways, including biochemical, neurological and cellular processes related to electromagnetism, correlated quantum information flow, and perhaps other means for modulating activity and information flow across hierarchical levels of biology.

Homeostasis "refers to the ability of the body or a cell to seek and maintain a condition of equilibrium or stability within its internal environment when dealing with external changes. It is involved in the maintenance of the constant internal environment which includes the function of kidney, liver, skin, etc." (Biology-Online Dictionary).

Therefore, according to Muehsam's definition, the body's biofield would be responsible for modifying all bodily processes, from molecular to cellular to organismic, as new information impinges on the body from the environment, so as to maintain an optimal environment for bodily function. The definition also includes the terms "interpersonal" and "cosmic", which imply that the biofield not only regulates optimal function of the body, but also transmits information to the external environment and to the biofields of other creatures. If the biofield modulates information flow between systems through a mechanism such as electromagnetism, the laws of physics predict that changes in the properties of one biofield will induce changes in a neighboring biofield. This is illustrated by the high school physics experiment in which one magnet is brought towards another on a horizontal surface on which iron filings have been sprinkled. It is immediately obvious by the change in pattern of the iron filings, that the presence of the second magnet has altered the lines of magnetic force produced by the first magnet (Figure 3.2A,B). As will be discussed in the next section, this raises the possibility that as one person approaches another, the biofield of the person being approached may change. Likewise, if one person is giving Reiki to another, the Reiki may amplify the biofield of the practitioner so that it has a greater impact on the recipient (Oschman, 2000). If the biofield is electromagnetic in nature, then altering the biofield will also induce corresponding changes in electrically mediated neurological and cellular processes, and hence in organ function and disease states. This is because electric currents create electromagnetic fields, and so they are part of the same system. When a charged particle, such as an electron, proton, or ion is in motion, as occurs during a nerve impulse, magnetic lines of force rotate around the particle. If these lines of magnetic force are altered by the presence of another external field, then the corresponding current, or ion movement, will change.

The biofield definition also proposes "quantum information flow" as a possible means by which the biofield transmits information. Quantum information is information stored in very small structures called quantum bits or *qubits*. Qubits can be made from any quantum system that has two states, for example the spin of an electron. Because of the principle of superposition, qubits can be in both

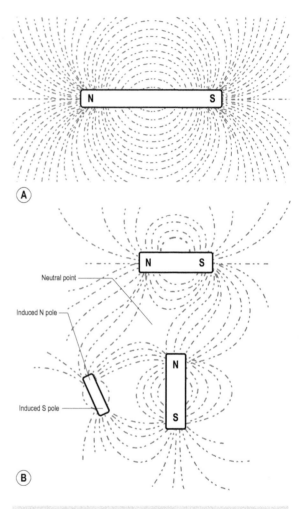

Figure 3.2
Diagram depicting electromagnetic field of a bar magnet (**A**) and how the field is changed by the presence of another magnet (**B**).
(From: http://www.uq.edu.au/_School_Science_Lessons/UNPh29.html#29.1.1H)

their possible states at once. If this concept is applied to two particles, this means that the two particles are in both states at the same time. However, due to the Copenhagen Interpretation of quantum mechanics, as soon as the particles are observed, one particle adopts one state and the other particle, the other state. This is called the "collapsing effect". If the particles are separated from each other, this effect is maintained across space. This system of two particles acts as if they are one and their system has two possible states. They are said to be "quantum entangled". In the case of entangled particles, the collapsing effect is transmitted from one to the other faster than even light, instantaneously. Einstein called it "spooky action at a distance." These concepts are accepted by scientists and have been confirmed at the microscopic level (Hensen et al., 2015; Herbst et al., 2015). Hensen et al. used a pair of diamond chips with a gap in each diamond's atomic matrix, which trapped a single electron. The diamonds were placed 1.3 km apart. The team then randomly measured one of two properties and found a correlation between the two particles that could not be explained by hidden variables. Herbst et al. separated two quantum-entangled photons even farther. Using a massive detector between the Canary Islands of La Palma and Tenerife, it separated the photons by 143 km.

Currently, three UK universities (University of Southampton, Queen's University Belfast and University College London) have formed a consortium with European universities and British photonics technology company M Squared to test the limits of superposition, the law that allows microscopic particles such as atoms and electrons to be in two places at once. The experiment will involve a tiny particle of glass, one-thousandth of the width of a human hair. However, there is currently no proof that superposition, quantum entanglement and spooky action at a distance hold true for larger scale systems, such as computer chips and sensors. Even more importantly, there is absolutely no evidence that quantum phenomena can account for distance Reiki. Many Reiki practitioners, most of whom are not scientists but some whom are, are eager to explain distance healing in terms of quantum physics. For example, holistic psychotherapist and author, Daniel J. Benor (2000) states:

While distant healing appears to contradict our ordinary sense of reality and the laws defined by Newtonian science, there are theoretical paradigms that appear to offer explanations for healing. These studies of absent healing introduce Newtonian medicine to the action of mind from a distance, "nonlocal consciousness," as Larry Dossey terms it. <u>This is consonant with the theories of modern physics, that postulate interactions between certain particles from any distance. These hypotheses have been supported by research</u>.

It should be noted that none of the "supporting research" references are scientific papers. Dean Radin (2015), author and Chief Scientist of the Institute of Noetic Sciences, also makes the point, but to a much lesser degree, that quantum physics could explain distance healing:

. . . given the well-accepted evidence for quantum nonlocality, which demonstrates the existence of "spooky action at a distance" (as Einstein described it), and especially the growing evidence for quantum coherence effects in living systems, possible physical mechanisms for DHI (Distant Healing Intention) are no longer inconceivable.

Due to the lack of supporting experimental evidence that quantum phenomena apply to systems above the microscopic scale, these explanations of distance healing are premature.

Is the Body Biofield Electromagnetic?

The human body emits low-level light, heat, and acoustical energy and also has electrical and magnetic properties. Although all of these emissions can be considered to be part of body biofield, no agreement has been reached in the scientific community on the definition of the biofield in terms of its components. Most research has focused on electromagnetic aspects of the biofield. It is known for certain that the heart and the brain, through their electrical activity, produce electromagnetic fields that extend out from the body. These electromagnetic fields form a large part of the body's biofield. The heart's electromagnetic field is about one hundred times as strong as that of the brain, and can be detected at three or more feet away from the body using a sensitive magnetometer, called a superconducting quantum interference detector (SQUID). A diagram of the structural pattern of the heart–brain field, based on a figure produced by the Institute of HeartMath, is shown in Figure 3.3. Both fields oscillate at

Chapter 3

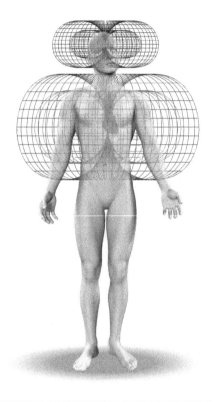

Figure 3.3
The structural pattern of electromagnetic energy generated by interaction between biofields of the heart and brain.

frequencies governed by the electrical activity of the brain (brainwaves of various frequencies) and the electrical activity of the heart (heart rate variability (HRV), or how the heart rate changes with time with various rhythms). Recordings obtained from several channels of a SQUID while monitoring a person's heart field are shown in Figure 3.4A. The vertical axis shows field strength (0.5 pico (10^{-12}) Teslas per division) and the horizontal axis represents time (1 second per division). This recording segment is only 6 seconds long and the distinct spikes that occur about every second correspond to the heartbeats. Every time the heart beats, there is a surge of electrical activity that causes a periodic response in the field being monitored. These spikes are not seen when there is no person being recorded

by the SQUID (Figure 3.4B). Figure 3.5 shows a 1-minute recording of the heart field of a volunteer. On this scale, a repeating wave pattern is visible with about 17 waves per minute. These waves are periodic fluctuations in the electromagnetic field resulting from HRV, natural variations in the heart rate rhythm. This frequency of periodicity of the signal is consistent with the respiratory component of HRV; each in-breath causes a slight increase in heart rate and corresponding boost in the strength of the heart field, and each out-breath causing a decrease in heart rate, and drop in field strength, which added together form a wave. The recordings were obtained using the SQUID at Scripps Center for Integrative Medicine (Figure 3.6A,B) by Ann Baldwin.

Interest in the biofield as an electromagnetic entity started in the 1970s when Harold Sexton Burr, Professor of Yale School of Medicine, published a book called *Blueprint for Immortality: the Electric Patterns of Life* (Burr, 1972). This book reported a series of studies on the role of electricity in development and disease, based on the idea that there is a blueprint for each organism that directs its assembly and maintenance. Scientists at that time considered that any energy field surrounding an organism would be too weak to detect. Since then, as mentioned above, ultrasensitive detectors have been developed that are routinely used to measure and monitor such fields. It is clear that Burr's "electric patterns of life" are at least partially electromagnetic, but other forces, as yet unknown, may contribute to the body's biofield.

How could Reiki influence the electromagnetic component of the biofield? Is Reiki electromagnetic? How does Reiki travel through the body? In 1990, John Zimmerman proposed a hypothesis to answer these questions (Zimmerman, 1990). He proposed that the regular pulsing of the Earth's magnetic field at a frequency of 7.8 Hz (Schumann frequency) entrains the brain waves of a relaxed, experienced healer who is focusing their attention on healing another being. Schumann resonance is an electromagnetic phenomenon produced by pulses of lightning traveling around the earth, bouncing back and forth between the ionosphere and the earth's surface

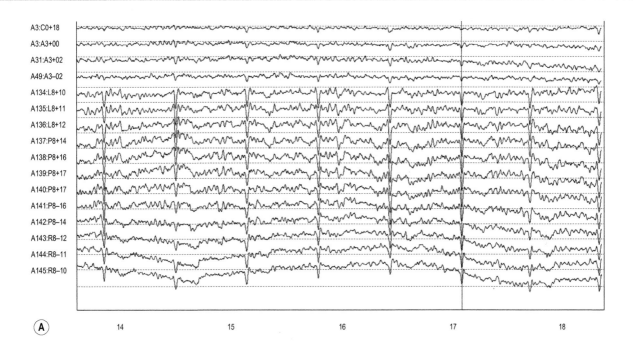

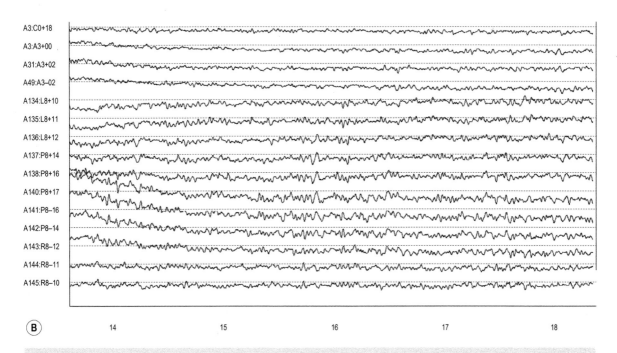

Figure 3.4
Electromagnetic field of beating heart (**A**) and electromagnetic background noise (**B**) recorded for 6 seconds using SQUID.

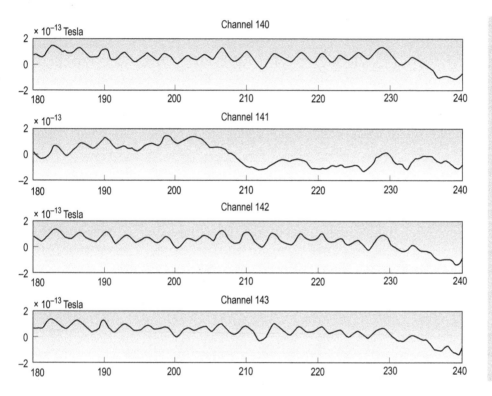

Figure 3.5
Electromagnetic field of beating heart recorded for one minute using SQUID.

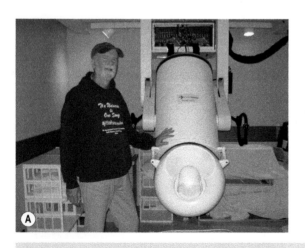

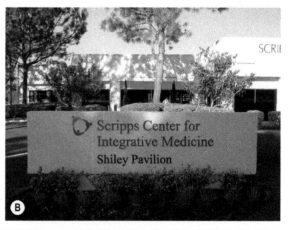

Figure 3.6
William Rand with Superconducting Quantum Interference Detector (**A**), at Scripps Center for Integrative Medicine (**B**).

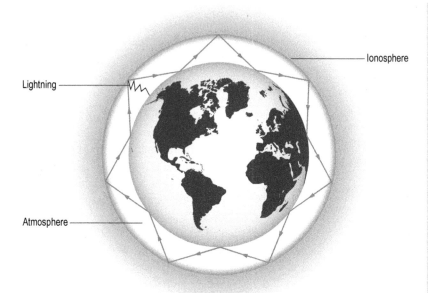

Lightning

Ionosphere

Atmosphere

Figure 3.7
Depiction of Schumann Resonance (7-10 Hz): electromagnetic pulses generated from lightning. (From: Bentov I. Micromotion of the body as a factor in the development of the nervous system. In Sannella L. (Ed.), Kundalini: Psychosis or Transendence? Integral Publishing, Lower Lake, CA, 1976 (appendix A).

(Figure 3.7). The lightning causes the space between the ionosphere and earth's atmosphere to vibrate or resonate at frequencies usually in the range of 7–10 Hz, known as extremely low frequency (ELF). Brain waves arise because of the rhythmic synchronized spread of direct current though large groups of neurons in the brain. Brain waves vary in frequency; a pacemaker in a part of the brain called the thalamus regulates the frequency. There are short periods, lasting from 5 to 25 seconds, when the brain waves are in a "free run" period and are susceptible to entrainment by external fields; that is, they adopt the frequency of the external field, which in this case is the Schumann frequency. The Schumann resonance matches the frequency of α brainwaves (which correlate with a meditative state) but is thousands of times stronger than the electromagnetic field normally created by brainwaves. As a result, entrainment of the α brainwaves by the Schumann resonance would greatly increase the strength of the associated electromagnetic field of the brainwaves. It should be noted, however, that the idea of bodily systems being entrained by external rhythms, instead of just by internal pacemakers, is still controversial. Oschman (2000) has described the research supporting the idea that brain waves can be entrained by external rhythms.

Zimmerman also hypothesized that the healer consciously or subconsciously adjusts their respiration rate to an exact sub-harmonic of the Schumann frequency so that their body biofield synchronizes with the brain waves. The person being healed then allows their brain waves to become synchronized with the healer's biofield. When this occurs, effective ELF healing energies from the healer's hands are emitted, which affect the biochemistry and cell physiology of the patient being healed. In support of this hypothesis, there is evidence that artificially generated ELF electromagnetic frequencies can promote healing. For example, a frequency of 7 Hz can initiate bone growth and 10 Hz, ligament healing (Siskin and Walker, 1995). Pulsed electromagnetic field devices are currently being marketed to improve bone healing. A systematic review found that patients treated with electrical stimulation as an adjunct for bone healing have significantly less pain and experience lower rates of radiographic nonunion or persistent nonunion (Aleem et al., 2016).

Becker (1992) further developed Zimmerman's model, suggesting that it is the pineal gland in the brain that responds to the Schumann rhythm. According to Oschman (2000), 20–30% of the cells in the pineal gland are magnetically sensitive. Sandyk (1992) proposed that the presence of α brainwaves could be used as a neurophysiological marker for the activity of the pineal gland. Therefore, there does seem to be a functional link between ELF electromagnetic radiation, the pineal gland, and α brainwaves. Becker also proposed that the electrical currents of the brainwaves are conducted through the body by the perineural system, a sheath of cells that surrounds each nerve (Becker, 1991). Becker identified the existence of perineural currents that are stimulated when nerve endings are exposed by tissue injury and alert the rest of the body to the location of the injury. The brain is the source of negatively charged particles that form the basis of such currents. In this way, the brainwaves regulate the sensitivity and activity of the whole nervous system.

Pulling all this information together, Oschman (2000) developed a diagrammatic model to explain the internal pathways involved in the body's responses to external magnetic rhythms, and how those responses lead to projection of healing energy from the hands (Figure 3.8). He summarized it as follows:

Micropulsations of the geomagnetic field, caused by the Schumann resonance, are detected by the pineal and magnetite-bearing tissues associated with the brain. During the "free-run" period, when the brainwaves are not being entrained by the thalamus, the Schumann resonance can take over as the pacemaker, particularly if the individual is in a relaxed or meditative state (Schumann signals are thousands of times stronger than brainwaves). The brainwaves regulate the overall tone of the nervous system and the state of consciousness. The electrical currents of the brainwaves are conducted throughout the body by the perineural and vascular systems. The biomagnetic field projected from the hands can be much stronger than the brainwaves (Seto et al., 1992) indicating that an amplification of at least 1,000 times takes place somewhere in the body. Alternatively, the body may simply act as an effective antenna or channel for the Schumann micropulsations. The projected fields scan or sweep through the frequencies medical researchers are finding useful for "jump-starting" injury repair in a variety of tissues.

Is Reiki Electromagnetic?

To test the model of energy healing proposed by Oschman, it is necessary to determine whether Reiki practitioners produce measurable electromagnetic fields from their hands when healing. Zimmerman (1990) used a SQUID to measure the electromagnetic fields produced by the hands of Therapeutic Touch practitioners as they healed a person in a room with "moderate" magnetic shielding. It is essential to use magnetic shielding to prevent external electromagnetic sources from interfering with the signal recorded from the practitioner. Therapeutic Touch is an energy healing modality that is very similar to Reiki. In this experiment, it was reported that four out of seven healers showed detectable changes in the amplitude and/or frequency of their biomagnetic fields as they attempted to heal the other person. However, the results presented consisted of a single scan from the hand of just one practitioner before and during healing (Figure 3.9). The range of frequencies detected in the scan was 0.3 to 30 Hz, which is similar to those associated with healthy tissue and organs. No scales of amplitude or of time were provided in the figure and so it cannot be compared with recordings from other sources. This single recording is widely cited as proof that energy healers produce electromagnetic fields from their hands. In a more extensive study, Seto et al. (1992) used an electromagnetic sensor designed to minimize external background noise to measure electromagnetic fields from the palms of 37 subjects who claimed to emit external Qi. The detector, despite having a sensitivity of less than 100 picoTesla (pT), could not measure the electromagnetic signal from the heart. On the other hand, it was stated that magnetic fields 1,000 times greater than that of the cardiac biofield, in a frequency range of 4–10 Hz were detected, from the hands of three out of 37 of the subjects. However, no corresponding electric current was detected in the hands of the participants, suggesting that the electromagnetic field was not really emanating from the subjects but probably from an external source.

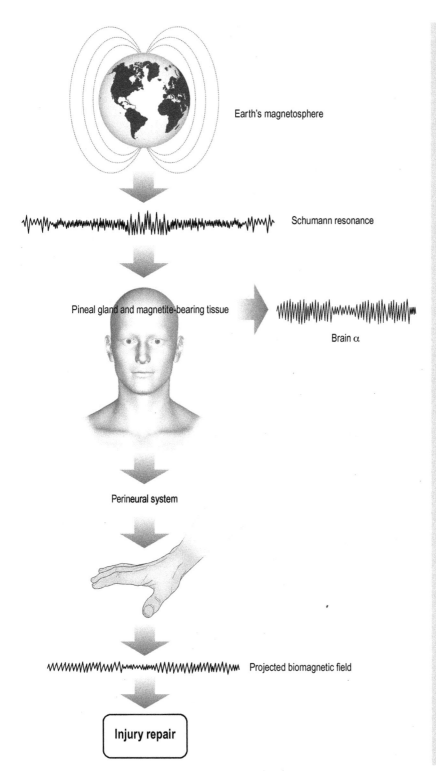

Earth's magnetosphere

Schumann resonance

Pineal gland and magnetite-bearing tissue

Brain α

Perineural system

Projected biomagnetic field

Injury repair

Figure 3.8
Diagram showing possible mechanism for Reiki Energy Flow by R.O. Becker.

(From: Becker RO. *Cross currents: the perils of electric pollution, the promise of electromedicine.* Jeremy P. Tarcher, Los Angeles, CA, USA, 1999, p. 80, (Figs 3–4).)

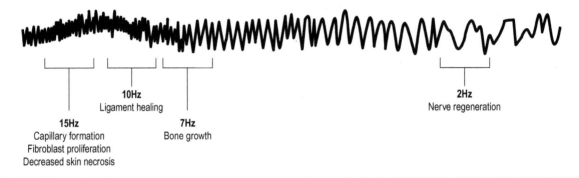

10Hz
Ligament healing

2Hz
Nerve regeneration

15Hz
Capillary formation
Fibroblast proliferation
Decreased skin necrosis

7Hz
Bone growth

Figure 3.9
Electromagnetic signal recorded by Dr John Zimmerman, at the University of Colorado, Denver, from the hand of a practitioner of therapeutic touch. The frequency is not steady but sweeps up and down from 0.3 to 30 Hz, with most activity between 7 and 8 Hz.

Due to the paucity and uncertainty of the data obtained from these early studies, Baldwin et al. (2013) decided to repeat the experiment with Reiki practitioners using modern equipment and up-to-date magnetic shielding. The SQUID that was used was located at the Scripps Center for Integrative Medicine, San Diego, California. In this experiment, the electromagnetic field from the hands and heart of three Reiki masters was measured when they were: (1) not practicing Reiki, (2) sending Reiki to a distant person, and (3) sending Reiki to a person in the room. Measurements were also made on four Reiki-naïve volunteers. These measurements were repeated after they received Reiki training and were instructed to self-administer Reiki. For all subjects, under all conditions, sensors closest to the heart and the hands of the subjects produced spikes of 2 pT that corresponded to the electromagnetic field produced by the heartbeat (Figure 3.4). Therefore, this instrument was at least 50 times more sensitive than that used by Seto et al. (1992). However, none of the recordings of Reiki Masters as they sent Reiki showed electromagnetic field intensities any greater than their baseline recordings. This is illustrated in Figures 3.10A (Reiki Master baseline recording) and 3.10B (Reiki Master sending Reiki). In each case, the vertical axis represents electromagnetic field intensity in Tesla and the horizontal axis, time in seconds.

It could be argued that perhaps the Reiki Masters did not show increased field intensity when sending Reiki because they were unconsciously sending Reiki even at baseline. However, the Reiki Master baseline recordings were no different from the baseline recordings of Reiki-naïve subjects. These results, using modern equipment and extremely effective electromagnetic shielding, indicate that practicing Reiki does not appear to produce high-intensity electromagnetic fields from the heart or hands. On the other hand, as mentioned previously, it is possible that energy healing is stimulated when the practitioner tunes into an external environmental radiation, such as the Schumann resonance. The ability of the Reiki practitioners to connect with environmental radiation would have been blocked by the strong electromagnetic shielding surrounding the SQUID. An ideal detector of Reiki energy would need to function without electromagnetic shielding in an environment free from external sources of electromagnetic radiation and would require sensitivity in the range of 100 pT (if Seto's results are to be believed). At present, such an instrument is not on the market, but a recent publication reports favorable results from a portable diagnostic device for cardiac magnetic field mapping in shielded and unshielded environments (Mooney et al., 2017). Further clinical testing of more advanced noise-removal algorithms is required before it can be approved for diagnostic use.

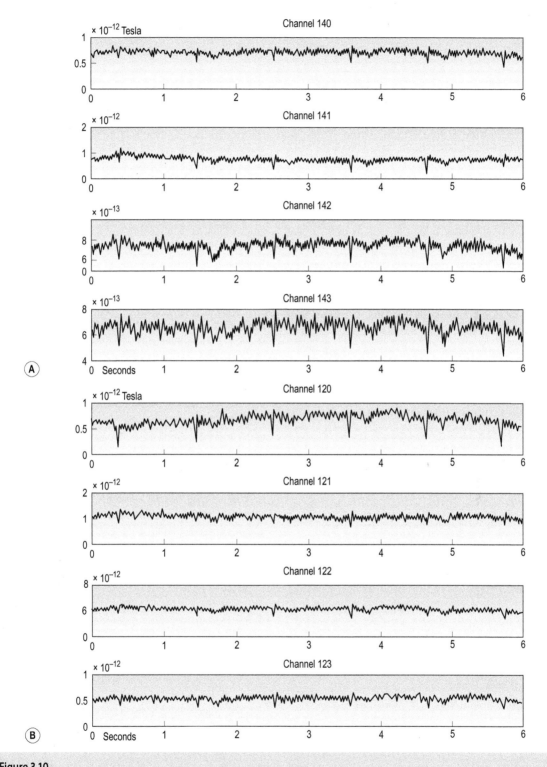

Figure 3.10
(**A**) Electromagnetic field of heart of Reiki master while NOT sending Reiki (channels 140–143). (**B**) Electromagnetic field of heart of Reiki master while sending Reiki (channels 120–123).

In an interesting pilot study, a portable three-axis digital gaussmeter, which could detect 10^{-7} Tesla (100,000 pT) levels of electromagnetic fields, was used to monitor Reiki practitioners (n = 17) and healers from several different healing traditions (n = 15). Initially, the biofield of each hand was monitored and then each healer was instructed to transmit biofield therapy. Significant increases in extremely low frequency (ELF) fluctuations of the signal were observed compared to baseline controls for both hands of practitioners as they transmitted their therapy. In addition, significantly larger increases in ELF fluctuations were observed with more experienced practitioners. Thus, changes in ELF magnetic fields were correlated with the practitioner's sense of biofield manipulation (Connor et al., 2006). This study indicates that Reiki might influence fluctuations in the biofield rather than altering the mean intensity.

Summary

Presently, the biological mechanism by which Reiki mediates its beneficial effects is not known. The most rational model proposed so far is the Oschman theory, which postulates that the flow of Reiki in the body of a practitioner is triggered by an environmental source, such as Schuman radiation, which then entrains and amplifies the brainwaves. The electric currents of the brainwaves travel through the body via perineural sheaths, and perhaps the vascular system, and create changes in the body's projected electromagnetic biofield. Reiki practitioners take advantage of the changes they experience in their hands to induce alterations in the biofield of the person they are healing. Changes in the client's biofield automatically lead to alterations in the body's intrinsic neural and cellular currents, thus modifying mental and bodily functions. The projected fields from the hands of the Reiki practitioner scan or sweep through the extremely low frequencies medical researchers are finding useful for "jump-starting" injury repair in a variety of tissues. A problem with this model is that there is very little evidence that the hands of Reiki practitioners actually do project pulsing electromagnetic radiation. Hopefully, with the advent of the new technology that is on the horizon, more accurate and convincing data can be obtained from Reiki practitioners during the healing process. It is important that research aimed at testing possible mechanisms of Reiki and monitoring its clinical outcomes continues because the results will provide a solid scientific basis from which to improve and extend the practice of Reiki. The subsequent chapters in this book will demonstrate that, before an exact mechanism is known, it is definitely worthwhile to practice Reiki because substantial evidence reveals that Reiki benefits almost everyone.

References

Aleem IS, Aleem I, Evaniew N, Busse JW, Yaszemski M, Agarwal A, Einhorn T, Bhandari M. Efficacy of Electrical Stimulators for Bone Healing: A Meta-Analysis of Randomized Sham-Controlled Trials. *Scientific Reports* 2016; 6: 31724.

Baldwin AL, Rand W, Schwartz GE. Practicing Reiki does not routinely appear to produce high intensity electromagnetic fields from the heart and hands of Reiki practitioners. *Journal of Alternative and Complementary Medicine* 2013; 19(6): 518–526.

Becker RO. Evidence for a primitive DC electrical analog system controlling brain function. *Subtle Energies & Energy Medicine* 1991; 2: 71–98.

Becker RO. Modern bioelectromagnetics and functions of the central nervous system. *Subtle Energies & Energy Medicine* 1992; 3: 53–72.

Benor DJ. Distant Healing. *Subtle Energies & Energy Medicine* 2000; 11(3): 249.

Biology-Online Dictionary. www.biology-online.org/dictionary

Burr HS. *Blueprint for immortality*. CW Daniel, Saffron Walden, UK, 1972.

Connor M, Schwartz GE, Tau G. Oscillation of amplitude as measured by an extra low frequency magnetic field meter as a biophysical measure of intentionality. Toward a Science of Consciousness 2006. April 4-8, Tucson, Arizona. Abstract # 208. http://www.consciousness.arizona.edu/abstracts.htm.

Crawford CC, Sparber AG, Jonas WB. A systematic review of the quality of research on hands-on and distance healing: clinical and laboratory studies. *Alternative Therapies in Health and Medicine* 2002; 9(3): A96–104.

Demir M, Gulbeyaz C, Kelam A, Aydmer A. Effects of distant Reiki on pain, anxiety and fatigue in oncology patients in Turkey: a pilot study. *Asian Pacific Journal of Cancer Prevention* 2015; 16:4859–4862.

Hensen B, Bernien H, Dreau AE, Reiserer A, Kalb N, Blok MS, Ruitenberg J, Vermeulen RFL, Schouten RN, Abellán C, Amaya W, Pruneri V, Mitchell MW, Markham M, Twitchen DJ, Elkouss D, Wehner S, Taminiau TH, Hanson R. Loophole-free Bell inequality violation using electron spins separated by 1.3 kilometres. *Nature* 2015; 526: 682–686.

Herbst T, Scheidl T, Fink M, Handsteiner J, Wittmann B, Ursin R, Zeilinger A. Teleportation of entanglement over 143 km. *Proceedings of the National Academy of Sciences of the United States of America* 2015; 112(46): 14202–14205.

Kawakita K, Okada K. Acupuncture therapy: mechanism of action, efficacy, and safety: a potential intervention for psychogenic disorders? *BioPsychoSocial Medicine* 2014; 8: 4.

Kozyrev NA. Possibility of experimental study of the properties of time. JPRS 45238, translation, US Department of Commerce, from Russian, Pulkovo, O. VOZMOZHNOSTI EKSPERIMENTAL NOGO ISSLEDOVANIYA SVOYSTV VREMENI, September 1967, pp. 1–49.

Mooney JW, Ghasemi-Roudsari S, Reade Banham E, Symonds C, Pawlowski N, Varcoe BTH. A portable diagnostic device for cardiac magnetic field mapping. *Biomedical Physics and Engineering Express* 2017; 3: 015008.

Muehsam D, Chevalier G, Barsotti T, Gurfein BT. An overview of biofield devices. *Global Advances in Health and Medicine* 2015; 4: 42–51.

Oschman JL. *Energy Medicine: The Scientific Basis.* Churchill Livingstone, Harcourt Publishers Ltd, Edinburgh, UK, 2000.

Radin D, Schlitz M, Baur C. Distant Healing Intention Therapies: An Overview of the Scientific Evidence. *Global Advances in Health and Medicine* 2015 Nov; 4(Suppl): 67–71.

Rubik B, Muehsam D, Hammerschlag R, Jain S. Biofield Science and Healing: History, Terminology, and Concepts. *Global Advances in Health and Medicine* 2015 Nov; 4(Suppl): 8–14.

Sandyk R. Alpha rhythm and the pineal gland. *International Journal of Neuroscience* 1992; 63 (3–4): 221–227.

Seto A, Kusaka C, Nakazato S, Huang WR, Sato T, Hisamitsu T, Takeshige C. Detection of extraordinary large biomagnetic field strength from human hand. *Acupuncture & Electro-Therapeutics Research International Journal* 1992; 17: 75–94.

Shore AG. Long-term effects of energetic healing on symptoms of psychological depression and self-perceived stress. *Alternative Therapies in Health & Medicine* 2004; 10(3): 42–48.

Siskin BF, Walker J. Therapeutic aspects of biomagnetic fields for soft tissue healing. In: Blank M, ed. *Electromagnetic Fields: Biological Interactions and Mechanisms* 1995; 250: 277–285.

Stoeger WR, Yasskin PB. Can a macroscopic gyroscope feel torsion? *General Realtivity and Gravitation* 1979; 11(6): 427–431.

Stone E. An account of the success of the bark of the willow in the cure of agues. *Philosophical Transactions Royal Society* 1763; 53: 195–200.

Swanson C. Kozyrev: Of Time and Torsion. In: *Life Force, the Scientific Basis: Breakthrough Physics of Energy Medicine, Healing, Chi and Quantum Consciousness.* Poseidia Press, Tucson, AZ, USA, 2010.

vanderVaart S, Berger H, Tam C, Goh YH, Gijsen VMGJ, de Wildt, Adio A, Koren G. The effect of distant Reiki on pain in women after elective Caesarian section: a double-blinded randomized controlled trial. *BMJ Open* 2011; 1: e000021.

Vasudev S, Shastri S. Effect of distance Reiki on perceived stress among software professionals in Bangalore. *International Journal of Indian Psychology* 2016; 3(4): 58.

Yurth DG. Torsion Field Mechanics: Verification of Non-local Field Effects in Human Biology. Conference: 6th International Symposium of the New Energy Society, Salt Lake City, UT, USA, 2000.

Zimmerman J. Laying-on-of-hands healing and therapeutic touch: a testable theory. *BEMI Currents, Journal of the Bio-Electro-Magnetics Institute* 1990; 2: 8–17.

Chapter 4

Optimizing the Use of Reiki with Your Patients

Link to Research Findings – When is Reiki Most Likely to Work?

As with any therapy, Reiki is most effective if both the patient or client and the practitioner have confidence that it will help the situation. As outlined in Chapter 2, research shows that Reiki is effective for reducing acute and chronic pain, anxiety, and depression and for improving well-being. Pain, anxiety, or depression can accompany many common diseases and disorders, such as arthritis, fibromyalgia, irritable bowel syndrome, chronic respiratory diseases, multiple sclerosis, shingles, headaches, musculoskeletal injury and pain, and broken bones. Pain, anxiety, and depression often overlap; chronic pain is depressing and likewise, major depression may feel physically painful. If the practitioner makes it clear to the client that the goal is to reduce the severity of their symptoms, rather than to necessarily cure the disease, this will prevent unrealistic expectations and disappointment on the part of the client. In the case of people with chronic diseases, particularly those staying in hospital, Reiki can have an uplifting effect, beyond just treating symptoms. Giving and receiving Reiki can bring compassion and humanity back into the patient's experience. During a typical day, patients may experience treatments from many different healthcare workers, each one focusing on their own particular job, rather than on treating the patient as a whole person. This benign neglect can make a patient feel lonely, uncared for, and unloved. At a time when patients can feel passive in their care, Reiki brings them a sense of empowerment. By choosing to receive Reiki, patients can actively participate in their healing process. Family members may also decide to take Reiki training so that they may take an active role in hastening their relative's recovery.

In hospitals, there are several practical situations in which Reiki has been shown to be exceptionally beneficial. One example is using Reiki for surgery: to reduce the anxiety felt pre-surgery, decrease the level of pain felt pre- and post-surgery, and minimize the need for pain relief medications post-surgery. Such medications often have side effects. Another added bonus is that patients who receive Reiki spend less time in hospital. Hospitals with Reiki programs usually provide patients with a session on the morning of surgery and an additional 15–20-minute session is given prior to their transport to the operating room. Some patients even receive Reiki in the operating room. Follow up sessions are given immediately after surgery and one or two days post-surgery. Patients who respond well to the Reiki treatments can be referred for Reiki training so they can practice Reiki self-treatments on a continuing basis.

A second example is offering Reiki to patients who have just had a heart attack, a very painful and anxiety-causing event. Reiki helps in many ways. Firstly, it reduces the patient's anxiety. Anxiety causes increased blood pressure and heart rate, both of which can exacerbate cardiac problems, so less anxiety will protect the heart from further damage. Secondly, receiving Reiki usually decreases the incidence of depression and negative thoughts, both of which are known to be risk factors for cardiovascular problems. Thirdly, Reiki may improve the quality of sleep. Research has shown that people with poor sleep habits may be at a higher risk of developing cardiovascular disease. Better quality and quantity of sleep allows the body to rest and provide the energy needed for healing damaged tissue. Fourthly, heart attack patients often feel quite severe pain and they notice a reduction in pain sensation following Reiki sessions. Last, but not least, Reiki has been shown to improve heart rate variability (HRV), allowing the heart to respond more quickly and appropriately to the patient's needs. This gives the patient an extra boost regarding their chances of a full recovery.

Another example in which Reiki has shown to be extremely effective is in the care of patients with cancer. However, it should be made clear to patients from the start that Reiki, by itself, will not cure the cancer. Reiki is not an alternative treatment, but a therapy that complements the use of radiation, surgery, and chemotherapy. Multiple studies have shown that Reiki is invaluable in reducing the pain, muscle tension, insomnia, fatigue, anxiety, and depression that always accompany the disease to some degree. These symptoms are often made worse by chemotherapy and that is another situation in which Reiki can be very helpful. Reiki works by soothing the patient through the unpleasant side effects of chemotherapy, such as weakness and nausea. Reiki is perfectly safe and has no side effects. Reiki can be given as often as desired, and many patients appreciate Reiki sessions several times a week. In addition, caregivers and relatives who devote a large proportion of their life looking after their cancer patient benefit from Reiki sessions. Reiki gives caregivers a respite from their worries, replenishes their energy, and widens their perspective.

Hospices provide another situation in which Reiki is particularly effective. People undergoing palliative and/ or hospice care usually enjoy the gentle, peaceful feeling of being touched by a Reiki practitioner. They also experience relief from pain, anxiety, and fear. By providing comfort and a sense of calm, Reiki enhances the quality of their final days. Reiki practitioners often find that patients are more calm and compliant with them than with other medical personnel because Reiki practitioners are not attached to any particular outcome. For example, Elise M. Brenner, PhD, Reiki hospice volunteer, related the following story in *Spirit of Change Magazine*, Spring 2010:

One day, upon entering the room of Agnes, one of the hospice patients who suffers from dementia, I found her engaged in a mini-battle with a care attendant. The latter was determined to finish getting Agnes dressed, while Agnes was equally determined not to be dressed. There was waving of arms and bitter complaints from Agnes. The care attendant valiantly pursued her goal, despite the ongoing protests, and ultimately Agnes was successfully clothed. Each was unhappy when it was over. I commented that Agnes' hair was getting long as I began to brush it. Unexpectedly, the care attendant told me that the hairdresser had tried to cut it twice, but that Agnes had tried to bite her so Agnes' hair had

remained uncut. I took Agnes in her wheelchair to a quiet spot to begin Reiki.

Agnes calmed down from her agitated state, but not first without a few biting comments about her recent struggle over getting dressed. As we sat together with the Reiki healing energy flowing, I was overcome by a sweeping thought. Unlike the care attendant and the hairdresser, I had the privilege of not being attached to the outcome of my interactions with Agnes. It was both a liberating and a humbling realization.

Patients receiving Reiki as a part of their palliative care often find that their spirit becomes stronger and they are able to accept thoughts of their death with less fear. Reiki practitioners are trained to focus on their intention that the Reiki energy goes to the client's "greatest good". This style of care is particularly appropriate for patients who are in hospice care because all effort is focused towards their physical and emotional comfort rather than on achieving a particular outcome.

Finally, another way in which Reiki can be used to advantage in hospitals does not involve the patients, but instead focuses on the nurses and other caregivers. Hospital nurses, who are prone to burnout, often practice Reiki on themselves because they find it to be a very effective tool for maintaining general well-being. Nurses who are taught Reiki experience immediate stress relief and relaxation after just a few minutes of self-treatment while on the job. It is not just the nurses who benefit from their self-care. A three-year study, carried out by the National Nursing Research Unit at King's College London and Southampton University aimed to determine which particular staff attitudes and behaviors most affected patient experiences (Maben et al., 2012). National Nursing Research Unit director and lead study author, Jill Maben, said:

This study strongly suggests that patient experiences are better when staff feel they have a good working environment, support from co-workers and their manager and low emotional exhaustion.

As will be shown in Chapter 8, Reiki is an excellent remedy for low emotional exhaustion.

Giving a Reiki Session

It is very important when giving Reiki treatments in hospitals or elsewhere to ensure that the patient understands what Reiki is and to only give a Reiki session at the patient's request. Even though there is no medical contraindication for receiving Reiki, permission should always be obtained from the patient's nurse or physician. Practitioners should never diagnose, suggest changes in treatment or guarantee a full recovery. Also, if the issue comes up, it is important to explain that Reiki is *not* a religion and that members of many religious groups including Christians, Muslims, Hindus, and Jews use Reiki and find it compatible with their religious beliefs. On the other hand, in their *Committee on Doctrine, United States Conference of Catholic Bishops*, 25 March 2009, the Catholic Bishops made the following statement:

Reiki therapy finds no support either in the findings of natural science or in Christian belief. For a Catholic to believe in Reiki therapy presents insoluble problems. In terms of caring for one's physical health or the physical health of others, to employ a technique that has no scientific support (or even plausibility) is generally not prudent.

This statement is correct in that it is imprudent to use a health-related technique that has no scientific support. However, as outlined in Chapter 2, the number and quality of peer-reviewed research studies that demonstrate statistically significant evidence in support of Reiki as a healing modality is growing year by year; this fact contradicts the Bishops' statement that Reiki has no scientific support or even plausibility. In spite of the Catholic Bishops' viewpoint, many practicing Catholics are open to giving and receiving Reiki. Since giving Reiki addresses spiritual, as well as emotional and physical, health, it is very important that Reiki is taught and introduced in a neutral way without invoking any deity. In this way, all Reiki students and recipients, including atheists, are allowed the freedom to incorporate it into their personal belief system as they see fit. Once the client, Reiki practitioner, and nurse or physician, if applicable, are comfortable with the choice of Reiki for the client to address a particular physical or emotional issue, there are several other factors that need to be considered because they will influence the client's experience and the effectiveness of the session.

1. Where should the Reiki session take place?

2. At what positions on the client's body should the practitioner place their hands?

3. How does the mental, emotional, and physical condition of practitioner affect their healing effectiveness?

4. Should the practitioner breathe more slowly than usual when performing Reiki?

5. How important is maintaining hydration for the client and the practitioner?

6. How does a practitioner ensure that their client is comfortable during the session?

These six questions will now be addressed in turn.

1. Venues for Reiki Sessions

If the client/patient is an outpatient, the following options are available for arranging Reiki sessions:

- Send client to a Reiki Center. Reiki Center locations can be found by researching online or by contacting a professional Reiki association. An example of a Reiki Center, the Reiki Center of Sedona, Arizona, USA is shown in Figures 4.1A–C. Like most centers, the Reiki Center of Sedona offers both training and private sessions.

- Send client to a private practitioner selected according to the criteria described in Chapter 1. A typical private practitioner Reiki room is shown in Figure 4.2.

- Give the client Reiki yourself in your office or clinic if you are trained to at least Level Two.

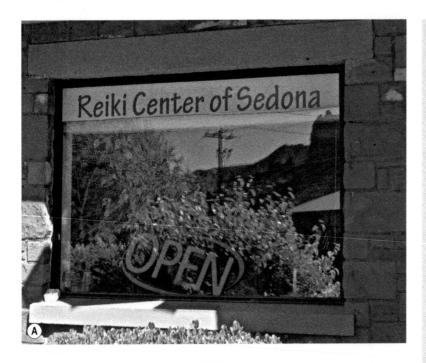

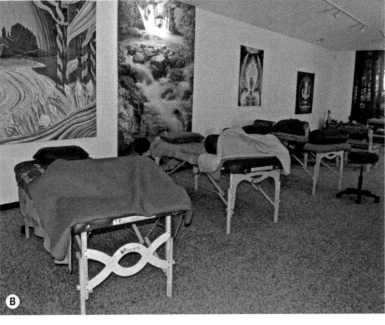

Figures 4.1A,B
The Reiki Center of Sedona, Arizona.
(Continued)

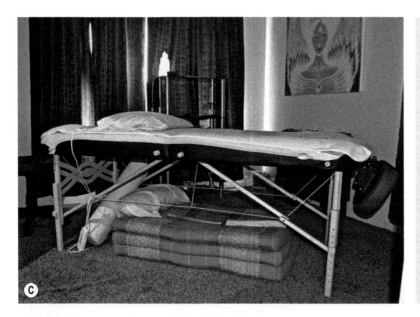

Figures 4.1C
The Reiki Center of Sedona, Arizona.

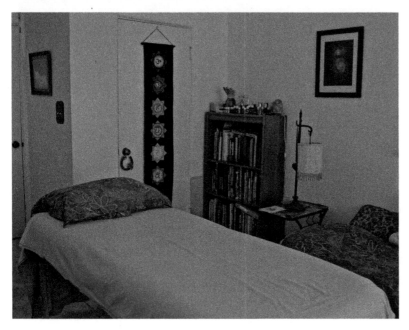

Figure 4.2
A typical private practitioner Reiki room.

Chapter 4

If the patient is in hospital:

- Request a Reiki practitioner from your hospital Reiki program to administer Reiki at the patient's bedside.

- Contact a private practitioner to visit the patient in hospital.

- Give the client Reiki yourself at their bedside if you are trained to at least Level Two.

It is important that any Reiki practitioner working in a hospital environment has received basic training in hospital protocols as described in Chapter 14. In particular, the practitioner has to be flexible regarding the specific needs of the patient and the medical staff, and be willing to curtail or temporarily interrupt their session, if necessary.

2. Practitioner: Use of Hand Positions

Mrs. Takata taught a standardized set of hand positions to be used on the client, or self, when giving Reiki. These positions are based on the locations of the seven main chakras (see Figure 1.1) and thus target the major organs and glands. Reiki is commonly given first to the front of each chakra, with the client lying supine (on their back), and then to the back of each chakra while the client lies prone (on their front). Photographs demonstrating the hand positions are shown in Figure 4.3 (treating a client) and Figure 4.4 (treating the self). Further details concerning the hand positions can be found in *Foundations of Reiki Ryoho* by Nicholas Pearson (see references for full citation). This series of hand positions is very useful to ensure that all major parts of the body experience the Reiki energy. However, adaptability is key to a successful treatment. For example, a patient may have suffered burns and might not want to be touched, in which case the practitioner holds their hands a few inches from the surface of the patient's body. A client or patient might be unable or unwilling to lie prone, in which case the practitioner concentrates on the front of their body, or asks the patient if they can lie on their side, so that their back area can be accessed more

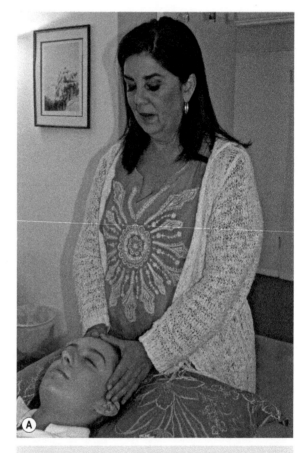

Figure 4.3A–H
Hand positions used by a Reiki practitioner treating a client.
(Continued)

easily. There may be a limited time available for the session, in which case the practitioner focuses on the areas that they sense need the most attention. As Reiki practitioners become more experienced, they are more able to feel sensations in their hands, such as heat, cold, pulsing, or tingling that indicate an area will benefit from Reiki. Most practitioners use a combination of standardized hand positions and intuitively guided hand positions to ensure that the client receives the best treatment that they need. To end a treatment, some practitioners place their hands on the soles of the feet of the client, which provides the client with

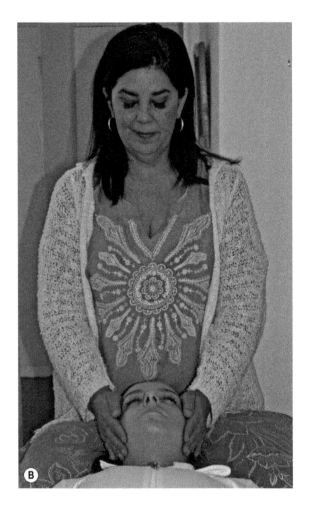

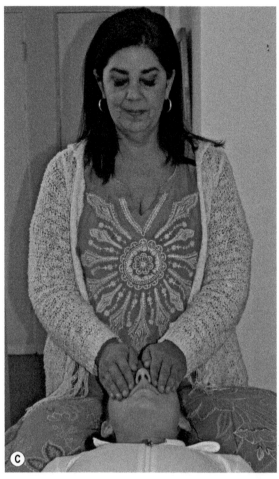

a grounding feeling of returning to Earth after their profound relaxation.

There is a differing viewpoint between Reiki practitioners about whether or not to guide the Reiki to specific parts of the body. On the one hand, most practitioners believe that Reiki is intelligent and "knows where to go". On the other hand, some practitioners believe that even though Reiki is intelligent, it makes sense to optimize its effectiveness by focusing on the areas that are causing the most concern. Usui himself agreed with this idea. In a translation of *Reiki Ryoho Hikkei*, the Reiki workbook that Usui gave to his Reiki students (published in *An Evidence Based*

History of Reiki, International Center of Reiki Training, Southfield, MI, 2015), Usui states:

The purpose of curing can be fulfilled just by gazing, or blowing, or pressing, or stroking the affected part, for instance, the head, if there's a brain trouble, or the stomach, if there's stomach trouble, or the eyes, if there's an eye trouble, etc.

Some Reiki practitioners with knowledge of human physiology may use Reiki to strengthen the immune system by concentrating on the heart chakra (thymus) and then on the left upper abdomen (spleen). The thymus and spleen are both organs of the immune system. Practition-

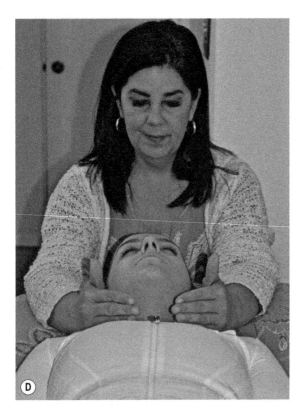

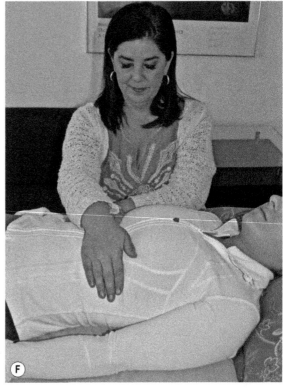

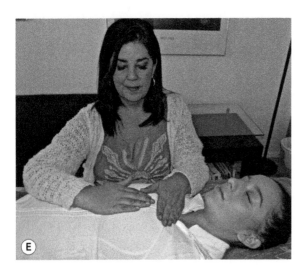

ers may attempt to regulate blood pressure by placing one hand on the back of the head and the other on the left or right carotid arteries in the neck; then they will switch to the other carotid. The carotid sinus baroreceptors, which are situated in the internal carotid arteries, regulate blood pressure. If a client or patient complains of lack of energy, the practitioner may place their hands on the throat chakra (thyroid) and the solar plexus at the center of the upper abdomen (adrenal glands). The thyroid gland makes and stores hormones that help regulate the heart rate, blood pressure, body temperature, and the rate at which food is converted into energy. Thyroid hormones are essential for the function of every cell in the body. The adrenal glands, situated on top of the kidneys, manufacture and secrete steroid hormones such as cortisol, estrogen, and testosterone that are essential for life, health, and vitality. Cortisol plays an important role in blood sugar metabolism

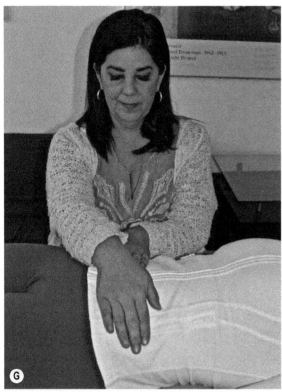

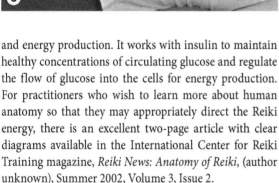

(G)

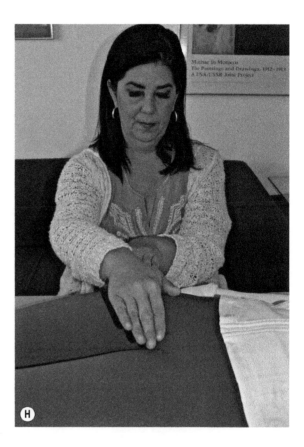

(H)

and energy production. It works with insulin to maintain healthy concentrations of circulating glucose and regulate the flow of glucose into the cells for energy production. For practitioners who wish to learn more about human anatomy so that they may appropriately direct the Reiki energy, there is an excellent two-page article with clear diagrams available in the International Center for Reiki Training magazine, *Reiki News: Anatomy of Reiki*, (author unknown), Summer 2002, Volume 3, Issue 2.

3. Practitioner: Mental, Emotional and Physical Condition

Mikao Usui taught that when a person practices Reiki, they act as a passive conduit, allowing the Reiki energy to flow through them without affecting the energy in any way. According to this precept, the mental, emotional, and physical condition of the practitioner should not influ-

ence their ability to provide Reiki to their client. This hypothesis has not yet been tested. There is no research on whether the health, stamina, or mood of the Reiki practitioner influences their effect on clients. However, a study by Rubik et al. (2006), did report a correlation between the physical, social, and emotional well-being of Reiki practitioners and the degree of recovery of heat-shocked bacteria after receiving Reiki from the practitioner for 15 minutes. In this experiment, cultures of *Escherichia coli* (*E. coli*) K12 bacteria, grown in dishes, were used to assess the efficacy of Reiki practitioners. *E. coli* is a bacterium commonly found in the gut of warm-blooded organisms. Most strains of *E. coli* are not harmful but are part of the healthful bacterial flora in the human gut. The K12 strain is so sensitive that it cannot even survive in the human gut, and so it is totally harmless to humans. Because growth is a measure

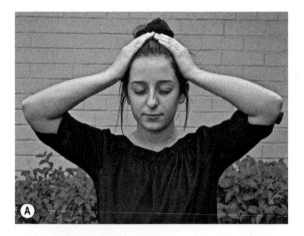

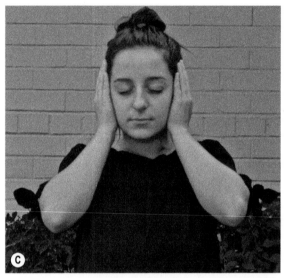

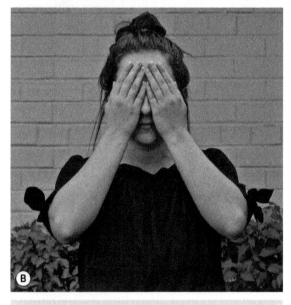

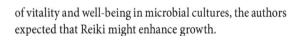

Figure 4.4A–M
Reiki practitioner treating self. (Continued)

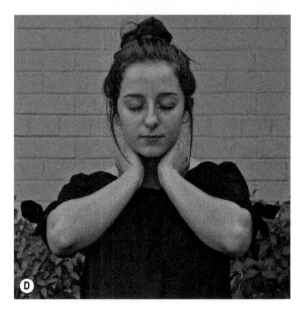

of vitality and well-being in microbial cultures, the authors expected that Reiki might enhance growth.

The bacteria were first heat-shocked to thwart their growth, and the numbers of bacteria in a given dish were counted automatically. Each of 14 Reiki practitioners gave Reiki to three dishes of bacteria in turn for 15 minutes and the numbers of bacteria were counted once more. The practitioners did not hold any particular intention to increase or decrease bacterial growth. Each practitioner completed a questionnaire before and after giving Reiki that rated their physical, mental, emotional, social, spiritual, and overall well-being. Matching dishes of bacteria from the same cultures that did not receive Reiki acted as controls.

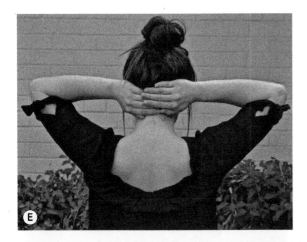

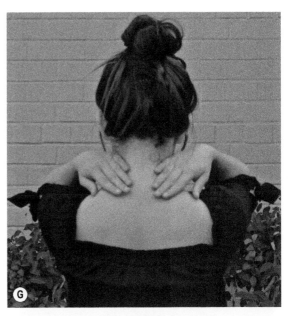

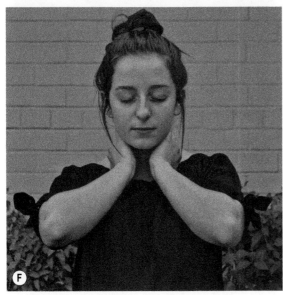

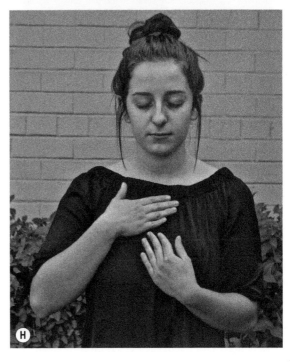

On average, the bacteria count was no greater for the Reiki-treated group than for the control group. However, the practitioners whose bacteria showed a greater increase in number after Reiki compared to the control condition, had started the session with significantly higher ratings of social and emotional well-being than those whose bacteria did not grow as well as the controls. Interestingly, this effect was amplified if the practitioners each gave Reiki to a person with a sprained ankle for 30 minutes prior to treating the bacteria (healing context). A correlation of initial

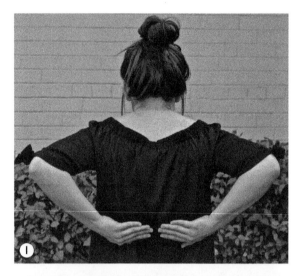

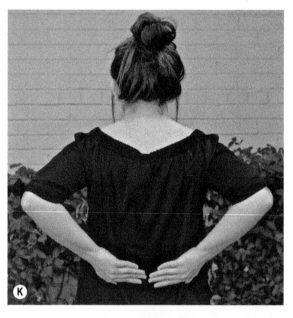

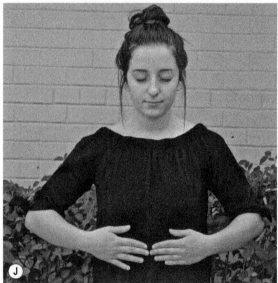

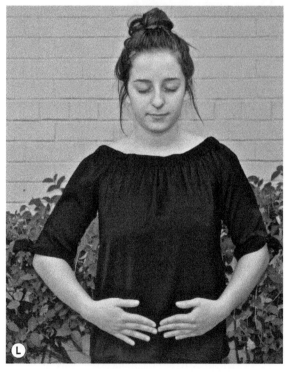

physical well-being with change in number of viable bacteria after Reiki compared to control was also seen. The authors concluded that the initial level of well-being of the Reiki practitioners correlated with the outcome of Reiki on bacterial culture growth. In addition, this time the average bacteria count post treatment was significantly greater for the Reiki-treated group than for the control group of bacteria (Figure 4.5). However, as can be seen in the figure, the initial count of the Reiki group was significantly lower than

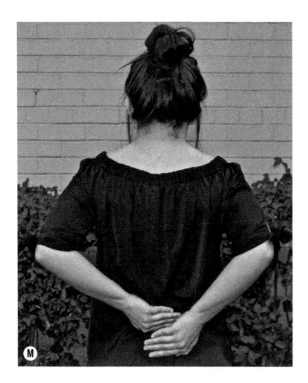

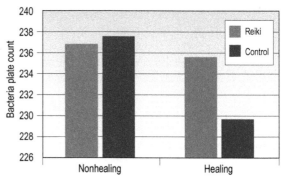

Figure 4.5
Mean bacteria count comparing Reiki and control groups in non-healing and healing contexts where "healing" indicates practitioner treated a human prior to the bacteria.
(From Rubik B, Brooks AJ, Schwartz GE. In vitro effect of Reiki treatment on bacterial cultures: Role of experimental context and practitioner well-being. *Journal of Alternative and Complementary Medicine* 2006; 12(1): 7–13.)

that of the control group. This poses the question that if the initial count of the Reiki group was as high as that of the control group, would the Reiki treatment have increased it further? Nevertheless, it does appear that the well-being and the state of the Reiki practitioner (i.e. whether or not they completed another Reiki treatment immediately prior to giving Reiki to the bacteria) did influence the healing outcome in this case.

4. Practitioner: Regulation of Breathing

Mikao Usui taught breath control to his Reiki students in the form of the "Gassho" breath, where the term Gassho, as used in Usui Reiki Ryoho, means "palms placed together in front of the chest" or "prayer position", and is often thought of as bringing unity to the body. The Gassho Breathing Technique is very simple:

- Sit either on the floor or upright in a chair in a relaxed position with your hands in prayer position.

- Concentrate on breathing in and out slowly through your nose.

- With each in-breath, imagine that Reiki energy is entering your crown and filling your entire body.

- With each out-breath, visualize that you are exhaling Reiki from every pore in your body and off out into infinity.

Practicing the Gassho Breathing Technique before giving a Reiki session brings with it many benefits:

- Makes one relaxed and calm but alert.

- Makes one think clearly.

- Improves one's memory.

- Helps one see things in perspective.

- Is healthy for the heart.

Chapter 4

It is fascinating that Mikao Usui realized a century ago before the advent of physiological monitoring technology, that this type of breathing has such far-reaching physical, mental, and emotional benefits. In addition, he understood that practicing the Gassho Technique prior to giving a Reiki session would bring stillness to the practitioner's mind and body, thus enabling them to open up to the Reiki flow. During the last 20 years or so, it has been discovered that breathing a little deeper and slower than usual (at about 6 breaths per minute) while recalling a pleasurable sensation (such as Reiki flowing through the body), or experiencing a positive emotion, such as appreciation, gratitude, and compassion, profoundly alters the autonomic nervous system (ANS) (Moss, 2004). The ANS is the part of the nervous system responsible for control of the bodily functions not consciously directed, such as the heartbeat and digestive processes. The practice of Vinyasa yoga, which involves slow, deep breathing, affects the ANS similarly (Tay and Baldwin, 2015).

The ANS consists of two components: sympathetic nerves that speed up heart rate and parasympathetic nerves that slow it down. During mental stress, the sympathetic nerves are highly activated and heart rate increases, whereas during relaxation, parasympathetic nerve stimulation predominates and heart rate decreases. Respiration rate is closely coupled to the relative degree of stimulation of the sympathetic and parasympathetic nerves. During stress, when sympathetic stimulation is high, respiration is fast, whereas during relaxation, when parasympathetic stimulation is high, respiration slows down. This relationship is illustrated in Figure 4.6. It can be seen that breathing at 5–6 breaths per minute, such as during Gassho meditation, creates a balance between sympathetic and parasympathetic stimulation that maximizes coherence, or synchrony between respiration and heart rate. When a person is in a state of coherence, their heart rate increases as they breathe in and decreases as they breathe out, as shown in Figure 4.7. Looking at the middle panel, the uppermost plot shows respiration (6.52 breaths per minute), with each hump representing one breath, rising with the in-breath and falling with the out-breath. The lowermost plot shows the corresponding HRV, or the change in heart rate with time. Focusing on a single breath (one

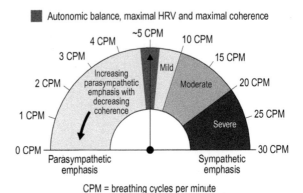

Figure 4.6

Diagram showing how respiration rate is correlated with sympathetic/parasympathetic balance.

(From: Coherence and the New Science of Breath. Copyright 2006 COHERENCE LLC)

hump), it is obvious that the corresponding heart rate increases with the in-breath and decreases with the out-breath, in perfect synchrony. This is coherence. The sympathetic/parasympathetic balance that is created during coherence leads to optimal cardiac function, improved oxygenation of the blood, enhanced cognitive ability and focusing skills, and a broadened emotional perspective. These are all qualities that aid a Reiki practitioner in providing a caring, compassionate, and effective Reiki session to their client. By contrast, research has shown that mental stress and negative emotions such as frustration, anger, anxiety, and worry lead to heart rhythm patterns that appear incoherent—highly variable and erratic. Overall, if a person is feeling negative emotions there is less synchronization in the reciprocal action of the parasympathetic and sympathetic branches of the nervous system. This de-synchronization, if sustained, taxes the nervous system, impeding the efficient synchronization and flow of information throughout the brain, making it difficult to remember things and to make rational decisions. Lack of coordination between the sympathetic and parasympathetic nervous branches also leads to imbalanced emotions, reinforcing the existing negative emotions that first

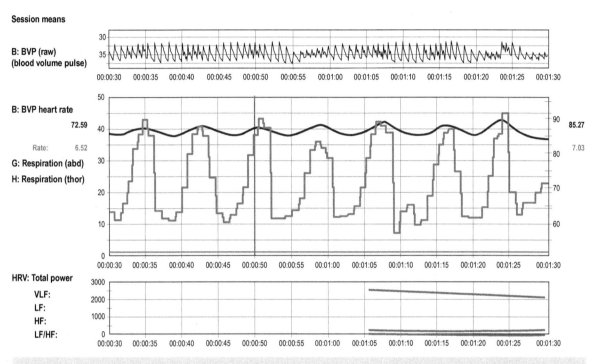

Figure 4.7
Pulse and heart rate variability of a person in a coherent state.

triggered the imbalance. Remembering to practice the Gassho Breathing Technique before providing Reiki will ensure restoration of an optimal autonomic balance in the practitioner as shown by the HRV recordings of a person when they practice Gassho Breathing (Figure 4.8A) and when they do not (Figure 4.8B). The Gassho HRV recording shows a waveform typical of a coherent state, whereas the non-Gassho recording demonstrates the much more random pattern associated with normal breathing. Recent research from the Institute of HeartMath strongly suggests that if a person is in a coherent state when they interact with another individual, then that individual will also become more coherent (McCraty, 2017). Therefore, if a Reiki practitioner becomes coherent by practicing Gassho Breathing prior to giving a Reiki session, their client is also likely to benefit from increased coherence.

5. Hydration of Client and Practitioner

The most common physiological response of a client after they have received Reiki is that they feel hot. Reiki practitioners also very often experience the same reaction. That is why it is important that both the client and the practitioner drink a glass of water after the session is over. It is also advisable for the practitioner to offer their client or patient some water before their session, just in case they are already dehydrated. Keeping the body hydrated ensures that blood volume is maintained so that blood pressure does not fall and so that adequate circulation to the brain, in particular, is sustained. If blood flow to the brain is impaired even for a few minutes, this can lead to feelings of weakness and dizziness. When one is hydrated, the heart pumps a sufficient volume

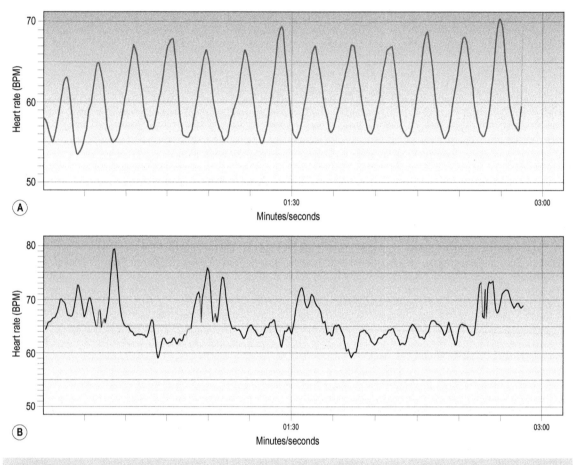

Figure 4.8
Heart rate variability of a person (**A**) practicing and (**B**) not practicing Gassho Breathing.

of blood with each beat so that the heart rate does not need to increase to maintain normal cardiac output. This means that the heart works more efficiently and does not waste energy. Thirst is not the best indicator of hydration. By the time a person feels thirsty, they are already dehydrated. A much better indicator is the color of the urine. Pale and clear indicates good hydration, whereas if it is dark the person should drink more water. Drinks containing electrolytes, such as sports drinks, are unnecessary after a Reiki session. They are only required if the person is engaging in vigorous exercise. Drinks containing caffeine make dehydration worse because caffeine is a diuretic and causes one to lose more fluids. Some medications, such as nonsteroidal anti-inflammatory drugs (NSAIDs), opiate pain medications, and some antidepressants, can also act as diuretics and so ensuring good hydration is even more important for clients or patients who are taking these medications. Further details about hydration and health are described in an excellent review (Popkin et al., 2010).

6. Comfort of Clients

The basic ways in which Reiki practitioners can ensure that their clients and patients are at ease during their session have been covered in Chapter 1. In this chapter, further details will be provided with regard to temperature, music, and chair Reiki.

Temperature. To ensure that clients and patients are comfortable during their Reiki session, the room should be set to a comfortable temperature such as is usual in a work place. The Occupational Health and Safety Administration (OSHA) recommends employers maintain workplace temperatures in the range of 68–76° Fahrenheit (20–25° Centigrade) and keep humidity in the range of 20–60%. Blankets (and socks) should be made available for clients who are sensitive to cold.

Music. Most clients enjoy hearing soft music as they receive Reiki, but they should always be given the choice to decline before the session begins. There are hundreds, maybe thousands, of recordings that are classified as Reiki music and most practitioners have selections from various musicians that they personally enjoy. When working with a new client, it is prudent to ask them if they are comfortable with the music selection and the volume before starting Reiki. Of course, for practitioners working in hospitals, the option of playing soft music may not be available. It 1w might be argued that lying down on a massage table listening to soft, pleasant music might by itself reduce a client's stress and anxiety, and that there is no need for Reiki. A small study compared the effects of Reiki with music and music alone on 37 people who were living with human immunodeficiency virus (HIV) (Bremner et al., 2016). The Reiki with music group, but not the music-only group, had six weekly, 30-minute Reiki sessions. Both groups received a meditative CD with instructions to listen for 30 minutes a week. Baseline and six and 10 week follow-up measures included established experimental questionnaires for assessing depression and anxiety, and visual analog scales for pain

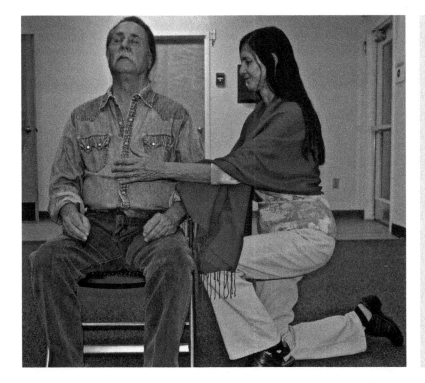

Figure 4.9
Reiki practitioner giving a person Reiki as he sits in a chair.

and stress. Significant improvements in relief of pain and stress were found in the Reiki with music group, but not in the music-alone group. Both groups did experience reductions in anxiety and depression over the 10-week period. This small study shows that music alone can relieve depression and anxiety, but that only the combination of Reiki and music can effectively reduce patients' pain and stress.

<u>Chair Reiki</u>: Often situations arise which may call for a Reiki session but there is no bed or Reiki table available. In those cases, it is perfectly acceptable to seat the client on a chair for their Reiki session. A simple straight-backed dining chair is all that is needed. The same Reiki hand positions can be used as when treating a client on a Reiki table (Figure 4.9). However, it is important that the practitioner is also comfortable as they work on the client, making sure to keep their back straight and bending only at the knees, not the hips.

References

Bremner MN, Blake BJ, Wagner VD, Pearcey SM. Effects of Reiki with music compared to music only among people living with HIV. *Journal of the Association of Nurses in AIDS Care* 2016; 27(5): 635–647.

Maben J, Peccei R, Adams M, Robert G, Richardson A, Murrells T, Morrow E. Patients' experiences of care and the influence of staff motivation, affect and well-being. Final Report. NIHR Service Delivery and Organization Program, 2012.

McCraty R. New frontiers in heart rate variability and social coherence research: techniques, technologies, and implications for improving group dynamics and outcomes. *Frontiers in Public Health: Hypothesis and Theory* 2017; 5: article 267.

Moss D. Heart rate variability biofeedback. *Psychophysiology Today: The Magazine for Mind–Body Medicine* 2004; 1: 4–11.

Pearson, N. Foundations of Reiki Ryoho: A Manual of Shoden and Okuden. Healing Arts Press, Simon and Schuster, 2018.

Popkin BM, D'Anci KE, Rosenberg AH. Water, hydration and health. *Nutrition Reviews* 2010; 68(8): 439–458.

Rubik B, Brooks AJ, Schwartz GE. In vitro effect of Reiki treatment on bacterial cultures: Role of experimental context and practitioner well-being. *Journal of Alternative and Complementary Medicine* 2006; 12(1): 7–13.

Tay K, Baldwin AL. Effects of breathing practice in vinyasa yoga on heart rate variability in university students: a pilot study. *Yoga & Physical Therapy* 2015; 5(4): 214.

Chapter 5
Reiki and Emotional Stress

How the Autonomic Nervous System Controls Stress Response

The part of the nervous system that is stimulated when one is anxious or fearful is the autonomic nervous system (ANS). The ANS innervates the heart and other organs and transmits messages from the brain to the organs and vice versa. In this way, it is possible for the heart, lungs, kidneys, and liver to function without any conscious input. There are two types of nerves involved, sympathetic and parasympathetic. Sympathetic nerves act like an accelerator, speeding up the heart and getting the body ready for action (fight-or-flight response). Parasympathetic nerves act like a brake, slowing down the heart and putting the body into 'rest and digest' mode. Autonomic nervous dysfunction is thought to play a significant role in anxiety and depression. Previous research indicates that individuals suffering from anxiety or depression often show decreased parasympathetic activity, increased sympathetic arousal and increased heart rate (Thayer et al, 1996).

Influence of the Limbic System on the Stress Response

The fight-or-flight response that is mediated through the ANS, is triggered by the limbic system. The limbic system is a collection of brain structures that integrate the various bodily sensations, thoughts, and memories experienced or recalled at a particular moment, into a complex electrical signal. This signal travels to a part of the limbic system called the hypothalamus that is responsible for activating the stress response. The stress response is mediated by stimulation of the sympathetic nerves and by attenuation of the parasympathetic nerves of the ANS. In addition, the endocrine system is activated to produce norepinephrine (noradrenaline), epinephrine (adrenaline), and the stress hormone, cortisol, from the adrenal glands on the top of each kidney. When a person is relaxed, the signals entering the hypothalamus cause it to stimulate the parasympathetic,

and attenuate the sympathetic components of the ANS, and also to inhibit release of stress hormones. It is important to note that the stress response is not a bimodal phenomenon, meaning that it is not either "on" or "off", but operates over a wide spectrum, reflecting the precise degree of anxiety or relaxation that a person may feel at any given moment. The role of the limbic system in modulating the stress response is illustrated in diagrammatic form in Figure 5.1. The signal from the limbic system influences the degree with which the hypothalamus sets off the "fight or flight" response via the endocrine system and the ANS. A more detailed diagram is shown in Figure 5.2. This diagram illustrates that just smelling a rose will affect the limbic system and hence the degree of activation of the stress response through the ANS. Exactly how the ANS is influenced will depend on the sensory preferences and memories of the individual. For example, one person might associate the smell of a rose with peace and tranquility, whereas another might be reminded of visiting an unpleasant relative whose house always smelled of roses. In the first case, the parasympathetic branch of the ANS would be preferentially activated, whereas in the second example, the sympathetic branch would be dominant.

When smelling a scent, the aroma first stimulates olfactory nerves in the nasal cavity; these nerves lead to the olfactory bulb. The neural signal is received by mitral cells in the olfactory bulb and transmitted through efferent nerves to the olfactory cortex. The olfactory cortex is linked directly to the amygdalae, two walnut shaped structures that are part of the limbic system. Although there is a left and a right amygdala, these structures are usually referred to as "the amygdala", and this is the terminology that will be used from here on. The amygdala is the most connected structure in the brain and there is a continual back and forth movement of information between the amygdala and all other parts of the limbic system and the cortex (Figure 5.3). For example, the amygdala connects with the hippocampus, another part of the limbic system, which is responsible for storing *factual* or declarative memories.

Chapter 5

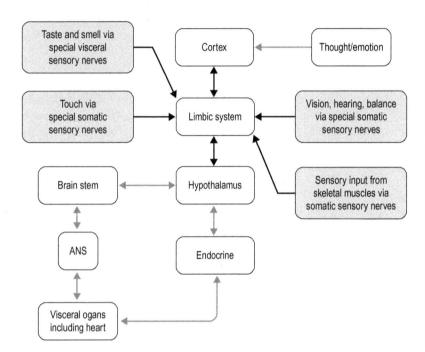

Taste and smell via special visceral sensory nerves → Cortex ← Thought/emotion

Touch via special somatic sensory nerves → Limbic system ← Vision, hearing, balance via special somatic sensory nerves

Brain stem ↔ Hypothalamus

Sensory input from skeletal muscles via somatic sensory nerves

ANS

Endocrine

Visceral ogans including heart

Figure 5.1
Physiology of mind–body interactions.

In the case of a person smelling a rose, a possible factual memory that could be evoked might be the location of the person the last time they smelled a rose. The amygdala itself stores *emotional* memories, such as how the person might have *felt* the last time they smelled a rose if it were during a particularly moving event. The amygdala is also connected to the thalamus, a part of the limbic system, situated just above the brainstem. The thalamus is known as the "gateway to the brain". All information entering the brain, *apart from olfactory information*, first passes through the thalamus that then directs the signal to the prefrontal cortex and other parts of the cortex where it is consciously perceived. In the case of odors, the information goes directly to the amygdala before reaching the thalamus. This is important because the main function of the amygdala is to trigger the hypothalamus to initiate the fight-or-flight response, and so smelling a particular dangerous odor may set off the fight-or-flight response before the smell is even consciously perceived. On the other hand, information perceived by sight, hearing, touch, or taste will be consciously acknowledged before the signal reaches the amygdala. Without the amygdala there would be no stress response.

How is the Amygdala Controlled?

The degree to which the amygdala is stimulated by a thought or sensation will be affected by any associated emotional and/or factual memories. Favorable memories will tone down the response of the amygdala, leading to a diminished stress response with very little sympathetic nervous activity and high parasympathetic (rest-and-digest) nervous activity. On the other hand, fearful or unpleasant memories will have the opposite effect on the ANS, resulting in an amplified stress response. Some people are naturally over anxious and that is usually because they have an overactive amygdala. The body produces a chemical called gamma-aminobutyric acid (GABA) which binds to receptors on the amygdala and suppresses its response to stimuli. Some people who are over anxious either do not produce sufficient GABA, or do not have an adequate number of GABA receptors on the amygdala. These people may rely on drugs termed "GABA-substitutes," such as Valium and Librium, to control their anxiety. These drugs, also known as benzodiazepines, calm down the amygdala

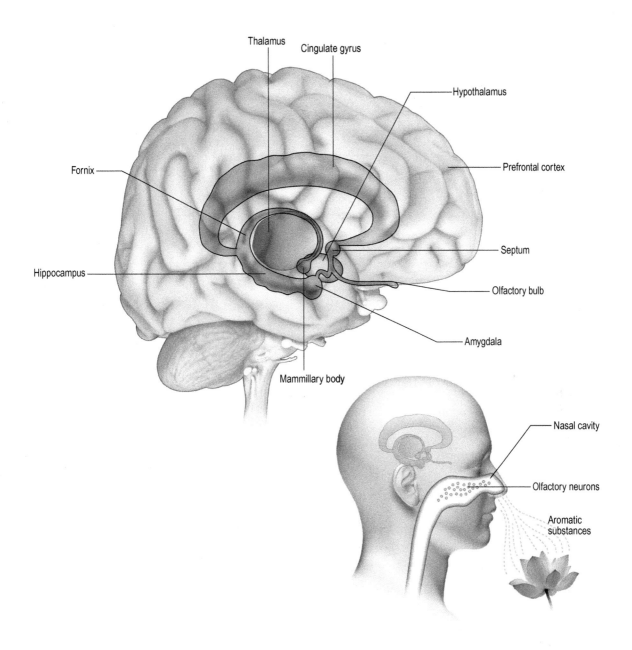

Figure 5.2
Diagram of the limbic system.

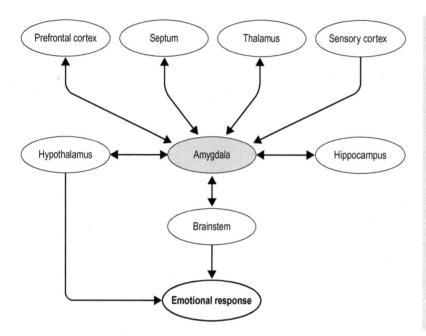

Figure 5.3
Diagram of integrated response of limbic system.

by binding to its GABA receptors, and thus are a solution for those people whose body produces insufficient GABA. However, benzodiazepines do have side effects, the most common of which is daytime grogginess or drowsiness. At higher doses, benzodiazepines may impair physical coordination and balance, increasing the risk of falls and other accidents. Some benzodiazepines can dull memory and the ability to learn and retain new information. All these side effects are more serious in older people. In addition, partly because GABA receptors adapt to the drug's presence, they become even more underactive when the GABA is withdrawn. Therefore, benzodiazepines can cause physical dependence and withdrawal reactions such as restlessness, irritability, insomnia, muscle tension, weakness, aches and pains, blurred vision, and a racing heart. It is for these reasons that an alternative therapy that is effective and without side effects is needed for the 18% of the adult US population who suffer from anxiety and other forms of emotional stress. In this chapter, evidence will be presented that receiving Reiki can help regulate the fight-or-flight response, possibly by stimulating the vagus nerve (parasympathetic). Another possibility is that Reiki might

increase GABA production, as was shown in two patients with depression and low back pain following a course of Hatha yoga (Streeter et al., 2012). However, at present, this idea is totally hypothetical. If Reiki can help regulate the fight-or-flight response, it is reasonable to suppose that receiving Reiki would also help control anxiety and depression. In Chapter 8, evidence will be presented that Reiki is indeed a viable and effective alternative to drugs for reducing anxiety.

Heart Rate Variability: An Indicator of Stress

Heart rate variability (HRV), which is the second-by-second change in heart rate as a function of time, reflects the interaction between sympathetic and parasympathetic ANS activity. When the sympathetic nerves increase in activity, heart rate increases, and when the parasympathetic nerve stimulation becomes dominant, heart rate decreases. A recording of healthy HRV is shown in Figure 5.4 (upper plot). The lower plot shows the corresponding electrocardiogram; each spike represents a ventricular contraction, or heartbeat. When heart rate increases, the time between

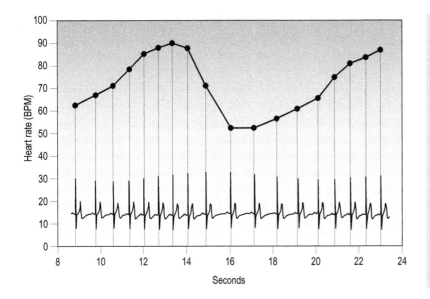

Figure 5.4
Recording of heart rate variability from a healthy person.
(From: Science of the Heart. Exploring the role of the heart in human performance. An overview of research conducted by the HeartMath Institute., 2016. Figure 3.1.)

each heartbeat is shorter (heartbeats are close together) and when heart rate decreases, the time between each heartbeat is longer (heartbeats are further apart). This variability in heart rate ensures that the brain and the rest of the body receive the exact amount of blood, and hence oxygen and nutrients, that they require at any given time. It also makes certain that the heart does not work harder than it needs by pumping faster or harder than required. When one is not physically or emotionally stressed, the sympathetic and parasympathetic ANS components are able to work together, sympathetic increasing when the heart rate is too low, and parasympathetic increasing when the heart rate is too high. The heart rate oscillates around its mean resulting in a high HRV; this is healthy because it means that the heart can quickly adapt to changes in the body's needs. The sympathetic and parasympathetic components cooperate, just like the accelerator and the brake when a car is being driven through stop-and-go traffic. The accelerator is engaged when the car ahead is sufficiently far away for forward travel to be safe, and the brake is applied when the car ahead is too close. Accurate timing is required for safe, efficient movement. The heart is similar. Heart rate should increase when the need for extra circulation arises, but should decrease as soon as that need is fulfilled.

On the other hand, when a person is physically, mentally, or emotionally stressed, the sympathetic ANS component goes into overdrive because one goal of the stress response is to increase the blood circulation to the muscles, heart, and brain to equip the body for "fight-or-flight". Sympathetic stimulation achieves this goal by increasing average heart rate and cardiac contractility, like stepping on the accelerator. The stress response locks the heart into overwhelming sympathetic activity and reduces HRV because the parasympathetic nerves are inhibited and can no longer regulate the heart rate and cardiac contractility. This response will benefit a person in the short-term if they need to run to escape from a stressful situation. However, in many, if not most cases, the stressor is long-term and psychological, such as chronic anxiety, depression, or frustration. In these cases, there is no need for the heart to work overtime to increase blood circulation because the person will not solve the problem by physically running away, but the heart rate increases anyway and so the heart wastes energy. In addition, as will be described later in this section, the absence of the regulatory effect of the parasympathetic nerves impairs memory and cognitive function and also increases emotional arousal, making the person even more anxious.

Chapter 5

To summarize, when one is emotionally balanced and at ease, sympathetic and parasympathetic nerves are metaphorically having a conversation, neither one overwhelming the other; heart rate oscillates around its average value and HRV is high (Figure 5.5A). In Figure 5.5A, the heart rate as shown varies from 58 to 75 bpm (17 bpm difference). The rhythmic oscillation is reflected in the spectrum average that shows one main frequency of oscillation of about 0.07 Hz, or 4.2 cycles per second. Heart rate oscillations between 3.0 and 9.0 cycles per second usually reflect a good balance, or "coherence", between sympathetic and parasympathetic activities. The amplitude of this peak is relatively high (910 ms^2/Hz), indicating a powerful oscillation. The coherence ratio is the percentage of time that the HRV is engaged in rhythmic oscillation so the ANS is balanced regarding sympathetic and parasympathetic activity. In this case, the coherence ratio is 100%, indicating perfect coherence.

When one is feeling even somewhat physically, mentally, or emotionally stressed, the sympathetic nerves become more stimulated than the parasympathetic nerves. Heart rate does not oscillate rhythmically but varies randomly and to a much lesser degree; HRV is low (Figure 5.5B). In Figure 5.5B, the heart rate as shown varies from 73 to 77 bpm (4 bpm difference). Most of the HRV frequency spectrum is not concentrated at a single frequency but is more spread out among different frequencies. The peak frequency is of small amplitude (50 ms^2/Hz) and is in the very low frequency range (further to the left in the spectrum seen in Figure 5.5B compared to Figure 5.5A). Heart rate oscillations at very low frequencies are associated with overwhelming sympathetic activity rather than a balance between sympathetic and parasympathetic. In this recording, the high coherence ratio was only 37%, indicating that during the recording time, sympathetic and parasympathetic activities were only in balance for 37% of the time.

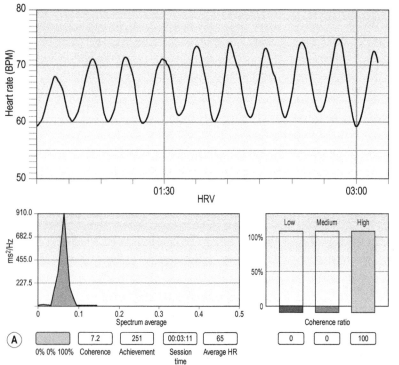

Figure 5.5A
Heart rate variability of a person when emotionally balanced.
(Continued)

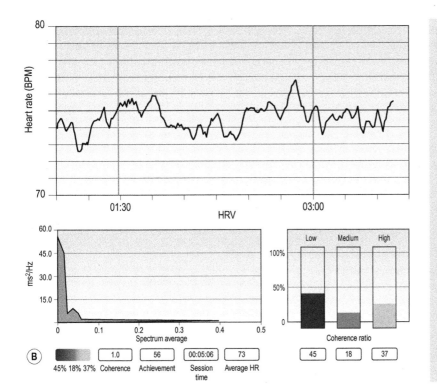

Figure 5.5B
Heart rate variability of a person
when emotionally stressed.

In some cases, such as Parkinson's disease, the ANS will be locked into the parasympathetic system and average heart rate will be low. Once again, the heart rate will not rhythmically oscillate around the mean because sympathetic stimulation will be impaired, and HRV will be low.

Clinical Use of Heart Rate Variability as a Marker for Stress

Heart rate variability is easy to measure and indicates by its magnitude and by its oscillation frequency spectrum whether or not a person is experiencing balance between the sympathetic and parasympathetic components of their ANS. For those reasons, HRV is an ideal clinical marker for emotional stress and anxiety. Previous research indicates that individuals suffering from anxiety or depression often show decreased overall HRV and parasympathetic activity, increased sympathetic arousal, and increased heart rate (Thayer et al., 1996; Chalmers et al., 2014). Inter-

estingly, people who are "worried", rather than diagnosed with anxiety disorder, show an even more robust correlation with low HRV (Chalmers et al., 2016). One way to increase HRV is to practice HRV biofeedback techniques. HRV biofeedback involves training people to adjust their breathing rate to a resonant frequency; a breathing rate (usually slower than normal breathing) at which HRV is maximized. When this occurs, parasympathetic activity is increased and there is improved regulation of emotionally mediated reflexes throughout the body (Lehrer et al., 2003). Recent research has shown that if a person who is anxious or depressed practices HRV biofeedback, they experience two benefits: HRV increases and their anxiety and/or depression is significantly reduced.

One biofeedback study (Karavidas et al., 2007), conducted on 11 depressed patients, showed significant improvements in two measures of depression and an increase in HRV after a 10-week period of practice. Another

Chapter 5

biofeedback trial (Siepmann et al., 2008), conducted on 14 depressed patients, resulted in significantly reduced depression, decreased heart rate, and increased HRV. Therefore, it appears that the ability to regulate one's HRV and, in particular, to increase the parasympathetic component of HRV, is strongly correlated with improved mood. Therefore, if Reiki does indeed enhance HRV and parasympathetic activity, then it would be likely to reduce anxiety and depression. Scientific studies that report the effects of Reiki on HRV will be discussed later in this chapter.

How Heart Rate Variability Influences Cognitive and Emotional Function

The studies listed in the previous paragraph provide evidence that HRV is connected to improved emotional function and stability. Recent research has also shown that high HRV is associated with enhanced cognitive function in middle-age adults (Zeki et al., 2018). The authors suggest that because this association was observed as early as middle age, it may be possible to develop preventive strategies early in life to delay the progression of cognitive impairment. Basically, they are postulating that if a person can adopt practices to increase their HRV when they are young, then they will reduce the chances of developing dementia later on. However, the mechanism by which such improvements may occur is not currently known. Future studies are needed to explore underlying pathways including brain-imaging experiments.

As a start to understanding the connection between HRV and brain function, Thayer and Lane (2000) have proposed a model by which dynamic connections between the limbic structures and the cortex of the brain may explain how the parasympathetic (rest and digest) contribution to HRV is linked to higher-level cognitive functions and emotional self-regulation. This model is quite complicated and will not be discussed in this chapter. On a very simplistic level, the Institute of HeartMath has diagrammed a model to demonstrate the cognitive-HRV connection (Figure 5.6) and the emotional regulation-HRV connection (Figure 5.7). Both figures focus on the connections, including neural (sympathetic and parasympathetic), between the heart and the brain and emphasize the communication from the heart to the brain. Of course communication occurs in both directions but about twice as much information is transmitted from the heart to the brain as from the brain to the heart. In Figure 5.6, the HRV pulse is shown passing through the medulla and then to the thalamus. When the signal consists of ordered, or coherent, heart rhythms, the thalamus is aided in its task of synchronizing cortical activity, or ensuring that each region of the cortex is cognizant of activities in other parts of the cortex. When the signal consists of disorganized heart rhythms, this function is impaired. Evidence for this effect is partly based on experiments showing that memory and performance of cognitive tasks improves as the HRV pattern becomes more coherent. Figure 5.7 shows the HRV signal passing through the amygdala. Ordered, or coherent, heart rhythms inform the amygdala that a person is calm and in charge, whereas a disordered HRV signal indicates to the amygdala that the person is stressed and ready for the fight-or-flight response. Evidence for this idea is based on Karl Pribham's Theory of Emotion. The amygdala receives information from every part of the body. Basically, the amygdala can be thought of as a filing cabinet full of information. Each time a new piece of information arrives, the amygdala searches through its files to find a match. For example, a disordered HRV signal may arrive that is similar to one that normally appears when a person is anxious. This information will be added to the other signals that are arriving from different parts of the body, cortex, and limbic system and if this other information is consistent with the HRV signal, a feeling of anxiety will develop and will be consciously acknowledged in the cortex. However, at this point, it is possible for the HRV signal to be consciously and deliberately adjusted by the individual. For example, if the person mentally recalls a pleasant experience, the parasympathetic nerves will become stimulated and the HRV signal will become more coherent. On receiving this modified signal, the amygdala will find the match that is consistent with a feeling of pleasure, and the sense of anxiety will be lessened.

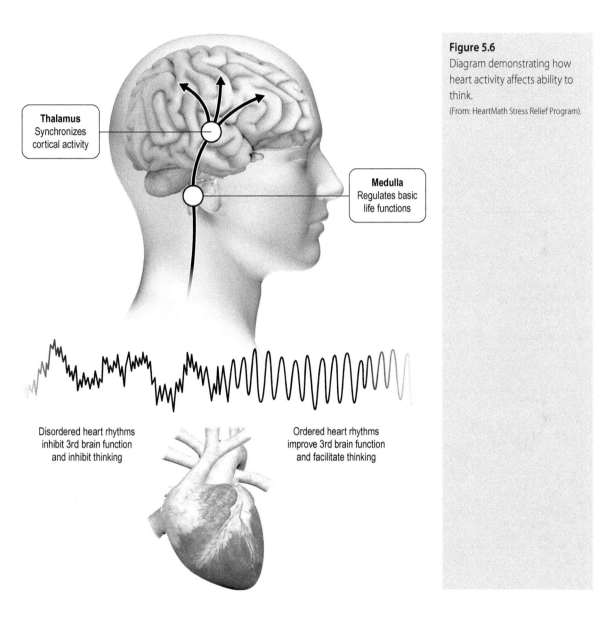

Figure 5.6
Diagram demonstrating how heart activity affects ability to think.
(From: HeartMath Stress Relief Program).

Thalamus
Synchronizes cortical activity

Medulla
Regulates basic life functions

Disordered heart rhythms inhibit 3rd brain function and inhibit thinking

Ordered heart rhythms improve 3rd brain function and facilitate thinking

Effects of Reiki on Stress Response of Patients and Clients

There are currently four published, peer-reviewed papers that investigate the effect of Reiki on heart rate and/or HRV in human patients or clients (Mackay et al., 2004; Friedman et al., 2010; Diaz-Rodriguez et al., 2011; Pizzinato et al., 2012) and two in animals (Baldwin and Schwartz, 2006; Baldwin et al., 2008). In addition, a further paper describes the physiological responses (heart rate, HRV, and blood flow in cutaneous blood vessels in the fingers) of Reiki Masters as they self-administer Reiki (Baldwin and Schwartz, 2012). These papers will be discussed in this chapter. Another nine papers address the effects of Reiki

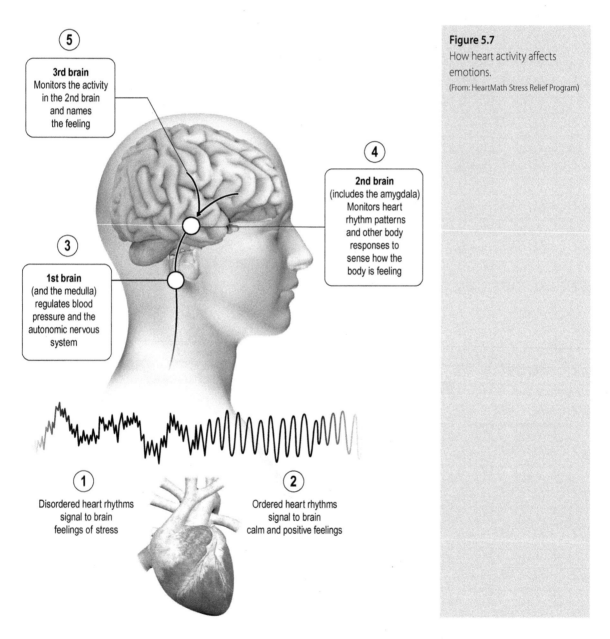

5

3rd brain
Monitors the activity
in the 2nd brain
and names
the feeling

4

2nd brain
(includes the amygdala)
Monitors heart
rhythm patterns
and other body
responses to
sense how the
body is feeling

3

1st brain
(and the medulla)
regulates blood
pressure and the
autonomic nervous
system

1

Disordered heart rhythms
signal to brain
feelings of stress

2

Ordered heart rhythms
signal to brain
calm and positive feelings

Figure 5.7
How heart activity affects
emotions.
(From: HeartMath Stress Relief Program)

on generalized stress and/or anxiety in terms of patients' answers to established scientific questionnaires before and after receiving Reiki. These nine studies will be described in Chapters 8 and 9. Experiments in which physiological, numerical data, such as heart rate or HRV, are obtained from participants receiving or giving Reiki are more valu-able when judged as evidence for efficacy, than those in which participants are asked to complete questionnaires related to their emotions or sensations. This is because physiological measurements are objective, whereas answers to questionnaires are subjective in nature and may easily change according to other factors not relevant to the experimental goals. For example, a participant may indicate a more positive response on a questionnaire after receiving Reiki than they actually sense, because they may feel a need to please the experimenter or the Reiki practitioner. However, subjective assessment tools do provide useful information that cannot be gleaned from numerical data. Records of comments made by Reiki recipients add a more personal dimension to scientific research and may raise some important questions for further research that might otherwise go unnoticed. Studies that combine objective physiological measures with more subjective patient and client outcomes really provide the most accurate picture of how receiving Reiki affects the mind and body.

Evidence that Reiki Reduces Emotional Stress: Objective Data

The seven reports presenting objective data were all pilot studies and they only involved small numbers of participants; thus, the results do not have the credence of large-scale studies. In addition, the participating populations varied widely: healthy humans in three studies; mentally, emotionally, and/or physically debilitated humans in another two studies; and rats that had been subjected to environmental noise in two further studies. Nevertheless, even though the participant numbers were low and the participant populations were varied, the results were surprisingly consistent. The effects of Reiki in these experiments included increasing overall HRV, increasing the parasympathetic component of HRV, as well as decreasing heart rate and blood pressure. All these responses to Reiki reflect improved stimulation of the parasympathetic "rest and digest" component of the ANS, and reduced activity of the sympathetic fight-or-flight component; both these responses are necessary for alleviating feelings of anxiety and other forms of emotional stress.

Healthy Participants

In one of the studies on healthy humans (Pizzinato et al., 2012), 27 people had their HRV measured before and after a single 40-minute rest period on one day, and before and after a single 40-minute Reiki session the following day.

On average, the participants' overall HRVs significantly increased after the rest period *and* after the Reiki session, but the change was shown to be statistically significantly greater when they received Reiki compared to rest. High HRV, provided there is no arrhythmia, or pathological irregularity in the heartbeat, is a strong indicator of good physical and emotional health. This was the first reported experiment to determine the effects of Reiki on HRV in healthy humans. Problems with the study included the short duration (140 seconds) of the HRV recordings. It is usually recommended to measure HRV for 5 minutes to obtain an accurate short-term assessment of this parameter. In addition, very little information was provided about the participants, the Reiki practitioner, or the way in which the Reiki sessions were conducted.

In the other study on healthy humans (Mackay et al., 2004), 45 test-subjects (both males and females in the age range 23–59) were randomly assigned to one of three groups: Reiki, sham Reiki, or rest. Each group had a 15-minute rest period to establish baseline measurements followed by a 30-minute treatment period of Reiki, sham Reiki, or rest, and ending with another 10-minute rest period. The Reiki practitioner placed their hands over the subject's body (but not touching) in a series of six hand positions chosen to correspond with key chakras, over clothing, for a 30-minute period. The hands were placed over the participants' eyes, temples, occiput (back of head), chest, knees, and the soles of the feet. The only point at which the practitioner touched the participant was underneath the head to reach the occiput. The sham Reiki treatment was provided by a person who was not trained in Reiki and who simply mimicked the hand positions of the Reiki practitioner. Each subject was monitored for various cardiovascular measures including heart rate, blood pressure, and respiration rate. In both Reiki and sham Reiki groups, the heart rate and respiration rate decreased compared to baseline while the parasympathetic component of HRV increased. All these responses indicate that both Reiki and sham Reiki increased parasympathetic activity, the "rest and digest mode". The control group showed no change in any parameter. Therefore, just the presence of a person paying attention to the participant resting on a Reiki table can produce a physiologically significant relaxation response in the recipient. However, the decrease in heart rate was significantly greater in the Reiki group compared to the sham Reiki group, and the mean blood pressure was significantly reduced by Reiki but not by sham Reiki or by rest. In addition, in the Reiki group only, there was an observed increase in skin temperature, which could have been caused by increased blood flow to the skin, enabled by the reduced constriction of small arteries, suggesting a decrease in sympathetic activity of the ANS. Therefore, Reiki itself has a significant relaxation effect that goes beyond the placebo response one might have in response to another person offering their attention and gentle touch. Increased blood flow to the skin has also been reported in Reiki masters when they self-administer Reiki (Baldwin and Schwartz, 2012). This study will be described in more detail later in this chapter.

Stressed Participants

In one study (Diaz-Rodriguez et al., 2011), Reiki was performed on healthcare professionals diagnosed with burnout syndrome (BS) to determine whether it lessened their symptoms of anxiety. It was hypothesized that Reiki would produce a parasympathetic response as indicated by changes in HRV, increases in body temperature and salivary flow rate and a decrease in the concentration of the stress hormone cortisol, present in the saliva. Twenty-one female healthcare professionals, with a mean age of 44 years, attended two treatment sessions held one week apart. In the first session, the participants were randomly assigned to either a group that received a Reiki treatment from an experienced Reiki Master, or a group that received sham Reiki performed by a nurse with no Reiki experience. The Reiki Master held their hands for about 5 minutes over the participant's body in each Reiki hand position, and the nurse just mimicked the hand positions. Both treatments lasted 30 minutes. Measurements of HRV, body temperature, and salivary flow rate were taken before and after the treatment. The second session was the same as the first except that each participant received the alternate treatment compared to the first session. Reiki, but not sham Reiki, produced a statistically significant increase in

HRV, a decrease in the low frequency component of HRV consistent with reduced sympathetic activity, and an elevation of body temperature. The high frequency component of HRV, which reflects parasympathetic activity was not affected by either treatment, nor were the salivary flow rate and cortisol concentrations. These results indicate that Reiki treatment produces a mild but significant relaxation response, over and above that associated with attention or touch, in nurses with BS.

In another study (Friedman et al., 2010), Reiki was performed on patients recovering from acute coronary syndrome, which usually means a heart attack, to determine whether it would improve their HRV. There is evidence to show that patients with a higher HRV have a better chance of survival after a heart attack. Medications that improve parasympathetic activity, such as beta-adrenergic blockers, also produce better outcomes. If Reiki also enhances parasympathetic activity, it might improve survival after a heart attack without the patient having to resort to beta-blockers. The 49 patients (mean age of 60) were randomized to one of three treatment groups: a resting control group; a group that listened to slow, classical music; and a group that received light touch Reiki from nurse Reiki practitioners. Treatments were started within 72 hours of the acute cardiac event. The duration or frequency of the treatments was not reported in the paper. All subjects lay supine in bed from baseline through intervention, underwent continuous electrocardiographic (ECG) monitoring, and their emotional states were assessed using a subjective 10-point Likert scale. Continuous ECG recordings were obtained from 12 control patients, 13 music patients, and 12 Reiki patients. The parasympathetic component of HRV (shown as HF) increased significantly in the Reiki treatment group, did not appreciably change in the control group, and decreased slightly in the music group. The average time interval between consecutive heartbeats (RR Interval) increased significantly more in the Reiki group than in the music group but not when compared to the resting control group. An increase in inter-beat interval is equivalent to a decrease in heart rate. Reiki treatment, but not music or rest, was associated with increases in positive emotional states and decreases in negative emotional states. This study sheds light on a possible mechanism for the effects of Reiki therapy, i.e. parasympathetic stimulation, by using a combination of directly measured vagal response via HRV and emotional status via the 10-point Likert scale. The results demonstrate a direct relationship between physiology and emotional well-being. However, a sham Reiki light touch treatment was not part of the study so the touch effect cannot be ruled out as contributing to the relaxation effect of the Reiki.

Animal Studies

Scientific studies in which animals are used as participants, instead of human subjects, make an invaluable contribution to clinical research. That is because, unlike humans, animals do not arrive with opinions about the research based on past experiences, or with expectations about whether or not the research is likely to be successful. In this way, laboratory animals are basically clean slates because they do not introduce uncontrolled psychological variables into the experiment. Laboratory animals are also housed identically and fed the same diet and so do not complicate the experiment with additional uncontrolled environmental variables. With regard to Reiki research, there are currently only two published studies in which animals were used as experimental subjects (Baldwin and Schwartz, 2006; Baldwin et al., 2008). More research using animals is needed in order to obtain the high quality, accurate, and unambiguous data necessary for eventually elucidating the mechanisms by which Reiki mediates its beneficial effects on mind and body. Evidence of mechanisms, whatever those mechanisms may be, would greatly improve the status of Reiki in the medical and scientific communities, leading to more funding and support for establishing Reiki centers and for developing teaching programs.

The Reiki study by Baldwin et al., 2008 was performed on rats that were exposed to artificially generated white noise for 30 minutes on eight days, consecutively. The noise level was 90 dB which is about as loud as a power lawn mower. This level of noise, which is similar to that found in some facilities that are used for housing research animals, has been shown to cause deleterious physiological changes in rats (Baldwin et al., 2006; Baldwin and Bell, 2007), as well as increased heart rate and blood pressure (Burwell and Baldwin, 2006). The goal of the Reiki experiment was to determine whether application of Reiki to noise-stressed rats would reduce their heart rates and blood pressure. Three male rats were used that were each implanted with an electronic telemetric device that could monitor heart rate and blood pressure. On all eight days, baseline data were recorded for 15 minutes prior to the intervention. For the first three days, the rats were just exposed to noise without Reiki. Their heart rates and blood pressure increased during the noise, as shown in Figure 5.8. For the last five days of noise exposure, each rat received 15 minutes of Reiki from one of the level-three practitioners prior to the noise and 15 minutes of Reiki during the noise. The Reiki practitioners positioned the palms of their hands facing the cage, about four feet away from the front of the cage. Two weeks after the Reiki treatments, the experiment was repeated but with students, untrained in Reiki, performing sham Reiki. The sham Reiki practitioners were asked not to think about the rats, whereas the Reiki practitioners focused their full attention on the rats to which they were sending Reiki. There was no direct contact or talking to the animals in either case. After Reiki and before exposure to noise, the rats showed significant decreases in heart rate compared to baseline. In this case, the degree to which heart rate decreased after Reiki depended directly on its initial baseline value. Reiki, but not sham Reiki, significantly reduced the rise in heart rate produced by exposure of the rats to noise. Neither Reiki nor sham Reiki significantly affected blood pressure. These findings help substantiate that Reiki produces homeostasis, in this case, by reducing heart rates in rats that are stressed by noise, as well as in rats that have a higher than average heart rate before being exposed to noise.

Another Reiki study (Baldwin and Schwartz, 2006) was performed on 16 rats, 12 of which had been exposed to 15 minutes per day of 90 dB white noise for three weeks. Four of the noise-exposed rats also received 15 minutes of Reiki each day before the noise. Another

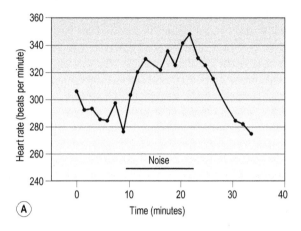

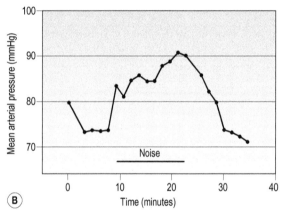

Figure 5.8

Changes in heart rate of rats subjected to noise.

(From: Baldwin AL, Wagers C and Schwartz GE. Reiki improves heart rate homoeostasis in laboratory rats. *Journal of Alternative and Complementary Medicine* 2008; 14(4): 417–422. Figure 4.)

four rats received sham Reiki, and the remaining four did not receive any additional treatment. A further control group of four rats were not exposed to noise and did not receive Reiki or sham Reiki. After three weeks, a fluorescent dye was injected into the circulation of each rat. The rats were examined to determine whether their intestinal circulation had become leaky to the dye, indicating tis-

sue injury. As shown in Figure 5.9, the rats that received noise but not Reiki or sham Reiki demonstrated the most leakage as measured by number and size of the leaks, whereas the rats that were not exposed to noise showed very little leakage. The rats that received Reiki or sham Reiki showed significantly less leakage to the dye than those that received noise only. Most importantly, the rats that received Reiki showed significantly less leakage than those that received sham Reiki. These results mean that although having a person (sham Reiki practitioner) sit with the rats before and during the noise did reduce the leakage somewhat, Reiki had a significant ameliorating effect on the leakage above and beyond the placebo response.

Self-Administered Reiki

A study by Baldwin and Schwartz (2012) examined ANS changes in Reiki Masters while practicing without a recipient. On the basis that Reiki appears to cause a relaxation effect by stimulating the parasympathetic nerves and inhibiting activation of the sympathetic nerves, it was hypothesized that Reiki practitioners would experience reduced heart rate, increased HRV, and increased blood volume in the cutaneous blood vessels of the fingers. One group of 31 Reiki Masters and another group of 32 control subjects without Reiki training were included in the study. Measurements were made for 5 minutes before, during, and after self-practice (or viewing a calming picture for the control).

Pulse sensors were clipped to the ears for heart rate and HRV and a laser Doppler perfusion imager scanned the index, middle, and ring fingers to detect changes in cutaneous blood volume. The effects of Reiki on blood flow regulation will be considered in detail in Chapter 6. Only the heart rate and HRV results will be discussed in this chapter. Reiki self-practice did *not* significantly affect heart rate or HRV on average. This is contrary to the hypothesis and opposite to the responses seen in other studies focusing on the responses of recipients of Reiki compared to baseline. It is possible that Reiki may affect practitioners and recipi-

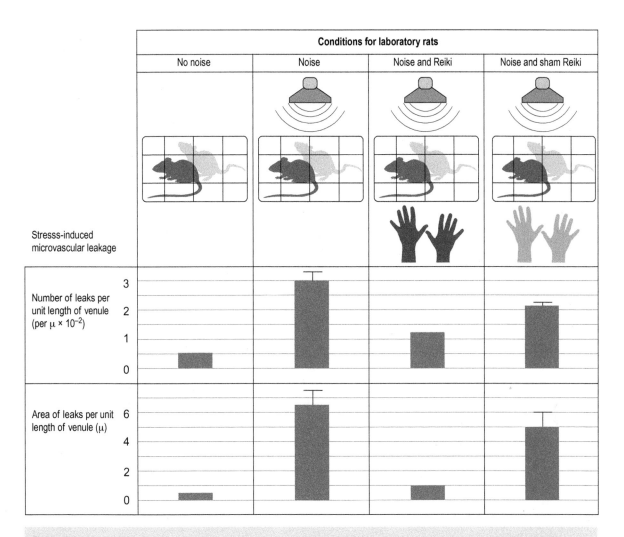

Figure 5.9

Effects of Reiki on stress-induced leakage of small blood vessels in rats.

From: Baldwin AL and GE Schwartz. Personal interaction with a Reiki practitioner decreases noise-induced microvascular damage in an animal model. *The Journal of Alternative and Complementary Medicine* 2006; 12(1): 15–22. Figure 3.)

ents differently and that practitioners do not experience a simple physiological relaxation response, perhaps because they are focusing on sending Reiki. Another explanation for this result is that the Reiki masters in this study may not have all incorporated the Usui "Gassho" breathing technique while they self-administered Reiki. If they had breathed more deeply and slowly as they performed Reiki, they would have approached their resonant frequency and shifted to an ANS balance with higher HRV (Lehrer et al., 2003).

Chapter 5

Case Study

KR came for a Reiki session because she was feeling anxious and depressed. She was approaching menopause and was also worried about her son, even though she said there was no reason for her to be worried. I scanned her body with my hands and experienced quite intense heat and a tingly sensation in my hands at all her major chakras. When I started the Reiki, I felt a lot of sensual activity in my hands at her heart chakra so I spent most of the session working on that area. At the end of the session, I scanned her body once more and the chakras felt less active. After the session, KR mentioned, without any prompting, that she had felt heat in her heart area during the Reiki. KR returned one week later for another session. She said that she was finding it easier to put the worry aside. Once again, I felt fairly high activity over all the chakras during the pre-scan but when I started the Reiki I did not feel such high activity in the heart area compared to the previous week. This time I felt more activity at the second and third chakras. The second chakra is associated with the reproductive organs and creativity, and the third chakra with the solar plexus, adrenal glands, and personal power. I intuitively felt a sense of stability and power coming from her. After the session was over, she mentioned that she had felt activity in the trunk area and started to cry. She said she felt guilty about worrying too much about her son and having negative thoughts. At this point, I taught her how to breathe more deeply and slowly so that she could calm herself down and release the worry. KR returned for a third session a week later. She said that the breathing made her feel much better. As I scanned her body and then performed Reiki, the sensation in my palms, as I held them over the chakras, was calmer and quieter than the weeks before. After the session was over, she said that she felt healed and she felt that the Reiki had treated her whole body. KR decided that she wanted to learn Reiki herself and the next month took first level Usui Reiki. Three years later, she became a Reiki Master and is still practicing. This case study is a good example of how Reiki sometimes appears to make things worse before they get better. In these cases, it is thought that the Reiki may be bringing suppressed emotions to the surface so that they can be processed and released.

References

Baldwin AL, GE Schwartz. Personal interaction with a Reiki practitioner decreases noise-induced microvascular damage in an animal model. *Journal of Alternative and Complementary Medicine* 2006; 12(1): 15–22.

Baldwin AL, RL Primeau, WE Johnson. Effect of noise on the morphology of the intestinal mucosa in laboratory rats. *Journal of the American Association for Laboratory Animal Science* 2006; 45(1): 74–82.

Baldwin AL, Bell IR. Effect of noise on microvascular integrity in laboratory rats. *Journal of the American Association for Laboratory Animal Science* 2007; 46(1): 58–65.

Baldwin AL, Wagers C, Schwartz GE. Reiki improves heart rate homoeostasis in laboratory rats. *Journal of Alternative and Complementary Medicine* 2008; 14(4): 417–422.

Baldwin AL, Schwartz GE. Physiological changes in energy healers during self-practice. *Complementary Therapies in Medicine* 2012; 20: 299–305.

Burwell AK, Baldwin AL. Do audible and ultrasonic sounds of intensities common in animal facilities affect the autonomic nervous system of rodents? *Journal of Applied Animal Welfare Science* 2006; 9(3): 179–200.

Chalmers JA, Quintana DS, Abbott MJ, Kemp AH. Anxiety disorders are associated with reduced heart rate variability: a meta-analysis. *Frontiers in Psychiatry* 2014; 5: Article 80, 1–11.

Chalmers JA, Heathers JAJ, Abbott MJ, Kemp AH, Quintana DS. Worry is associated with robust reductions in heart rate variability: a transdiagnostic study of anxiety psychopathology. *BMC Psychology* 2016; 4: 32–41.

Diaz-Rodriguez L, Arroyo-Morales M, Fernandez-de-las-Penas C, Garcia-Lafuente F, Garcia-Royo C, Tomas-Rojas I. Immediate effects of Reiki on heart rate variability, cortisol levels, and body temperature in health care professionals with burnout. *Biological Research for Nursing* 2011; 13: 376–382.

Friedman RSC, Burg MM, Miles P, Lee F, Lampert R. Effects of Reiki on autonomic activity early after acute coronary syndrome. *Journal of the American College of Cardiology* 2010; 56: 995–996.

Karavidas MK, Lehrer PM, Vaschillo E, Vaschillo B, Marin H, Buyske S, Malinovsky I, Radvanski D, Hassett A. Preliminary results of an open label study of heart rate variability biofeedback for the treatment of major depression. *Association for Applied Psychophysiology and Biofeedback* 2007; 32: 19–30.

Lehrer PM, Vaschillo E, Vaschillo B, Lu SE, Eckberg DL, Edelberg R, Shih WJ, Lin Y, Kuusela TA, Tahvanainen KU, Hamer RM. Heart rate variability biofeedback increases baroreflex gain and peak expiratory flow. *Psychosomatic Medicine* 2003; 65(5): 796–805.

Mackay N, Hansen S, McFarlane O. Autonomic nervous system changes during Reiki treatment: a preliminary study. *Journal of Alternative and Complementary Medicine* 2004; 10(6): 1077–1081.

Pizzinato E, Muller J, Lingg G, Dapra D, Lothaller H, Endler PC. Heart rate variability in a study on Reiki treatment. *The Open Complementary Medicine Journal* 2012; 4: 12–15.

Siepmann M, Aykac V, Unterdorfer J, Petrowski K, Mueck-Weymann M. A pilot study on the effects of heart rate variability biofeedback in patients with depression and in healthy subjects. *Association for Applied Psychophysiology and Biofeedback* 2008; 33: 195–201.

Streeter CC, Gerbarg PL, Saper RB, Ciraulo DA, Brown RP. Effects of yoga on the autonomic nervous system, gamma-aminobutyric-acid, and allostasis in epilepsy, depression, and post-traumatic stress disorder. *Medical Hypotheses* 2012; 78(5): 571–519.

Thayer JF, Friedman BH, Borkovec TD. Autonomic characterics of generalized anxiety disorder and worry. *Biological Psychiatry* 1996; 39: 255–266.

Thayer JF, Lane RD. A model of neurovisceral integration in emotion regulation and dysregulation. *Journal of Affective Disorders* 2000; 61: 201–216.

Zeki A, Hazzouri AI, Elfassy T, Carnethon MR, Lloyd-Jones DM, Yaffe K. Heart rate variability and cognitive function in middle-age adults: the coronary artery risk development in young adults. *American Journal of Hypertension* 2018; 31(1): 27–34.

Chapter 6
Reiki and Blood Circulation

How Blood Flow is Regulated

The amount of blood flowing to different organs and other parts of the body is highly regulated according to need. For example, during exercise, more blood is required by the heart and skeletal muscles and less by the digestive system. The heart pumps blood into the main artery (aorta) which then splits into smaller arteries, and then even smaller arteries (arterioles) and then into tiny blood vessels called capillaries with diameter of about one-tenth the width of a human hair (Figure 6.1). The capillaries form networks that infiltrate tissues and organs so that sufficient nutrients and oxygen from the blood can reach every cell. The capillaries then converge to form small veins (venules) which converge further into larger veins that eventually lead into the main vein (vena cava) that feeds into the heart. By the time the blood returns to the heart, it is depleted of oxygen, so it is then pumped by the heart into the pulmonary artery that leads to the capillaries in the lungs. At this point, the blood is replenished with oxygen that enters the blood from the lungs through the capillary walls. The blood returns to the left atrium (LA) of the heart through the pulmonary vein and is pumped into the left ventricle (LV) ready to be ejected once more into the aorta for its next circuit through the body. The volume of blood per second flowing through the whole circulation depends on the mean arterial pressure; the higher the pressure, the greater the flow. It also depends on the total resistance of the circulatory system to flow. In terms of fluid flow through a simple tube, the narrower the tube, the greater is the resistance and the slower the flow. For example, if a hose is connected to a tap and the tap is turned on full, the water flows quickly. However, if the hose is pinched, thereby reducing the diameter, the flow is immediately reduced. The tap would have to be connected to a much greater water pressure to still maintain the same flow rate when the hose is pinched. Likewise, for each blood vessel or network of blood vessels in the circulatory system, the same relationship applies. If the networks of blood vessels are constricted, blood pressure will need to increase in order to preserve the same blood flow as when they are dilated.

So during the fight-or-flight response, how does the body cause more blood to flow through the vessels associated with the skeletal muscles than with those serving the intestines? There are extrinsic, neural, systemic mechanisms that affect the whole body, and intrinsic, local mechanisms that influence specific organs, muscles, and other body systems. Sometimes they work together both reducing or both increasing blood flow, and sometimes in opposition, in which case the system that is able to operate the most efficiently in a given region will overcome the other.

Extrinsic Mechanisms of Blood Flow Regulation

Extrinsic mechanisms include sympathetic nerves and circulating hormones; there are no parasympathetic nerves surrounding or innervating blood vessels. Arteries and arterioles have thick walls that consist largely of circumferentially oriented smooth muscle cells in the tunica media (Figure 6.2). Sympathetic nerves surround the arterioles and, when stimulated, release noradrenaline. Noradrenaline and adrenaline are also released into the bloodstream by the adrenal glands. These substances can bind to two types of receptors on smooth muscle cell membranes: alpha-adrenergic and beta-adrenergic. Adrenaline has a higher affinity than noradrenaline for beta-receptors. The alpha-adrenergic receptors cause the smooth muscle cells to contract, hence constricting the blood vessels, whereas the beta-adrenergic receptors produce relaxation of smooth muscle cells and consequential dilation of the blood vessels. Alpha-adrenergic receptors are present in *most* blood vessels, whereas beta-adrenergic receptors are only found in the arterioles of skeletal muscle, the liver, the heart (coronary arterioles), and the skin. Alpha-adrenergic receptors are also present in these same arterioles. Another type of smooth muscle cell receptor, the sympathetic cholinergic receptor, is present in arterioles in the skin. When acetylcholine and possibly other as-yet-unidentified glandular substances bind to sympathetic cholinergic receptors, the arterioles tend to dilate.

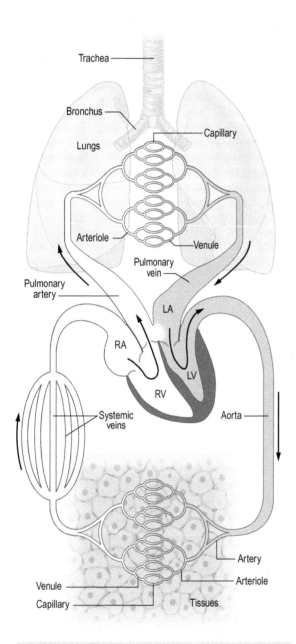

Figure 6.1
Diagram of the cardiovascular system.

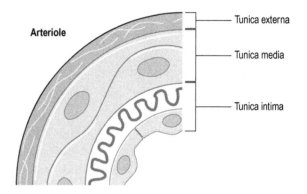

Figure 6.2
Diagram showing structure of wall of small artery.
(From: https://opentextbc.ca/anatomyandphysiology/chapter/20-1-structure -and-function-of-blood-vessels/.Figure 3)

During the fight-or-flight response, the presence of beta-receptors in the arterioles of the heart causes those arterioles to dilate, and ensures that blood flow goes preferentially to the heart to provide it with enough energy to pump more quickly and increase cardiac output. In the skin during the fight-or-flight response, the alpha-receptor response overwhelms that of the beta-receptors, and vasoconstriction occurs. The skin goes pale. There is no pressing need for the skin to have increased blood supply during an emergency, but the skeletal muscles do require extra nutritional blood flow. At the start of the fight-or-flight response, the skeletal muscle arterioles dilate and supply extra blood due to the relaxation response of the beta-adrenergic receptors. Once exercise is underway, one or more of the local, intrinsic regulatory mechanisms, such as the metabolic or the shear-dependent response takes over the process of maintaining vasodilatation. The local, intrinsic mechanisms are described in detail below.

Intrinsic Mechanisms of Blood Flow Regulation

According to Secomb (2008), "the regulation of blood flow is achieved by the combined effects of multiple interacting mechanisms, including sensitivity to pressure, flow rate, metabolite levels and neural signals". The major mediators of flow regulation, the arterioles and small arteries, are located some distance from the regions of tissue that they supply. For this reason, flow regulation requires that the metabolic and hemodynamic conditions within the tissue are sensed and that this information is transferred to the upstream arterioles. The three mechanisms by which blood flow to localized organs or areas is regulated are: (i) metabolic, (ii) myogenic, and (iii) shear-dependent.

Metabolic Response

In order for organs to function, it is essential that the nutritional needs are met and that waste products are efficiently removed. Low concentrations of extracellular oxygen, amino acids, vitamins, and glucose, and high concentrations of carbon dioxide, adenosine, potassium ions, and lactate signal that blood flow to the organ must be increased. Given that arterioles are the main mediators of blood flow regulation, a vital aspect of the metabolic response is the need for arterioles to receive information about the metabolic status of the tissue that they supply. Oxygen is a crucial metabolite, and arterioles *in vivo* react to oxygen levels, constricting as surrounding oxygen levels are increased and dilating as oxygen levels are decreased. When skeletal muscles are working during the fight-or-flight response, the metabolic mechanism is the principal means by which blood flow increases to provide the muscles with energy. Even though sympathetic nerves activate the alpha-adrenergic vasoconstrictor response, the arterioles still dilate because the metabolic response is much stronger.

Myogenic Response

Another way that bodily systems can control the amount of blood they receive is by the myogenic response. This response is generated by the stretching of circumferentially oriented smooth muscle cells within the walls of small arteries. When blood flow to an organ increases, and surpasses its usual rate, the arterioles expand, causing the smooth muscle cells to stretch; the stretching stimulates a contractile response that decreases blood flow to the organ. Thus, the organ does not receive more blood than it needs. The biophysical mechanism by which stretching of smooth muscle cells stimulates contraction has not been established but it depends on local levels of metabolites and signaling molecules, communications with other cells, and neural inputs.

Shear-Dependent Response

The term "shear stress" refers to the frictional force experienced by the inner surface of a tube as fluid flows through it. In terms of the circulation, the tube is the blood vessel and the fluid is blood (Figure 6.3). Shear stress (SS) is proportional to the viscosity of the blood and to the "rate of strain" or how quickly the flow velocity (u) changes from the middle of the blood vessel to the endothelium. (In Figure 6.3, "P" represents the blood pressure that does not have any direct effect on shear stress). Due to the dependence on rate of strain, the faster the blood flow and the narrower the blood vessel, the greater is the shear stress. All blood vessels are lined with a layer of cells called the endothelium. When this layer experiences increased shear stress, it releases a molecule called nitric oxide (NO) that diffuses into the arterial wall, binds to the smooth muscle cells and causes them to relax. This process makes the vessel dilate, increasing blood flow to the organ.

In a given situation for a particular organ, muscle, or body system, it is usual that a variety of these extrinsic and intrinsic mechanisms contribute to maintaining a healthy blood flow.

Effects of Reiki on Blood Flow in Fingers of Reiki Practitioners

How can Reiki assist in blood flow regulation? Problems with the circulation can be due to: (i) narrowing of arteries in the legs due to build up of fatty plaques within the artery wall (peripheral arterial disease), (ii) impaired ability of the endothelial lining of arterioles to produce the vasodilator, NO (diabetes and hypertension), and (iii) abnormal constriction of peripheral arteries (mainly in hands and feet) in response to emotional stress or cold (Raynaud's disease). Since Reiki practitioners very often report an increased

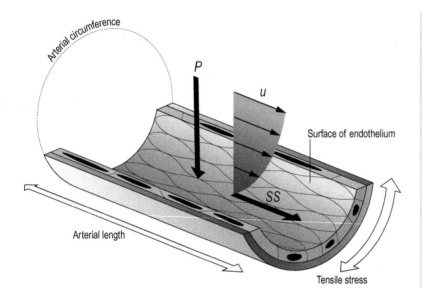

Figure 6.3
Diagram showing physical forces acting on artery wall during blood flow.
(From: Zaromytidou M, Siasos G, Coskun AU, Lucia M et al. Intravacular hemodynamics and coronary artery disease: New insights and clinical implications. Hellenic Journal of Cardiology 2016; 57(6): 389–400. Figure 1.)

sensation of warmth in their hands when they practice Reiki, it is probable that Reiki restores circulation to the hands and fingers during practice. The study by Baldwin and Schwartz (2012) demonstrates that Reiki does indeed restore blood flow to the fingers of Reiki practitioners as they practice Reiki. This article will be discussed in detail in this section of the chapter. There are currently no scientific studies to determine whether Reiki improves the peripheral circulation of people *receiving* Reiki. Although Reiki recipients often report feeling the heat of the practitioners' hands during a session, they rarely indicate that their own hands feel hot. It is possible that to successfully treat people with circulation problems, such as Raynaud's disease, it may be necessary for those people to study Reiki so that they can practice on themselves. More information about Raynaud's disease, its symptoms, and ideas for further research that is needed to qualify Reiki as an effective therapy for the disease, will be provided at the end of the chapter.

The Baldwin and Schwartz 2012 study examined changes in the cutaneous perfusion of blood in the fingertips of 31 Reiki Masters before, during, and after a self-Reiki treatment. Perfusion is a measure of blood flow within a tissue. The Reiki group included seven males and 24 females (ages 18–65; average age 50). Thirty-two subjects (10 males and 22 females, ages 20–75; average age 53) who had no training in Reiki acted as controls. The researchers hypothesized that during self-practice, Reiki practitioners would experience increased peripheral blood perfusion in their fingertips and that no difference would be observed in the control group. Each participant sat next to a Laser Doppler perfusion imager and placed their hand on the imaging screen as shown in Figure 6.4. The index, middle, and ring fingers were scanned for 5 minutes to monitor perfusion. If the subject was a Reiki practitioner, they were asked to practice Reiki on themselves for the next 5 minutes while their fingers were scanned. During scanning, it was essential that their hand be kept stationary. If the subject was in the control group, they were asked to gaze at a calming picture for 5 minutes while their hand was being scanned. After the Reiki practice or picture-gazing activity, a final 5-minute scan was performed. When the last scan was over, each Reiki Master was asked how they had felt during their self-practice. The reason for asking this question was

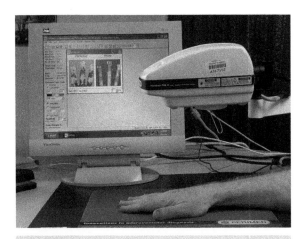

Figure 6.4
A person placing their hand on a laser Doppler perfusion imager.

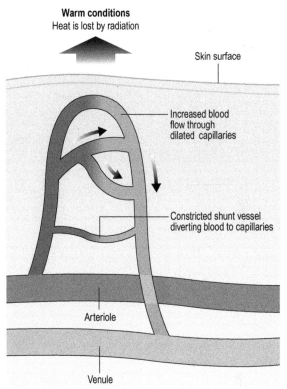

Figure 6.5
Diagram depicting the nutritive and the thermoregulatory circulations in the finger or palm.
(From: Flavahan NA. A vascular mechanistic approach to understanding Raynaud phenomenon. Nature Reviews Rheumatology 2015; 11: 146–158. Figure 4a.)

because although Reiki practitioners usually report feeling calm when delivering Reiki, they may feel less at ease practicing with one hand on the Laser Doppler perfusion imager.

Laser Doppler Scanning

The Laser Doppler process measures the total local microcirculatory blood perfusion including the perfusion in capillaries (nutritive flow), arterioles, venules, and shunting vessels. Shunting vessels, found in the skin of fingers and palms, are blood vessels that link the arterioles to the venules, bypassing the capillaries. The shunting vessels are in charge of thermoregulation, constricting to reduce blood flow in the skin, and thus heat loss, when the environmental or local temperature is low, and dilating when it is hot. A diagram depicting the nutritive and the thermoregulatory circulations is shown in Figure 6.5. The Laser Doppler technique is based on the emission of a beam of laser light carried by a fiber-optic probe. The laser light is scattered and partly absorbed by the tissue being scanned. Light hitting moving blood cells in the blood vessels undergoes a change in wave-

length (Doppler shift), while light hitting static objects is unchanged. The information is sensed by a returning fiber, converted into an electronic signal and analyzed. The perfusion can be calculated because the magnitude and frequency distribution of the Doppler-shifted light is directly related to the number and velocity of blood cells. Most people are more familiar with the Doppler shift as it relates to sound waves. For example, as an ambulance approaches, the sound that the siren makes is at a higher frequency than when the ambulance leaves, as illustrated in Figure 6.6. The Laser Doppler perfusion imager soft-

Chapter 6

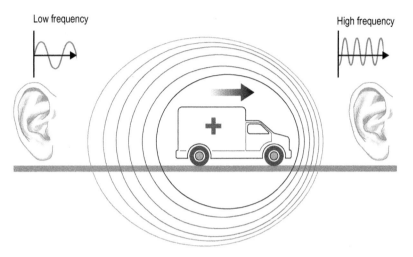

Low frequency

High frequency

Figure 6.6
Diagram to explain the Doppler effect.
(From: Steam Artwork, steamcommunity.com)

Perfusion

Photo

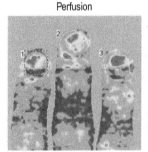

Perf: 0.63 V Int: 6.48 V

Figure 6.7
Sample image of blood flow in the hand from a Laser Doppler perfusion imager.

ware is designed to present the calculated perfusion data in terms of a digital image of the tissue being scanned. A typical image of the cutaneous blood flow in the hand is shown in Figure 6.7. The red to yellow to green to blue areas represent regions of highest to lowest perfusion, shown as the white to dark shaded areas in Figure 6.7. The photographic image of the same hand positioned next to the perfusion image shows the selected regions of interest (circles) at the fingertips. The incorporated software is able to calculate numerical values for the relative perfusions of each area.

Results

Cutaneous perfusion increased significantly in the Reiki group during self-administered Reiki, but this was not seen in the control group while they were gazing at the picture. These perfusion results are consistent with Reiki practitioners' reports of feeling warmth in their hands. Sample images of blood perfusion in the fingers before and during Reiki are shown in Figures 6.8A,B. A brighter shading is visible in the fingers during Reiki self-practice (Figure 6.8B) compared to results from the same individual before they started Reiki (Figure 6.8A). The perfusion results averaged over all participants in each group for each scan are shown in Figure 6.9. One other group who performed a different type of energy healing (reconnective healing) is included in the figure for comparison. Data points 4–7 reflect perfusion changes taking place during the 5-minute period of Reiki, reconnective healing, or gazing at the calming picture. Those points indicate a sharp increase in perfusion during Reiki, a much smaller increase during reconnective healing and a slight decrease during picture gazing. In fact, on average, perfusion of the fingertips increased by 13.7% for Reiki and 6.5% for reconnective healing, while there was a 3.8% decrease for the control. When analyzed separately, each of the three fingertips of the Reiki Masters showed similar results, including a sharp drop in perfusion

Perfusion   Photo

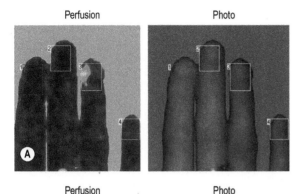

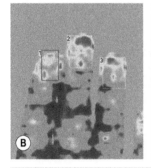
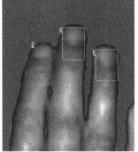

Perfusion   Photo

Figure 6.8
Sample images of blood flow in fingers (**A**) before and
(**B**) after performing Reiki on self.

at the onset of self-practice (point 4). This was also true for reconnective healing.

Discussion

The fact that self-practice of Reiki increased the observed blood perfusion in the fingers indicates that the Reiki caused the blood vessels in the skin of the fingers to expand or dilate. Scientific researchers have long known that the smooth muscle cells of some blood vessels in the finger skin possess special receptors (beta-adrenergic and cholinergic) that cause the blood vessels to dilate when stimulated by adrenaline (in the case of beta receptors), or by acetylcholine or some other as-yet-unknown glandular substance in the case of cholinergic receptors. It is possible that performing Reiki on one-

self may stimulate release of one or more of these substances in the bloodstream that causes dilation of blood vessels in the finger skin resulting in increased perfusion. The abrupt decrease in perfusion observed at the start of Reiki (Figure 6.9, point 4) is interesting because it indicates that the finger arterioles are constricting and implies that at the immediate onset of Reiki, the sympathetic nerves are stimulated to release adrenaline or noradrenaline that binds to the vascular smooth muscle cell alpha-adrenergic receptors. Therefore, self-practice of Reiki appears to evoke a two-phase perfusion response in the skin of the fingers: an initial decrease, followed by a marked increase above the initial perfusion state. The apparent sympathetic stimulation at the onset of Reiki may be a result of the focused attention that practitioners initially engage in when connecting to the Reiki energy.

Raynaud's Disease

According to the Raynaud's Association, Maurice Raynaud recognized the condition of interruption of blood flow to the fingers, toes, nose, and ears, later named "Raynaud's disease", in 1862. The blood flow is interrupted because blood vessels feeding the peripheral parts of the body constrict in response to cold temperatures or emotional stress. About 5–10% of Americans and 5–20% of Europeans suffer from Raynaud's disease. Women are four times as likely to be affected as men. Although this disease is not disabling, it does adversely affect quality of life. During an attack of Raynaud's disease, the affected areas of the skin usually turn white, then blue, and feel cold and numb. As circulation improves, the affected areas may turn red, throb, tingle, or swell. When people without Raynaud's are exposed to cold temperatures, sympathetic nerves are activated and some blood vessels in the fingers constrict, reducing blood flow to those areas. When people with Raynaud's are exposed to cold, the fall in blood flow to the fingers is much more marked, even though the sympathetic nervous activity is similar to that of people without the disease (Fagius and Blumberg, 1985). This result suggests that the adrenergic receptors in the smooth muscle cells of the arterioles are much more sensitive and/or pro-

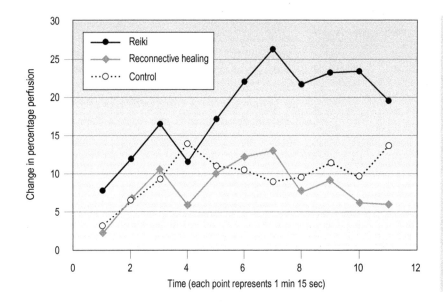

Figure 6.9

Graph showing how Reiki affects blood flow in fingers.

(From: Baldwin A, Schwartz GE. Physiological changes in energy healers during self-practice. Complementary Therapies in Medicine, 2012; 20: 299–305. Figure 4.)

lific in people with Raynaud's. This means that therapies need to be focused on improved release of vasodilators that can bind to the sympathetic cholinergic or beta-adrenergic receptors in the smooth muscle cells of finger skin arterioles to cause relaxation and improved blood flow. Further experiments using Reiki are needed to determine whether Reiki promotes blood flow by increasing activation of these receptors. For example, if chemical antagonists to these receptors are administered prior to Reiki self-practice, and improved blood flow to the fingers is no longer observed, this would imply that the Reiki works by stimulating those particular receptors. Another important line of research is to determine whether increased blood flow to the fingers occurs in Reiki recipients, as well as in Reiki practitioners.

Case Study

A Reiki practitioner, DW, who trained with the author, had the following comment regarding the effect of self-administered Reiki on the blood flow in her lower arms and hands.

The most remarkable thing that I have noticed with Reiki and circulation is how much it improved my own, after becoming a Reiki practitioner and giving myself treatments. I used to have cold hands often, and sometimes my forearms would "fall asleep" when driving. Now both are very rare occurrences for me. My feet also stay warmer in the winter than they did before Reiki.

References

Baldwin AL, Schwartz GE. Physiological changes in energy healers during self-practice. *Complementary Therapies in Medicine* 2012; 20: 299–305.

Fagius J, Blumberg H. Sympathetic outflow to the hands of patients with Raynaud's phenomenon. *Cardiovascular Research*, 1985; 19: 249–253.

Secomb T. Theoretical models for regulation of blood flow. *Microcirculation* 2008; 15(8): 765–775.

Chapter 7
Reiki for Relaxation and Well-Being

Defining Relaxation and Well-Being in Terms of Clinical Outcomes

Relaxation

Relaxation is defined by the Oxford English Dictionary as "the state of being free of tension and anxiety". This state is achieved by stimulating the parasympathetic nervous system (the "rest and digest" component of the autonomic nervous system (ANS)). As a result, biological changes occur, including decreases in oxygen consumption, respiratory rate, heart rate, and blood pressure. Herbert Benson, MD, cardiologist, and founder of the Mind/Body Medical Institute at Massachusetts General Hospital in Boston, defined these changes as the "Relaxation Response" (Benson and Proctor, 2010). Benson developed a specific protocol similar to Transcendental Meditation for eliciting the relaxation response:

Steps to Elicit the Relaxation Response

The following is the technique reprinted with permission from Dr. Herbert Benson's book, *The Relaxation Response* (1976), pp. 162–163.

1. Sit quietly in a comfortable position.

2. Close your eyes.

3. Deeply relax all your muscles, beginning at your feet and progressing up to your face. Keep them relaxed.

4. Breathe through your nose. Become aware of your breathing. As you breathe out, say the word, "one"*, silently to yourself. For example breathe in . . . out, "one", in . . . out, "one", etc. Breathe easily and naturally.

5. Continue for 10 to 20 minutes. You may open your eyes to check the time, but do not use an alarm. When you finish, sit quietly for several minutes, at first with your eyes closed and later with your eyes opened. Do not stand up for a few minutes.

6. Do not worry about whether you are successful in achieving a deep level of relaxation. Maintain a passive attitude and permit relaxation to occur at its own pace. When distracting thoughts occur, try to ignore them by not dwelling upon them and return to repeating "one".

With practice, the response should come with little effort. Practice the technique once or twice daily, but not within two hours after any meal, since the digestive processes seem to interfere with the elicitation of the Relaxation Response.

* It is better to use a soothing, mellifluous sound, preferably with no meaning or association, to avoid stimulation of unnecessary thoughts – a mantra.

Of course, the Benson Relaxation Response is not the only way that the parasympathetic nervous system can be stimulated to produce the biological effects associated with relaxation. As will be discussed in the following sections of this chapter, there is strong scientific evidence that receiving Reiki stimulates the parasympathetic nervous system, leading to similar clinical outcomes as produced by the Relaxation Response. In addition, when a person receives Reiki, absolutely no effort is required.

Chapter 7

Clinical Outcomes

Clinical outcomes are tested, proven and calibrated parameters that measure or assess a particular function or characteristic, in this case, relaxation. Clinical outcomes for relaxation reflect the relative activities of the sympathetic and parasympathetic components of the autonomic nervous system. A state of relaxation is achieved when the activity of the sympathetic nerves is diminished and the parasympathetic system is stimulated. The vagus nerve is the main (but not the only) nerve in the parasympathetic system. It connects the brain stem to the body and is largely responsible for the mind–body connection because it has neural connections to all major organs and glands except for the adrenal and thyroid glands. This nerve has profound control over heart rate and blood pressure. During relaxation, the vagus nerve becomes stimulated and releases the neurotransmitter, acetylcholine, which acts on the heart's pacemaker to slow down heart rate and reduce blood pressure. The vagus nerve is also instrumental in increasing heart rate variability (HRV) because during relaxation it periodically overcomes the sympathetic system for short periods and slows down the heart rate, thus allowing the heart to operate over a wider frequency range. With a high HRV, the heart can quickly change its beat from fast to slow, or vice versa, according to the needs of the body and brain. It is rather like driving a car in traffic, alternately using the accelerator and the brake to adapt to variations in traffic flow as opposed to keeping a steady speed regardless of the conditions. Obviously, adaptability leads to a safer, more efficient ride. **Decreased heart rate and blood pressure and increased HRV are well-established clinical outcomes for relaxation.**

A variety of relaxation methods have also been shown to suppress inflammation. **Therefore, low concentrations of various molecules associated with inflammation (cytokines) serve as clinical outcomes of relaxation.** Although the inflammatory response is vital for ridding the body of dangerous bacteria and foreign bodies, it is important to keep this response under control. Uncontrolled inflammation can lead to heart disease, insulin resistance, tumor growth, and organ damage. Relaxation helps control inflammation by inhibiting the genes responsible for expressing the inflammatory marker, nuclear factor kappa light chain enhancer of activated B cells, NF-κβ. Emotional stress may increase inflammation. For example, a group of elderly people who reported feelings of loneliness had more transcription factors for NF-κβ than elderly people who were not lonely. After the lonely group took an eight-week course in mindfulness-based stress reduction, they no longer felt lonely and had a reversal of pro-inflammatory gene expression (Creswell et al., 2012). Another study was performed on cancer patients who showed high levels of blood-borne pro-inflammatory markers (Irwin et al., 2014). A group of these patients underwent treatment with tai chi exercises. They demonstrated a reduction in expression of NF-κβ which decreased the inflammatory response. Further evidence that relaxation suppresses the inflammatory response is provided by other studies reviewed in the literature (Buric et al., 2017).

A likely mechanism for the regulatory effect of relaxation on inflammation is called the "cholinergic anti-inflammatory pathway". This pathway was discovered as a result of electrically stimulating the vagus nerve (van Maanen et al., 2009; Huston and Tracey, 2011) and is illustrated in Figure 7.1. When the vagus nerve is stimulated electrically, a signal is transmitted along it to the abdomen, and then through a second nerve to the spleen. This second nerve releases noradrenaline which stimulates adjacent immune cells (T cells) in the spleen to produce acetylcholine. The acetylcholine binds to another set of immune cells, the macrophages, and inhibits the activity of NF-κβ in the cell nucleus suppressing production of pro-inflammatory molecules called cytokines, such as tumor necrosis factor-α.

Normally it is not necessary to artificially stimulate the vagus nerve to control inflammation. As shown in Figure 7.2, sensory neurons in the vagus nerve detect inflammation in the body and transmit action potentials from inflamed regions to the brain stem. This signal leads to the generation of action potentials in the descending vagus nerve that are transmitted to the spleen, where pro-inflammatory cytokine production is inhibited. Inflammation is

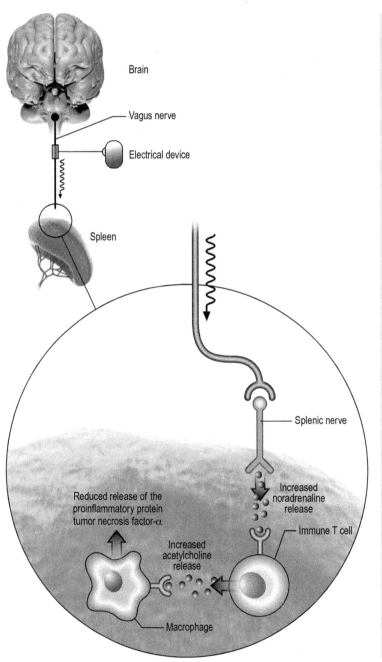

Brain

Vagus nerve

Electrical device

Spleen

Splenic nerve

Increased
noradrenaline
release

Immune T cell

Reduced release of the
proinflammatory protein
tumor necrosis factor-α

Increased
acetylcholine
release

Macrophage

Figure 7.1
The vagus nerve: the cholinergic
anti-inflammatory pathway.
(From: Fox D. The electric cure. Nature 2017; 545,
20–22.)

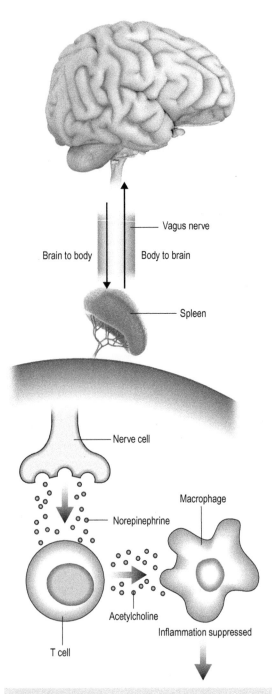

Figure 7.2

Mechanism by which the vagus nerve reduces inflammation.
(From Kevin Tracey, Feinstein Institute for Medical Research)

controlled. If a person is mentally or emotionally stressed, this controlling mechanism does not work so well because the sympathetic nervous system becomes highly activated leading to a pro-inflammatory response.

Respiration rate is another clinical outcome for relaxation. Whenever one is experiencing physical, mental or emotional arousal or stress, the sympathetic system is activated and body metabolism increases to mobilize energy stores. A higher metabolic rate causes tissues and organs to consume more oxygen from the blood to and release more carbon dioxide into the blood, which increases the acidity of the blood. These changes are sensed by chemoreceptors in the aorta and carotid arteries which stimulate the respiratory center to increase the rate and depth of breathing. Conversely, during relaxation, the vagus nerve is stimulated, less oxygen is needed and respiration is slower. **Thus, reduced respiration rate is a clinical outcome of relaxation.** Interestingly, the vagus nerve not only controls respiration but is also influenced by it. Vagal activation increases during exhalation, so by slowing down respiration through deep, intentional breathing, and lengthening the out-breath, the relaxation response can be elicited almost immediately. As mentioned in Chapter 4, Reiki founder Mikao Usui taught his students to breathe slowly when giving Reiki. At this point, there are no data published regarding respiration rates of people before and during a Reiki session. It would be interesting to see if they naturally slow down their breathing while receiving Reiki, since this would contribute to their relaxation response.

Two clinical outcomes of mental and emotional stress are skin conductance and salivary cortisol concentration. The skin conductance response (SCR) is an objective, transient indication of ANS arousal (sympathetic stimulation) in response to a stimulus. It is a common measure of emotional arousal in the laboratory. Specifically, the skin conductance response is a measure of the degree to which the skin can conduct an electrical current produced by applying a small voltage across two electrodes placed on the skin (Figure 7.3). It is important to note that the voltage applied to the electrodes is very small, and the current that can flow through them is very low and not noticeable. The more sweat on the skin, the greater is the number of sodium and chloride ions available to carry a current, and the higher is the skin conductance. Sympathetic arousal induces sweating. For that reason, the skin conductance response is a measure of sympathetic arousal that is often linked to stress. In fact, the lie detector is based on exactly this response. Conversely, the parasym-

pathetic stimulation and sympathetic diminution that accompanies relaxation results in less sweat production and a lower SCR. For this reason, **low SCR is a clinical output of relaxation.**

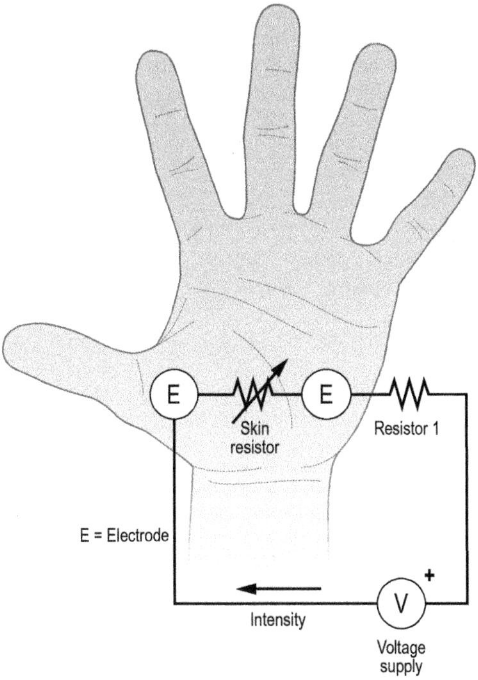

The stress hormone, cortisol, is released from the adrenal glands on top of the kidneys as part of the fight-or-flight response. First, the hypothalamus secretes corticotropin releasing hormone (CRH). In response, the pituitary releases adrenocorticotrophic hormone (ACTH) which reaches the adrenal glands through the bloodstream and then stimulates release of cortisol into the blood (Figure 7.4). Most secreted cortisol is bound to proteins in the blood, but a small amount is unbound. Unbound cortisol enters cells by passive diffusion, which allows measurement in bodily fluids, such as saliva. It is much more convenient and less invasive to measure concentrations of cortisol in the saliva than in the blood, and research shows that both measures are comparable. Salivary cortisol concentrations reflect momentary snapshots of the hypothalamus-pituitary-adrenal (HPA) axis activity, capturing acute cortisol production over the past 15–20 minutes. Cortisol is produced in response to stress because it provides the body with extra energy by:

i. Increasing production of glucose from protein amino acids in muscles.

ii. Assisting in breakdown of fats (from adipose tissue) into fatty acids to produce energy for synthesis of muscle protein.

Cortisol concentrations vary with circadian rhythm and are normally lowest around 3 AM, then begin to rise,

Figure 7.3
Diagram explaining skin conductance and its measurement.
(From: How Does a GSR Sensor Work? www.tobiipro.com)

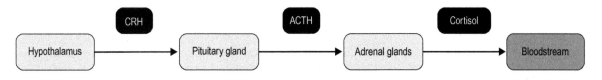

Figure 7.4
Diagram showing how the stress hormone, cortisol, is produced in the body.
(From: NIDDK Image Library)

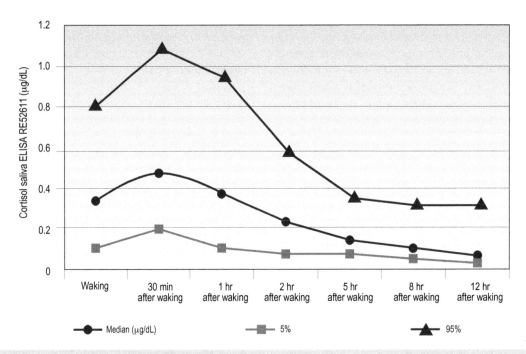

Figure 7.5
Graph showing daily rhythm of cortisol production in the body.

peaking at about 8 AM (Figure 7.5). Thus, it is important to either repeatedly sample salivary cortisol over time for each individual, or to take samples at the same specified time of day for each person in a group. In addition, cortisol concentrations vary with food intake and so patients or participants should be instructed to refrain from eating or drinking for 15–20 minutes prior to the test. **A salivary cortisol concentration in the daily range of about 0.1–0.5 µg/dL is a clinical outcome of relaxation.** High cortisol levels, in the daily range of about 0.35–1.1 µg/dL are indicative of stress, but levels that are too low, in the daily range of close to zero to 0.2 µg/dL, can cause weakness, fatigue, and low blood pressure.

Well-Being

Well-being is a much more multifaceted state than relaxation, although of course a certain amount of time spent in relaxation is essential for a person to maintain a state of

well-being. The term well-being is defined by the Oxford English Dictionary as: "the state of being comfortable, healthy or happy". However, a more complete and appropriate definition would be "the state of being comfortable, healthy *and* happy". In order to fulfill this definition, a variety of different aspects of well-being must be considered. For example, comfort and health cannot be achieved unless one has adequate physical, economic and social well-being. A person needs housing to protect against environmental hazards and extreme temperature, sufficient funds for nutritional food and drink, and a support network of friends and helpers. Even if these needs are fulfilled, a person may still not be happy. To achieve a state of happiness, one needs to feel satisfied with one's life and to enjoy a sufficient degree of emotional and psychological well-being. According to the Centers for Disease Control and Prevention, "well-being" is a valid population outcome measure that is meaningful to the public. They state that:

Well-being is associated with numerous health-, job-, family-, and economically-related benefits. For example, higher levels of well-being are associated with decreased risk of disease, illness, and injury; better immune functioning; speedier recovery; and increased longevity. Individuals with high levels of well-being are more productive at work and are more likely to contribute to their communities.

There is no sole determinant of individual well-being, but on the whole, well-being can be considered to include two aspects: "objective" and "subjective". Objective well-being depends on availability and access to basic resources such as safe housing, education, and economic security. Subjective well-being depends on good physical and psychological health, positive social relationships, as well as spiritual sustenance. Reiki, at least in the short-term, seems much more likely to directly affect *subjective* well-being rather than *objective* well-being because the latter depends on many other factors that are outside the control of a single individual and their friends and family. For that reason, only subjective well-being will be discussed in this chapter. However, it should be noted that if one decides to learn Reiki, rather than passively receiving Reiki sessions from a practitioner, objective well-being may also be improved. That is because Reiki is not just a technique, but a lifestyle. Living by the Reiki principles influences one's cognitive and emotional regulation skills such that one is more likely to jettison bad habits and to attract people who can offer positive support and guidance.

Clinical Outcomes

Subjective well-being is typically measured with self-reports. The Centers for Disease Control and Prevention has conducted multiple surveys to measure subjective well-being, using a variety of established questionnaires. Many questionnaires are scored using a Likert scale (named after the psychologist, Rensis Likert). Subjects choose from a range of five or seven possible responses to a specific question or statement; responses typically include "strongly agree", "agree", "neutral", "disagree", and "strongly disagree". Details of some widely used questionnaires can be found in the CDC Health Related Quality of Life article

(www.cdc.gov/hrqol/wellbeing.htm#) and a summary table is shown in Table 7.1. (The references cited in the table can be found in the CDC article online.) Briefly, the table lists five established and validated questionnaires that are appropriate for assessing subjective well-being:

i. General Well-Being Schedule (1971–1975) (GWB). This is an 18-item questionnaire that takes about 10 minutes to complete and addresses one's "inner personal state". It addresses degrees of anxiety, depression, general health, positive well-being, self control and vitality experienced over the last month.

ii. Quality of Well-Being Scale (QWB). This questionnaire contains 41 items, takes 10–15 minutes to complete and addresses general quality of life, including mobility, physical activity, social activity, and symptoms/problems.

iii. Satisfaction with Life Scale (SWLS). This is a five-item questionnaire that takes about 2 minutes to complete and addresses global cognitive judgments of satisfaction with life in general. A seven-point

Table 7.1.	
Survey	**Questionnaires/questions**
National Health and Nutrition Examination Survey (NHANES)	• General Well-Being Schedule (1971–1975).[43,44]
National Health Interview Survey (NHIS)	• Quality of Well-Being Scale.[45] • Global life satisfaction. • Satisfaction with emotional and social support. • Feeling happy in the past 30 days.
Behavioral Risk Factor Surveillance Systems (BRFSS)	• Global life satisfaction. • Satisfaction with emotional and social support.[47, 48]
Porter Novelli Healthstyles Survey	• Satisfaction with Life Scale.[49] • Meaning in life.[50] • Autonomy, competence, and relatedness.[51] • Overall and domain-specific life satisfaction. • Overall happiness. • Positive and Negative Affect Scale.[52]

(From: CDC Health Related Quality of Life article. Available at: www.cdc.gov/hrqol/wellbeing.htm#)

Likert scale is used to assess satisfaction, ranging from "strongly disagree" to "strongly agree" with the item in question.

iv. Meaning in Life Questionnaire (MLQ). This is a 10-item measure, taking 5 minutes to complete, with two subscales: presence, or how meaningful one considers one's life to be, and search, or desire to discover new or more meaning in one's life.

v. Positive and Negative Affect Scale (PANAS). This is a 20-item measure of positive and negative moods judged on a 1–5 scale that takes about 10 minutes to complete.

Other commonly used assessments of well-being are described below:

Quality of Life Scale (QOLS). This is a 16-item questionnaire that takes 5 minutes to complete and assesses material and physical well-being including relationships, social community activities (such as groups and clubs), civic activities (such as volunteer work), personal development, fulfillment, and recreation.

Rosenberg Self Esteem Scale (RSES). This is a 10-item questionnaire that takes about 5 minutes to complete and addresses self-esteem, scored on a Likert scale.

Well-Being Questionnaire (W-BQ12). This is a 12-item scale that measures general positive and negative well-being with a balanced set of positive and negative items.

Happiness Measure (HM). This two-item questionnaire measures intensity and frequency of happiness and relies on emotional well-being as an indicator of happiness. The first item presents a "happiness/unhappiness scale" with 11 descriptive phrases on a 0–10 scale. The second item assesses the percentage of time that the subject feels happy, neutral, and unhappy. Happiness Measure has the strongest correlation with daily life satisfaction compared to all other measures of well-being.

The Subjective Happiness Scale (SHS). This is a four-item measure that assesses global overall happiness, using a Likert scale. It is strongly correlated with other psychological well-being scales.

The Gratitude Questionnaire (GQ-6). This is a six-item questionnaire that uses a 1–7 Likert scale to assess proneness to experience gratitude in daily life. There is evidence that the GQ-6 relates to optimism, hope, spirituality, life satisfaction, empathy, and forgiveness.

The Flourishing Scale (FS). This scale consists of eight items that describe important aspects of human functioning, ranging from positive relationships to feelings of competence, to having meaning and purpose to life.

Effects of Reiki on Relaxation and Well-Being of Healthy People

There are currently six research studies focusing on the effects of Reiki on relaxation and/or well-being in healthy people. Two of these articles address relaxation (Witte et al., 2001; Mackay et al., 2004), two both relaxation and well-being (Bowden, 2010, 2011) and two well-being alone (Bukowski, 2015; Vitale, 2009). In this section, the results of these studies will be described in turn, together with details of the tests that were used to obtain the data in each case.

The purpose of the study by Witte et al. (2001) was to address deficiencies in Reiki research by objectively measuring its effects on physical and mental relaxation in 100 undergraduate students, ages 18–22. The hypothesis was that Reiki may induce relaxation more effectively than music, meditation, or being touched by a person without Reiki training. Equal numbers of students were assigned to each of the four possible protocols and were sent to stations that were identically set up and equipped. The Reiki and touch (placebo) practitioners held five hand positions on each subject for 5 minutes (totaling 20 minutes). It should be noted that the Reiki practitioner was only trained to level one and only had three months of experience. The Reiki and placebo practitioners were chosen to be of similar heights, build, age, and physical attractiveness and were similarly dressed. The students in the other two groups wore headphones and listened to either a relaxation meditation tape or to relaxing music for 20 minutes. Blood pressure and heart rate were measured before and after each procedure. In addition, subjects were asked to assess their physical and mental relaxation levels on a scale of 1–6 before and after their treatment. Most of the Reiki group (64%) was much more physically relaxed (by at least two steps in the scale) after treatment, compared to 24% of the placebo group, 36% of the meditation group, and 48% of the music group. Based on this finding, the authors concluded: "Reiki seems to be an effective means of inducing physical relaxation, even when limited to only five hand positions on the upper body of a seated subject for a total of 20 minutes." However, there was no significant difference between groups regarding mental relaxation. Between 40% and 48% of participants became more mentally relaxed regardless of treatment type. Similarly, systolic blood pressure decreased for all groups and the decrease was not significantly greater for any particular group. Interestingly, average diastolic blood pressure and heart rate actually increased slightly for the Reiki group, whereas both quantities decreased for the other groups. However, intergroup differences were not significant. Thus, although Reiki made students *feel* more physically relaxed than placebo-touch, music, or meditation, it did not show a more enhanced effect in reducing blood pressure and heart rate or reducing mental stress.

The article notes that students who were assigned to the Reiki group judged themselves to be more mentally relaxed at the start of the experiment than those in the other groups. Since Reiki is purported to "go where it is needed" this may be why students in the Reiki group did not show more of a decrease in mental stress compared to the other groups. Unfortunately, no actual pre and post values of blood pressure and heart rate were given, and so it is not known whether students assigned to the Reiki group also had lower pre-test blood pressure and heart rate. If this were so, then it would not be surprising that the average diastolic blood pressure and heart rate *increased* slightly on average after Reiki. If Reiki goes where it is needed, and brings systems back to balance, then some students with low diastolic blood pressure and heart rate, may have benefited from an increase in these values.

Strengths: The study was well designed and clearly articulated and could be replicated. The use of photos and well-defined charts make the study easy to read, even for a person with a limited scientific background.

Weaknesses: No clear consideration was given to the fact that there was no practitioner present during the meditation and music experiences, and how this might affect the outcome of those groups. In addition, the Reiki practitioner had minimal training and experience.

Future Research: More studies in which longer treatments are given by more experienced Reiki practitioners to a larger number of subjects would be useful. In addition, measurements should be made not just immediately after the treatment but also at a later time to determine whether Reiki confers any long-lasting benefits.

Similar to the study by Witte et al., the investigation by Mackay et al. addresses the effects of Reiki on heart rate and blood pressure in healthy people. Respiration rate and HRV are also monitored before and after treatment. The Mackay study has already been described in detail in Chapter 5 with regard to Reiki's effects on the emotional stress response. Here, the article will be considered in terms of Reiki's effects on relaxation, since heart rate, respiration rate, blood pressure and HRV are defined outcome parameters for relaxation. To recall, 45 test-subjects (both males and females in the age range 23–59) were randomly assigned to one of three groups: Reiki, sham Reiki, or rest. Each group had a 15-minute rest period to establish baseline measurements followed by a 30-minute treatment period of Reiki or sham Reiki or rest, and ending with another 10-minute rest period. The Reiki practitioner placed their hands over the subject's body (but not touching) in a series of six hand positions chosen to correspond with key chakras. Unfortunately, no information was provided regarding the training and experience of the Reiki practitioner. The average pre-treatment outcome values for the three groups were not significantly different except that heart rate was lower for the Reiki group. Although the absolute average values for all outcome parameters were given for the pre-measures, the effects of

Reiki, sham Reiki, and rest were only provided in terms of percentage change.

Cardiovagal tone is a computer-derived parameter that reflects the activity of the parasympathetic nervous system (rest and digest). Cardiac sensitivity to baroreflex represents the ease with which the heart responds to signals from the blood pressure sensors (baroreceptors) located in the aorta and carotid arteries. If a person is relaxed with high parasympathetic and low sympathetic activity, the CSB is high. This means that just the presence of a person paying attention to the participant resting on a Reiki table can produce a physiologically significant relaxation response in the recipient. However, the decrease in heart rate was significantly greater in the Reiki group compared to the sham Reiki group, and the mean blood pressure was significantly reduced by Reiki but not by sham Reiki or by rest. Therefore, Reiki itself has a significant relaxation effect beyond the placebo response. The control group did not show a change in any parameter, indicating that the relaxation responses to Reiki, and in some cases sham Reiki, were not caused by merely lying down and resting on a Reiki table.

It is interesting that, in this study, Reiki reduced heart rate and blood pressure to a greater degree than the other treatments, whereas in the study by Witte et al., Reiki had little effect on these parameters. This result is surprising because the Reiki group actually started off with a lower average heart rate than the other groups. However, we do not know how the average heart rate of this Reiki group before treatment compared to that of the younger Reiki group in the Mackay et al. study. It is possible that although the Reiki group had a lower pre-treatment heart rate than the other groups in the Witte et al. study, it was still higher than for the Mackay et al. study. Possible reasons for the apparent inconsistency in the cardiovascular responses to Reiki could be:

i.   The duration of treatment was 30 minutes in the Mackay et al. study rather than the 20 minutes in the Witte et al. study.

ii. The subjects were older in the Mackay et al. study and may have had higher initial heart rate and blood pressure since blood pressure is known to increase with age.

iii. The Reiki practitioner may have been more highly trained and experienced in the Mackay et al. study.

Unfortunately, information regarding measures of *actual* heart rate and blood pressure before treatment is missing from the Mackay et al. study. Neither is there any information included on the training and experience of the Reiki practitioner.

Strengths: This was a study in which participants were randomly assigned to one of three groups; if they were not assigned to the "rest only" group, they did not know whether they were receiving Reiki or sham Reiki. Each group included a fairly equal match of men and women. Multiple cardiovascular parameters were recorded over the duration of the study.

Weaknesses: The sample size was small. Some key information was missing, as described above and the authors noted some difficulties with the calibration of the method used for monitoring blood pressure.

Future Research: As for the study by Witte et al., more studies in which longer treatments are given by more experienced Reiki practitioners to a larger number of subjects would be useful.

The two studies by Bowden et al. (2010, 2011) focused on the effects of Reiki on the well-being and mood of psychology undergraduate students (35 in the first study and 43 in the second), in the age range 18–30. The tests used to assess well-being were the Depression, Anxiety, and Stress Scale (DASS-21) and the Pittsburgh Sleep Quality Index (PSQI). The DASS-21 is a 21-item measure of mental heath, focusing on depression, anxiety, and stress/tension. It takes about 5–10 minutes to complete. The PSQI is a 19-item questionnaire that assesses sleep quality over the previous month and takes 5–10 minutes to complete. A post-assessment version of the PSQI was also used to assess sleep quality over the previous week to estimate the effects of the treatment, whether or not it included Reiki. In the 2010 study, a measure of relaxation was also included, which was salivary cortisol concentration before and after treatment. In the first study, the participants were asked to perform one of three tasks involving relaxation and self-hypnosis for 20 minutes over 2–12 weeks (10 sessions) while a Reiki practitioner either sent them non-contact Reiki or did not, depending on their assignment. A Reiki practitioner was used who was trained to Usui Master level. She sat several feet behind each student and directed the Reiki by holding her hands 3–30 inches above their head or behind their back. For students assigned to the non-Reiki group, she sat impassively. The students were blind-folded so that they would not see the shadow of the practitioners' hands. The results trended towards a lower score in the DASS-21 test with Reiki compared to non-Reiki, but this was not statistically significant. It also happened that the participants who received Reiki started off with a higher DASS-21 stress score before treatment. Interestingly, in the Reiki group, there was a significant correlation between how stressed a person started (high score in DASS-21) and how much they improved. This finding is, once again, consistent with the idea that Reiki goes to where it is needed. No significant differences between the Reiki and non-Reiki groups were found for PSQI or for salivary cortisol.

In the second study (Bowden et al., 2011), the finding that in the Reiki group each participant's initial score on the DASS-21 test influenced their degree of improvement in stress reduction was further investigated. Participants were divided into two groups: high anxiety and depression (high mood) and low anxiety and depression (low mood) dependent on their score on a Hospital Anxiety and Depression scale. The participants performed a guided meditation, which they heard through headphones, for 25 minutes once a week over two to eight weeks (six sessions). During each session, the Reiki practitioner sat behind each participant in turn and either sent them non-contact Reiki or just sat impassively, depending on their assignment. It was hypothesized that students with higher levels of depression and/or anxiety would show a greater

degree of improvement than was observed with the mix of healthy participants of the first study. Results were compared between groups one week (post-treatment) and five weeks (follow-up) after the start of the experiment. The most important result was the sustained beneficial effect shown by the high mood (but not low mood) students following Reiki treatments. Statistically significant positive effects were seen on the stress and anxiety components of DASS-21 in the Reiki high mood group but not in the control high mood or in the low mood groups. This result was particularly significant for the stress score. As in the previous study (Bowden et al., 2010), no difference was seen in sleep quality (PSQI) between participants who received Reiki versus no Reiki, so this particular test does not seem to be a sensitive marker for effects of Reiki in healthy students.

Strengths: The Reiki-blinding method used in these experiments seemed to be successful. The majority of Reiki and control participants either believed that they were not in the Reiki group (6/20 Reiki; 11/19 Control) or were not sure (8/20 Reiki; 2/19 Control), suggesting that they were unable to detect the experimenter sending Reiki. The use of a consistent, single Reiki Master throughout the experiment reduces variability. Non-contact Reiki is a good choice in this case because it ensures that participants do not know for sure to which group they have been assigned. Therefore, the participants receiving Reiki do not expect a result any different from the control group.

Weaknesses: The participants were mostly female freshman students and so the results obtained may not apply to other populations. Although each participant received the same number of sessions, there was a wide variability in the number of weeks taken to deliver the sessions.

Future Research: These pilot studies indicate that Reiki reduces feelings of stress in young students who are prone to anxiety and depression and demonstrate the feasibility of conducting a larger, randomized, placebo-controlled trial.

The purpose of the study by Bukowski et al. (2015) was to determine the effects of a 20-week structured self-Reiki

Chapter 7

program on stress reduction and relaxation in college students. The 30 healthy university students (ages 18–25 years) accepted into the study completed two questionnaires designed to measure their expectation of the Reiki treatment: Reiki Baseline Credibility Scale and Reiki Expectance Scale. All participants, except for three, believed that Reiki is a credible technique for reducing stress levels. Except for two participants, they agreed that Reiki would be effective in reducing their stress levels. The participants also completed a Perceived Stress Scale (PSS-10) which is a 10-item questionnaire that asks participants to assess their responses to stressful situations experienced over the past month. The participants attended a Reiki 1 training class and then were instructed to perform self-Reiki twice weekly in their own homes for 20 weeks. The students completed the PSS-10 every four weeks and a Global Assessment Questionnaire (GAQ) at the end of the study. The GAQ asks participants how much they are in agreement, on a scale of 1–5, with the premise that they experienced a reduction in stress at the end of the study compared to the start. Each participant kept a log summarizing the outcome of each session in terms of perceived changes in stress levels or emotional state and these were submitted at the end of the study. Twenty students (15 women and 5 men) completed the study. The PSS data showed there was a significant decrease in stress levels each month compared to initial values. In addition, there was a statistically significant correlation between GAQ score and PSS assessed at the end of the study indicating that individuals were more likely to agree that there was an improvement in stress reduction, the lower their PSS score at the end of the study. The log entries supported this correlation, documenting increased ability to keep calm and relaxed, more perspective in stressful situations and good physical and mental health.

Strengths: Requiring the students to keep a weekly log of their stress levels after each Reiki session maximized the chances that they were compliant with their Reiki practice.

Weaknesses: The study had a small sample size and no control or sham-Reiki comparison groups. Therefore, the influence of factors such as expectancy and the placebo response on the results cannot be ruled out.

Future Research: This study provides some promising results consistent with previous findings that Reiki reduces stress in young people. Future investigations of self-Reiki with college students could be combined with a larger meta-analysis on the effects of Reiki on perceived stress.

The paper by Vitale (2009) also describes research on people who perform self-Reiki, in this case nurses. The objective was to determine whether self-practice of Reiki by nurses helps reduce their stress and improves their caring feelings for others. Eleven female nurses from the mid-Atlantic region, most of whom who were trained to Master level of Usui Reiki, were interviewed, using open-ended questions, about how their daily practice of Reiki enabled them to cope with job-related stressors. The questions included: "What is it like for you to do Reiki in self-care?" "What does doing a Reiki self-treatment mean to you?" "Is there anything else you want to add toward the overall experience of self-Reiki practice?" The nurses reported that although they practiced Reiki before starting work, they found it most useful to practice for short periods when given the opportunity during the day. Except for senior nurses who had their own offices, most of the nurses said that the only quiet, private place to practice was the bathroom. Inclusion of private spaces for brief meditative practice is missing from most hospitals. This problem highlights the lack of acknowledgement that time spent in meditative practices during the workday benefits one's mental health and actually improves job performance. Small, enclosed spaces in clinic and hospital buildings could fairly easily be created for Reiki practice perhaps by reassigning rooms previously used for other purposes.

Several characteristic themes emerged from analysis of the nurses' statements related to the benefits of Reiki self-treatment. These included spiritual connection, the ability to reach a calm and centered state, and the idea that a state of relaxation provides them with clarity of thought and a clearer perspective. They indicated that self-Reiki heightened their awareness of whether they were emotionally out of balance and gave them ability to quickly restore themselves to a tranquil state. The nurses perceived that caring for others provides an opportunity to care for themselves and that self-Reiki helps them "refuel and replenish" their ability to nurse.

Strengths: Qualitative data were analyzed using a rigorous, established method (Colaizzi method), in which significant statements are extracted from interviews and clustered into thematic categories which, in this case, related to the effects of Reiki self-practice on the nurses' working lives. This well-written paper provides new tools to measure the effects of Reiki self-practice in terms of assessing its personal energetic and spiritual dimensions.

Weaknesses: The study is limited to a small number of Caucasian nurses who were experienced in Reiki and so it is not possible to generalize the results.

Future Research: This promising pilot study could be extended to include greater numbers of nurses of varying gender and Reiki training levels. In addition, the use of Reiki self-care as a method for stress reduction could also be evaluated for other types of personnel working in clinical environments. Examples include physicians, physician's assistants, and physical, and occupational therapists.

Effects of Reiki on Relaxation and Well-Being of Hospital Patients

There are currently two published studies that report the effects of offering Reiki to hospital patients in terms of their relaxation and well-being. In one case, the patients were recovering from acute coronary syndrome, which usually means a heart attack (Friedman et al., 2010) and, in the other case, they were women with breast cancer who were undergoing chemotherapy (Orsak et al., 2015). Another paper (Salles et al., 2014) describes the effects of Reiki on people who, although not hospitalized, were diagnosed with hypertension. That study will be included in this section. The paper by Friedman et al. is already described in Chapter 5 as an example of how Reiki can reduce emotional stress, but it also fits in the category of "Reiki for Relaxation and Well-Being". The clinical outcome parameter used for relaxation is HRV and the

parameter for well-being is a 10-point Likert scale for emotional states. Forty-nine patients (mean age of 60) who had suffered a heart attack less than 72 hours previously, were randomized to one of three treatment groups: a resting control group; a group that listened to slow, classical music; and a group that received light touch Reiki from nurse Reiki practitioners. The rationale for choosing Reiki as a therapy for patients recovering from a heart attack was that medicines that enhance a patient's parasympathetic activity also improve their survival after a heart attack. Based on previous research (Mackay et al., 2004), it was hypothesized that Reiki would benefit these patients by improving their parasympathetic activity as indicated by changes in HRV. Emotional stress is a known risk factor for causing autonomic dysfunction and death after a heart attack and so, for this reason, the effects of Reiki on emotional states was also assessed. The parasympathetic component of HRV increased significantly in the Reiki treatment group, did not appreciably change in the control group, and decreased slightly in the music group. With regard to wellness, Reiki treatment, but not music or rest, was associated with increases in positive emotional states and decreases in negative emotional states. More specifically, Reiki treatment was associated with an increase in average Likert scale score for all positive emotional states (happy, relaxed, calm) and a decrease for all negative states (stressed, angry, sad, frustrated, worried, scared, anxious). The most positive change in emotional state was associated with Reiki, the intermediate change with music, and the least positive emotional change with resting control.

Strengths: The subjects were randomly assigned to each of the three treatment arms, thus minimizing the chances of differing populations (for example, with respect to age, gender, preference for a certain treatment) between groups. The Reiki treatment used standardized hand positions for all participants. Objective (HRV) and subjective (emotional states) measurements were used during the study to cover both physiological and psychological responses.

Weaknesses: This study only involved a small number of participants, did not provide any details about the frequency or duration of the treatments, and the participants knew which treatment they were receiving. A sham Reiki treatment, in which participants received light touch but not Reiki, was not part of the study so the touch effect cannot be ruled out as contributing to the relaxation effect of the Reiki.

Future Research: Further understanding of the mechanisms involved in the impact of Reiki on the physiological and psychological aspects of well-being requires comparison of Reiki with other control groups, including those who receive non-Reiki light touch and those who just experience the presence of another person quietly sitting in the room. Longitudinal studies are needed to evaluate whether Reiki treatment may offer a long-term, non-pharmacologic approach to improving HRV and optimizing the chances of a full recovery after acute coronary syndrome.

According to the World Cancer Research Fund and the American Institute for Cancer Research, breast cancer is the most commonly occurring cancer in women and the second most common cancer overall. There were over 2 million new cases worldwide in 2018. Belgium had the highest recorded incidence, standardized for age, followed by Luxembourg and the Netherlands. Chemotherapy is often given to patients to reduce the chances of the cancer spreading or returning. However, chemotherapy can cause debilitating side effects such as hair loss, anxiety, depression, nausea, fatigue, and heart failure. The study by Orsak et al., 2015 investigated whether Reiki treatment would improve the quality of life, mood state, and symptom distress of 36 women undergoing four sessions of chemotherapy for breast cancer. The clinical outcomes used in the research to assess well-being were "quality of life" (QOL), "symptom distress", and "mood states". Quality of life was assessed using the Functional Assessment of Cancer Therapy: Breast Cancer Version 4 scale, which consists of 36 items rated on a five-point Likert scale, with higher scores indicating higher QOL. Symptom distress was assessed using a 13-item questionnaire related to cancer symptoms such as nausea. Mood states were evaluated using the Profile of Moods Scale (POMS) short form questionnaire which consists of 40 words describing how one might feel right now in terms of anxiety, depression,

anger, vigor, fatigue, and confusion. Participants rated their symptom distress and moods using a five-point Likert scale. Patients completed the questionnaires at baseline prior to the start of chemotherapy and after chemotherapy sessions 1, 2, and 4.

This was a two-phase study. The first established the base levels for the outcome parameters by obtaining data from 10 patients undergoing chemotherapy. In the second phase, patients were randomly assigned to one of two groups. One group (15 patients) received 30 minutes of Reiki during chemotherapy and the other group (11 patients) had a companion present for 30 minutes. The companion group was included to account for the social support component that a Reiki practitioner may provide in addition to the Reiki itself. Six Reiki practitioners were used in the study, one master and five trained to level two. Standardized hand positions were used throughout. The companions were Reiki practitioners who engaged in patient-directed conversation with the patients but did not perform Reiki or touch the patients. It was hypothesized that both Reiki and companionship would make the side effects of chemotherapy more bearable, but that the effects of Reiki would be more marked. Results showed that neither Reiki nor companionship decreased symptom distress compared to standard care. Perhaps distress associated with chemotherapy-related symptoms is too persistent to be alleviated by these modalities. On the positive side and consistent with other studies, all patients found Reiki to be relaxing. Patients in both the Reiki and companion groups improved regarding quality of life and mood, whereas the standard care group did not. In addition, patients in the Reiki and companion groups reported reduced fatigue following chemotherapy compared to the chemotherapy alone group. Contrary to the hypothesis, patients in the companion group reported a higher QOL and mood than the Reiki group at the end of the study. However, the companion group also had a higher QOL than the Reiki group at the beginning of the study, which may explain the result.

Strengths: This study is unique in that it compares Reiki or the presence of a companion to standard care during the chemotherapy of women with breast cancer. Scientific method is maintained as shown by the inclusion of a control group, reproducible methodology, well-defined outcome scales, and detailed statistical analysis.

Weaknesses: The number of patients involved was small and the patients were not blinded as to their grouping. A major weakness of the experimental design was that the companion was allowed to speak with the patient throughout the 30-minute session, whereas conversation with the Reiki practitioner was limited to a few explanatory words at the start of the session. Therefore, the companions were able to offer more social support which is known to improve QOL and mood. In addition, since the companions were also Reiki practitioners, it is possible that they were unconsciously sending Reiki to the patients. If this were the case, the patients in the companion group would be receiving both Reiki and additional social support, whereas the patients in the Reiki group would be receiving only Reiki. A much better experimental design would have been to use non-Reiki practitioners as companions.

Future Research: The study is significant in demonstrating that complementary modalities such as Reiki and companionship can assist in the tolerance of conventional chemotherapy treatments, and that further studies with larger numbers of patients and comparison of early and late stage oncologic disease would be useful.

The study by Salles et al. (2014) is important because it investigated the effect of Reiki on blood pressure of patients diagnosed with hypertension. In January 2019, the American Heart Association reported that almost 100 million US adults had hypertension in 2016. In 2016, according to the Census Bureau, there were 250 million US adults in total, and so this means that 40% of American adults suffer from hypertension. Being diagnosed with high blood pressure does not necessarily mean that medications are indicated straight away; the first step is aiming for a healthier lifestyle. This is where Reiki comes into the picture. In the study by Salles et al., the immediate effect of Reiki was evaluated in 66 patients, of an average age of 60 years, who had been diagnosed with hypertension for an average of 12 years. The patients were randomly assigned to one of three groups: Reiki, sham Reiki, or rest. Blood pressure was measured before and after the 20-minute treatment or rest period. There was a statistically significant decrease in minimum, mean, and maximum BP for the Reiki group. Both rest and sham groups also showed a decrease in BP but to a lesser degree than the Reiki group, without statistical significance.

Strengths: This was a study in which participants were randomly assigned to the groups and those in the Reiki or sham Reiki groups were unaware of their group assignment. In addition, the data were coded so that the data analysts were unaware of the grouping and thus were not biased.

Weaknesses: There was only a single treatment of Reiki or sham-Reiki and the number of participants per group was small.

Future Research: The data support future research in which the effects of multiple Reiki treatments over weeks or months on larger populations are investigated. Such research is particularly important due to the huge numbers of adults who suffer from hypertension and the fact that high blood pressure, if left untreated, can increase the chances of heart disease.

Summary

A summary table of results of the Reiki studies addressing relaxation and/or well-being is shown in Table 7.2. This small group of research studies demonstrates that Reiki feels relaxing (as shown by comments from participants in two studies) and is physiologically calming, as indicated by an increase in the parasympathetic component of HRV in Reiki recipients in another study. Reiki also reduces blood pressure significantly more than for control groups. Two studies provide evidence that Reiki is most effective at reducing depression the more severe the depression, i.e. when there is a real need. Both of the studies involving sick patients in hospital demonstrated the power of Reiki compared to standard care or other therapies in improving mood states. Improved quality of

Table 7.2. Summary of Reiki research for relaxation and well-being

Study	Groups	Results	Faults
Witte et al., 2001	Reiki, Touch, Music, Meditation	• Reiki group more physically relaxed. • All groups showed ↓BP	• Inexperienced Reiki practitioner • No sham Reiki group
Mackay et al., 2004	Reiki, Sham Reiki, Rest	• Reiki group showed ↓HR and ↓BP	• Small sample size • No information about Reiki practitioner • Only % changes reported
Bowden et al., 2010	Non-contact Reiki, Non-contact Sham Reiki	• Only Reiki group showed correlation between initial depression DASS-21 score and improvement in DASS-21 score	• Limited to young, mainly female students
Bowden et al., 2011	Non-contact Reiki, Non-contact Sham Reiki	• Only Reiki high depression group showed significant improvements in DASS-21 score	• Limited to young, mainly female students
Bukowski, 2015	Self-Reiki only	• ↓PSS (Perceived Stress Scale)	• Small sample size • No control group • Limited to healthy, young students
Vitale, 2009	Self-Reiki only	• ↑ability to reach calm state • ↑clarity of thought • replenished ability to nurse	• Small sample size • Limited to Caucasian nurses
Friedman et al., 2010	Reiki, Music, Rest	Only Reiki showed: • ↑parasympathetic HRV • ↑+ve & ↓–ve emotional states	• Small sample size • No sham Reiki • No details on length/frequency of treatments • Participants not blinded as to group
Orsak et al., 2015	Reiki, Companion, Standard Care	• Reiki was more relaxing • Both Reiki and Companion groups: ↑QOL, ↑positive mood (POMS) and ↓fatigue	• Small sample size • Companions but not Reiki providers were allowed to talk to patients • Companions were also Reiki practitioners
Salles et al., 2014	Reiki, Sham Reiki, Rest	• All groups showed ↓BP but only statistically significant for Reiki	• Small sample size • Only one 20-minute treatment

life and decreased fatigue were other improvements experienced by Reiki recipients. In the two studies in which healthy participants practiced Reiki on themselves, Reiki was effective at reducing perceived stress. The most common problems associated with most of these studies were the small sample sizes and the limitation of participants to a narrow category as delineated by age, race, profession, etc. It is obvious that although these results are promising, further research using large, more heterogeneous populations is essential in order to make a solid case for using Reiki to enhance relaxation and well-being. In addition, there are several established parameters for well-being that have not yet been used for any of these studies so far; thus, there is untapped potential for further important research findings.

Case Study

SS has come for weekly Reiki sessions for the last two years. She is elderly and has suffered through many health problems, including breast cancer, inflammation of vocal chords and pneumonia. In addition, she is not very mobile and uses a walker for ambulation. She enjoys the weekly Reiki sessions because they help her relax, help her breathe more easily, and increase her energy. She has many friends and relatives of all ages with whom she likes to socialize and she feels that the Reiki sessions refuel and replenish her so she can enjoy those activities. One time she woke up feeling very tired and phoned her doctor to ask whether she should cancel her Reiki and massage appointments that day. Her doctor replied, "You can cancel anything but not the Reiki!"

References

Benson H, Proctor W. *Relaxation Revolution: The science and genetics of mind body healing.* Scribner, Simon and Schuster, Inc., New York, NY, USA, 2010.

Bowden D, Goddard L, Gruzelier J. A randomized controlled single-blind study of the effects of Reiki and positive imagery on well-being and salivary cortisol. *Brain Research Bulletin* 2010; 81: 66–67.

Bowden D., Goddard L, Gruzelier J. A randomized controlled single-blind trial of the efficacy of Reiki at benefitting mood and well-being. *Evidence-Based Complementary and Alternative Medicine* 2011; 2011: 381862.

Bukowski EL. The use of self-Reiki for stress reduction and relaxation. *Journal of Integrative Medicine* 2015; 13(5): 336–340.

Buric I, Farias M, Jong J, Mee C, Brazil IA. What is the molecular signature of mind-body interventions? A systematic review of gene expression changes induced by meditation and related practices. *Frontiers in Immunology* 2017; 8: 670.

Creswell JD, Irwin MR, Burkland LJ, Lieberman MD, Arevalo JM, Ma J, Breen EC, Cole SW. Mindfulness-based stress reduction training reduces loneliness and proinflammatory gene expression in older adults: a small, randomized controlled trial. *Brain Behavior and Immunity* 2012; 26(7): 1095-1101.

Friedman RSC, Burg MM, Miles P, Lee F, Lampert R. Effects of Reiki on Autonomic Activity Early After Acute Coronary Syndrome. *Journal of the American College of Cardiology* 2010; 56: 995–996.

Huston JM, Tracey KJ. The pulse of inflammation: heart rate variability, the cholinergic anti-inflammatory pathway and implications for therapy. *Journal of Internal Medicine* 2011; 269: 45–53.

Irwin MR, Olmstead R, Breen EC, Witarama T, Carrillo C, Sadeghi N, Arevalo JM, Ma J, Nicassio P, Ganz PA, Bower JE, Cole S. Tai chi, cellular inflammation, and transcriptome dynamics in breast cancer survivors with insomnia: a randomized controlled trial. *Journal of the National Cancer Institute Monographs* 2014(50): 295–301.

Mackay N, Hansen S, McFarlane O. Autonomic nervous system changes during Reiki treatment: a preliminary study. *Journal of Alternative and Complementary Medicine* 2004; 10(6): 1077–1081.

Orsak G, Stevens A, Brufsky A, Kajumba M, Dougall AL. The effect of Reiki therapy and companionship on quality of life, mood, and symptom distress during chemotherapy. *Journal of Evidence-based Complementary and Alternative Medicine* 2015; 20(1): 20–27.

Salles LF, Vanucci L, Siles A, DaSilva MJP. The effect of Reiki on blood hypertension. *Acta Paulista de Enfermagem* 2014; 27(5): 479–484.

van Maanen MA, Vervoordeldonk MJ, Tak PP. The cholinergic anti-inflammatory pathway: towards innovative treatment of rheumatoid arthritis. *Nature Reviews Rheumatology* 2009; 5(4): 229–232.

Vitale AT. Nurses' lived experience or Reiki for self care. *Holistic Nursing Practice* 2009; 23(3): 129–145.

Witte D, Dundes L. Harnessing life energy or wishful thinking? Reiki, placebo Reiki, meditation, and music. *Alternative and Complementary Therapies* 2001; 7(5): 304–309.

Chapter 8

Reiki for Anxiety and Depression

Defining Anxiety and Depression in Terms of Clinical Outcomes

Anxiety

According to the American Psychological Association:

Anxiety is an emotion characterized by feelings of tension, worried thoughts and physical changes like increased blood pressure. People with anxiety disorders usually have recurring intrusive thoughts or concerns. They may avoid certain situations out of worry.

Anxiety UK makes the point on their website (www.anxietyuk.org.uk/get-help/anxiety-information/) that:

whereas stress is something that will come and go as the external factor causing it (be it a work, relationship or money problems, etc.) comes and goes, anxiety is something that can persist whether or not the cause is clear to the sufferer.

Sometimes a seemingly small stressor can suddenly cause extreme distress to a person because their mind-body has already accumulated responses to multiple unresolved stressors and this additional, seemingly minor problem acts as a trigger. In such cases, the person experiencing the distress may have no idea what really caused it.

People who have been in a state of continual anxiety, in which they are excessively worried about a variety of events or activities more days than not, for at least six months, are said to suffer from generalized anxiety disorder (GAD) (as defined by National Institute of Mental Health, USA). People with GAD find it difficult to control their worry, which may cause impairment in social, occupational, or other areas of functioning. According to Dr. Andrew Weil, Founder and Director of the Center for Integrative Medicine, University of Arizona, about 3–4% of the US population has GAD during the course of a year.

Why are some people more prone to feeling anxiety than others? One reason that some people are naturally overanxious may be because they have an overactive amygdala, the part of the brain which triggers the fight-or-flight response. As described in Chapter 5, the body produces a chemical called gamma-aminobutyric acid (GABA) which binds to receptors on the amygdala and suppresses its response to stimuli. Some people who are overanxious either do not produce sufficient GABA, or do not have an adequate number of GABA receptors on the amygdala. Many people who suffer from anxiety rely on pharmaceutical drugs to alleviate their symptoms but all the drugs have side effects, many of which can be unpleasant and even dangerous. Another way that the fight-or-flight response can be regulated is by stimulating the vagus nerve (a major part of the parasympathetic component of the autonomic nervous system). Some scientific evidence is presented in Chapter 5 that Reiki may modulate the fight-or-flight response by stimulating the vagus nerve and reducing activity of the sympathetic nervous system. If Reiki can help regulate the fight-or-flight response, it is reasonable to suppose that receiving Reiki would also help control anxiety and depression.

Ashwini Nadkarni, MD, associate psychiatrist and instructor at Harvard Medical School, says:

Because Reiki is intended to induce relaxation in a manner similar to yoga or acupuncture and attenuate people's stress response – or the release of cortisol from their adrenal glands and activation of the sympathetic nervous system – it can be a creative and useful way to reduce stress.

Symptoms of Anxiety

Anxiety UK lists some of the most common physical symptoms of anxiety as follows:

- Increased heart rate

- Increased muscle tension

Chapter 8

- Tingling in the hands and feet

- Hyperventilation (overbreathing)

- Dizziness

- Difficulty breathing

- Wanting to urinate more often

- Feeling nauseous

- Tight band across the chest area

- Tension headaches

- Hot flushes

- Increased perspiration

- Dry mouth

- Shaking

- Choking sensations

- Palpitations

Some of the most common psychological symptoms of anxiety are:

- Thinking one may lose control

- Thinking one might die

- Thinking one may have a heart attack/be sick/faint/have a brain tumor

- Feeling that people are looking and observing one's anxiety

- Feeling detached from one's environment and the people in it

- Feeling that one wants to run away/escape from the situation

- Feeling on edge and alert to one's surroundings

Clinical Outcomes

Although anxiety is usually accompanied by increased heart rate and muscle tension, these physiological responses are not specific to feelings of anxiety. For that reason, in order to specifically evaluate the severity of anxiety, it is necessary to rely on subjective self-report questionnaires. Self-report measures have the advantages of brevity, ease of administration and scoring, and a decreased demand on human resources compared to interview-based assessments that require certified psychiatrists.

The two most commonly used questionnaires for evaluating anxiety are the State-Trait Anxiety Inventory (STAI) and the Beck Anxiety Inventory (BAI). The STAI is designed to differentiate between the temporary condition of "state anxiety" and the more long-standing quality of "trait anxiety" in adults. State anxiety refers to feelings of apprehension, tension, nervousness, and worry, which increase in response to psychological stress *at the time of stress*. State anxiety items include: "I am tense; I am worried" and "I feel calm; I feel secure." Responses for the "state" anxiety scale assess intensity of current feelings "at this moment" in terms of: 1) not at all, 2) somewhat, 3) moderately so, and 4) very much so. The trait anxiety scale evaluates the frequency of the same feelings over time, for example over the last six months. Trait anxiety items include: "I worry too much over something that really doesn't matter" and "I am content; I am a steady person." Responses for the trait anxiety scale assess frequency of feelings in terms of: 1) almost never, 2) sometimes, 3) often, and 4) almost always. The STAI has 40 items, 20 items allocated to each of the state anxiety and trait anxiety subscales. The STAI has been demonstrated to have adequate validity and reliability, with reliability coefficients ranging from 0.83 to 0.92 (Spielberger, 1989). For adults, this measure requires about 10 minutes to complete.

The Beck Anxiety Inventory (BAI) was developed by Aaron T. Beck to measure the somatic and panic-like symptoms of anxiety, which have been shown to be less characteristic of GAD. The BAI does not assess other primary symptoms of anxiety, such as worry and other cognitive aspects of anxiety. Somatic symptoms are those associated with sensations in the body such as muscle tension, dizziness, and heart racing. The BAI is a short list describing 21 anxiety symptoms such as "wobbliness in legs", "scared", and "fear of losing control."

Respondents indicate how much they have been bothered by each symptom over the past week. Responses are rated on a four-point Likert scale and range from 0 (not at all) to 3 (severely). It takes 5–10 minutes to complete. The total score ranges from 0–63. The following guidelines are recommended for the interpretation of scores: 0–9, normal or no anxiety; 10–18, mild to moderate anxiety; 19–29, moderate to severe anxiety; and 30–63, severe anxiety. The BAI has proven to be acceptably reliable with a test-retest reliability of 0.75 over an average time lapse of one week (Beck et al., 1988).

Another questionnaire that is specifically used to assess worry is the Penn State Worry Questionnaire (PSWQ). The PSWQ measures a general characteristic tendency to worry excessively. Oxford Dictionaries gives a simple definition of "worry" as: "feel anxious or troubled about actual or potential problems". This questionnaire is an especially useful instrument to assess the severity of the pathological worry characteristic of GAD. It has been shown to discriminate among the various anxiety disorders (GAD, panic disorder, obsessive-compulsive disorder, post-traumatic stress disorder and social anxiety disorder), since individuals with GAD score significantly higher on the PSWQ than any other anxiety disorder group (Molina and Borkovec, 1994). The PSWQ is a 16-item questionnaire that aims to measure the trait of worry, using Likert rating from 1 (not at all typical of me) to 5 (very typical of me).

The PSWQ has shown to possess high internal consistency and good test-retest reliability (Meyer et al., 1990).

Depression

According to the American Psychiatric Association:

Depression (major depressive disorder) is a common and serious medical illness that negatively affects how you feel, the way you think, and how you act. Fortunately, it is also treatable. Depression causes feelings of sadness and/ or a loss of interest in activities once enjoyed. It can lead to a variety of emotional and physical problems and can decrease a person's ability to function at work and at home.

Depression affects about one in 15 adults (6.7%) in any given year. Over a lifetime, one in six people (16.6%) will experience depression. Women are more likely than men to experience depression and some studies demonstrate that one-third of women will experience a major depressive episode in their lifetime. Depression can strike at any time but, on average, first appears during the late teens to mid-twenties. As stated by the Mental Health Foundation UK:

Depression is a common mental health problem that causes people to experience low mood, loss of interest or pleasure, feelings of guilt or low self-worth, disturbed sleep or appetite, low energy, and poor concentration.

Symptoms of Depression

Depressive symptoms can vary from mild to severe and may include:

- Feeling sad or having a depressed mood

- Loss of interest or pleasure in activities once enjoyed

- Changes in appetite – weight gain or loss unrelated to dieting

- Trouble sleeping or sleeping too much

- Loss of energy or increased fatigue

- Increase in purposeless physical activity (e.g. hand-wringing or pacing) or slowed movements and speech (actions observable by others)

- Feeling worthless or guilty

- Difficulty thinking, concentrating, or making decisions

- Thoughts of death or suicide

Symptoms must last at least two weeks for a diagnosis of depression. Patients generally receive as their standard treatment pharmaceutical drugs such as selective serotonin reuptake inhibitors, norepinephrine reuptake inhibitors, or other drugs that target specific neurotransmitters. However, research shows that about 20% of patients do not fill their prescriptions, and of those who do comply, 60% experience side effects such as constipation, diarrhea, and dizziness and may discontinue treatment (Xing et al., 2011). As an alternative, people with depression may benefit from talking therapies, such as counseling, cognitive behavioral therapy (CBT), and psychotherapy. A detailed review of 11 studies involving 1511 patients concluded that CBT worked as well as modern antidepressants for the treatment of moderate to severe depression (Amick et al., 2015). However, only 45% of patients responded to either treatment, where a "response" is defined as a 50% improvement from a baseline depression score. Nevertheless, since this response rate is better than nothing, the National Institute for Health and Care Excellence UK guidelines recommend that people in the UK with moderate to severe depression should be offered a combination of an antidepressant *and* a talking therapy such as CBT or interpersonal therapy. From these data, it is obvious that people who suffer from depression need additional therapies to use in conjunction with their standard treatment.

One theory regarding the cause of depression is that it is due to an overactive hypothalamus–pituitary–adrenal (HPA) axis stress response resulting in overproduction of the stress hormone, cortisol (Pariante, 2012). A diagram of the HPA axis is shown in Figure 8.1. It is not clear

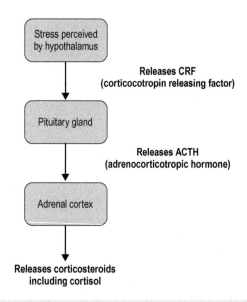

Figure 8.1
Diagram showing function of hypothalamus-pituitary-adrenal axis.

whether this means that depressed people have very high concentrations of cortisol in their bloodstream which overwhelms their brain and leads to depressive symptoms, or whether the overactive HPA axis is a compensatory mechanism that is elicited because their brain is resistant to cortisol. In fact, depression has been reported in people with disorders accompanied by high cortisol, such as Cushing's disease, and also in people with disorders linked to low cortisol, such as Addison's disease. Since, as illustrated by studies described in Chapters 5 and 7, Reiki appears to reduce perceived stress and enhance relaxation, there is a chance that it could be effective in alleviating depression, especially when used in conjunction with the standard methods of treatment. In addition, since Reiki operates by "returning the body to balance" and "working to the highest good", it is conceivable that patients would benefit from Reiki whether their circulatory cortisol concentrations were abnormally low or abnormally high.

Clinical Outcomes

There is no definitive diagnostic laboratory test that can establish whether a person has major depressive disorder. Just as for anxiety, all methods to evaluate depression rely on subjective questionnaires. However, all the questionnaires described below are widely used and have been rigorously tested for validity. All except one (the Hamilton Depression Rating Scale) are easy to administer because they need only to be completed by the patient.

Hamilton Depression Rating Scale (HAM-D)

When administering the HAM-D, a clinician interviews the patient and rates the severity of their depressive symptoms, such as low mood, insomnia, agitation, anxiety and weight-loss on a graded scale, ranging from "not present" to "severe". The questionnaire consists of 21 questions and it usually takes between 15 and 20 minutes to conduct the interview and score the results. It was originally published in 1960 by Max Hamilton, and is currently one of the most commonly used scales for rating depression in medical research. Analysis of 23 studies demonstrated that this test has a reliability coefficient of 0.79, which is adequate. There is a similar clinician-administered questionnaire for anxiety (HAM-A) that consists of 14 questions related to symptoms of anxiety, such as anxious mood, insomnia and gastrointestinal symptoms, but it has been criticized for its poor ability to discriminate between reduced anxiety and decreased depression.

Beck Depression Inventory (BDI)

The BDI is a 21-item questionnaire that covers aspects of depression such as irritability, hopelessness, feelings of guilt, and fear of being punished, as well as physical symptoms such as fatigue, weight loss and lack of interest in sex. Each item is rated on a four-point scale based on severity. A total score of 0–9 indicates that a person is not significantly depressed, 10–18 indicates mild to moderate depression, 19–29 indicates moderate to severe depression and a score of 30–63 suggests that a person is severely depressed. The BDI is commonly used for distinguishing between clinical depression and temporary unhappiness and is considered

both reliable and valid when administered to adults, with an excellent reliability coefficient of 0.92. It takes about 5–10 minutes to complete.

Quick Inventory of Depressive Symptomatology (QIDS-SR-16)

The QIDS-SR-16 questionnaire has proved to be useful for many years as a way to determine a patient's level of depression before, during, and after treatment. It is a 16-item questionnaire that covers symptoms of depression such as trouble sleeping, sadness, increased or decreased appetite, increased or decreased weight, indecision, problems concentrating, lack of self-worth, suicidal thoughts, lack of interest in activities of others, fatigue, and psychomotor agitation, or retardation. Each item is rated on a four-point scale based on severity. The QIDS-SR-16 has high reliability and validity with scores similar to those of the HAM-D. It takes about 5–10 minutes to complete.

Center for Epidemiological Studies Depression Scale (CES-D)

The CES-D questionnaire is a short (20 item) self-report scale that measures frequency of symptoms of depression in the past week on a four-point scale ranging from "rarely" to "most of the time". The symptoms selected for this questionnaire, such as "feelings of guilt and worthlessness" and "loss of appetite", have been used in previously validated longer scales. It has high validity and reproducibility but there is evidence that it may not be so useful for assessing major or clinical depression.

How Reiki Affects People with Anxiety and Depression

There are currently 11 research studies focusing on the effects of Reiki on anxiety and/or depression (Table 8.1). Five of these articles address anxiety or depression in people with additional maladies that are physical (Dressen and Singg, 1998; Shiflett et al., 2002; Vitale and O'Connor, 2006; Beard et al., 2011; Baldwin et al., 2017) and six others involve subjects for whom depression and/ or anxiety is their main issue (Shore, 2004; Richeson

Table 8.1 Summary of Reiki research: effects on anxiety and depression

Study	Groups	Results	Faults
Dressen and Singg, 1998 Chronic illness	• Reiki • Sham Reiki • Progressive muscle relaxation • Rest	• Only Reiki group showed: ↓ depression score ↓ state anxiety	• Patients self-selected for experiment (applied to advertisement)
Shiflett et al., 2002 Post-stroke rehabilitation	• Reiki (by Reiki Master) • Reiki • Sham Reiki • Standard care	• No effects of Reiki on overall depression scores • Reiki significantly improved depression item "ability to get going"	• Small sample size • Use of historical controls • Missing data from controls
Shore, 2004	• Reiki • Distance Reiki • Sham distance • Reiki	• Both Reiki groups showed: ↓ depression score ↓ perceived stress	• Small sample size • Subjects self-selected
Vitale and O'Connor, 2006 Hysterectomy	• Reiki • Standard care	• Reiki group showed ↓ state anxiety at discharge compared to control group	• Small sample size • No sham Reiki group included
Beard et al., 2011 Prostate cancer	• Reiki • Relaxation response therapy (RRT) • Wait list control	• Only RRT group showed: ↑ emotional well being ↓ anxiety if anxious initially	• Insufficient power for statistical significance – just trends • Subjects not blinded to treatment
Richeson et al., 2010 Elderly in communal dwelling	• Reiki • Wait list control	• Only Reiki group showed significant improvements in depression and anxiety scores	• Small sample size • No sham Reiki group included • Subjects and data collectors not blinded to grouping • One Reiki master on research team • Music during Reiki
Erdogan and Cinar, 2014 Elderly in nursing home	• Reiki • Sham Reiki • Standard care	• Only Reiki group showed significant: ↓ depression score with time in study	• Level of Reiki training of practitioners not given • Data collectors not blinded to grouping
Charkhandeh et al., 2016 Adolescents	• Reiki • Cognitive behavioral therapy • Wait list control	• Both Reiki and CBT groups showed significant: ↓ depression score	• No sham Reiki group included • Reiki sessions only 20 min versus 90 min for CBT • Not much information about Reiki sessions

(continued)

Table 8.1 Summary of Reiki research: effects on anxiety and depression (*continued*)

Study	Groups	Results	Faults
Bremner et al., 2016 HIV	• Reiki with music • Music	• Only Reiki w music showed acute (pre- vs post-session): ↓ depression score ↓ state anxiety ↓ stress • Both groups showed ↓ depression, anxiety and stress when comparing baseline with 10-week follow up	• Small sample size • No sham Reiki • HIV status self-reported
Kurebayashi et al., 2016 Stressed people seeking outpatient care	• Massage with Reiki • Massage with rest • No intervention	• Both groups showed: ↓ stress symptoms, ↓ state anxiety • There was a trend for massage with Reiki to be more effective at decreasing anxiety	• No information about Reiki practitioners • No sham Reiki • Only 10 min of Reiki after massage • Subjects not blinded to grouping
Baldwin et al., 2017 Knee surgery	• Reiki • Sham Reiki • Standard care	• Only Reiki group showed significant ↓ state anxiety 48 hours after surgery compared to pre-surgery	• Small sample size • By 48 hours post-surgery, 10 patients had left the study

et al., 2010; Erdogan and Cinar, 2014; Charkhandeh et al., 2016; Bremner et al., 2016; Kurebayashi et al., 2016). Six out of eleven of the clinical trials are pilot studies involving small numbers of participants; only five studies, three of which are pilot, compare results from Reiki and sham Reiki groups (Dressen and Singg, 1998; Shiflett, 2002; Shore, 2004; Erdogan and Cinar, 2014; Baldwin et al., 2017). Joyce and Herbison (2015) reviewed Reiki research studies published up to November 2014. Their initial selection criteria for inclusion in the review were: "Randomised trials in adults with anxiety or depression or both, with at least one arm treated with Reiki delivered by a trained Reiki practitioner". They also stipulated that studies in which subjects "were not assessed for anxiety or depression at baseline" be excluded. As a result of this criterion, four of the studies that are discussed in this chapter were excluded from their review (Dressen and Singg, 1998; Shiflett, 2002; Shore, 2004; Vitale and O'Connor,

2006). The reason that these studies are included in this chapter is that, although the subjects were not selected based on a clinical diagnosis of anxiety or depression at baseline, their test scores on established questionnaires for anxiety and/or depression *were* compared pre- versus post-treatment. Therefore, it is the opinion of this author that the subjects in these studies really did fulfill the criterion of "being assessed for anxiety or depression at baseline". In addition, the test scores revealed that, in two cases, the subjects, on average, were indeed suffering from mild to moderate depression prior to treatment (Shiflett et al., 2002; Shore, 2004). The previous review is also missing the five papers published during 2014 or later. The authors focus solely on three earlier articles that fit their criteria (Beard et al., 2011; Richeson et al., 2010; Bowden, 2011). The paper by Bowden is not reviewed in this chapter because it emphasizes mood and well-being rather than anxiety and depression and was already discussed in Chapter 7. Interestingly, the participants in the Bowden study had been assessed for depression at baseline (Bowden, 2011) using an established questionnaire similar to that used in the four studies that were excluded from the review by Joyce and Herbison.

This review will focus on the five publications in which results from Reiki and sham Reiki groups are compared. The purpose of the study by Dressen and Singg (1998) was to test the effects of Reiki on depression and anxiety in 120 self-selected patients who were chronically ill with a variety of medical conditions including headaches, coronary heart disease, and cancer. The patients were randomly assigned to one of four groups: Reiki, sham Reiki, progressive muscle relaxation (PMR) and control (no therapy). The Reiki sessions were given by Reiki Masters, and the sham Reiki by assistants who had not received Reiki attunement but who emulated the Reiki hand positions. All groups except the control group received 10 bi-weekly 30-minute sessions of their treatment. Each patient in each group was tested with a variety of questionnaires, including the BDI and the STAI before and after the 10-session treatment plan. The Reiki group was also tested three months later for follow-up. Reiki reduced depression and state anxiety to a significantly greater degree than any of the other treatments and these effects were maintained over the three-month follow-up period. The decrease in depression was described as "dramatic" and was greater in men than in women, possibly because the men, on average, started off with a greater degree of depression than the women. The authors postulated that men tend to give and receive physical touch less often than women, and perhaps the gentle, nurturing, non-sexual touch of Reiki lifted their spirits.

Strengths: A large sample of men and women were recruited and randomly assigned to groups within a placebo-controlled experiment. The experiment was long-term and each person except those in the control group received multiple treatments. Reiki treatments were provided by Reiki Masters and sufficient detail was provided about how sessions were conducted to allow repetition.

Weaknesses: The patients were not randomly selected but responded to an advertisement; thus, they were self-motivated and may not be typical of most other patients. Variability in the seriousness of a patient's illness was an uncontrolled confounding variable.

Future Research: Since this sample of patients was suffering from chronic illness, the results regarding effectiveness of Reiki in reducing depression and anxiety are not generalizable. Further experiments, using a similar experimental design and similar testing instruments, but with otherwise healthy people are needed to determine whether this very promising result is reproducible and generalizable.

The purpose of the paper by Shiflett et al. (2002) was to determine whether Reiki would reduce depression in 30 people recovering from subacute ischemic stroke (post-stroke rehabilitation) in a hospital. Ischemic stroke refers to impairment of blood flow to the brain, possibly by a blood clot, whereas hemorrhagic stroke refers to blood loss to the brain due to bleeding. There were three conditions: Reiki given by Reiki Master, Reiki given by first level Reiki practitioner and sham Reiki. Twenty additional subjects were identified as no-treatment historical controls from hospital records. The Reiki and sham Reiki practitioners both received Reiki training from the Reiki Master, but unbeknownst to them, the sham Reiki practitioners did not receive the Reiki attunement, and thus supposedly could not transmit Reiki. All practitioners were aware that there was a 50:50 chance that they would receive the attunement. The 30 experimental subjects received between six and ten 30-minute treatments over a two-and-a-half week period in addition to standard rehabilitation. They were blinded as to their group assignation. The outcome parameter used to test for depression was the Center for Epidemiologic Studies Depression Scale (CES-D). It was found that Reiki did not significantly reduce depression scores, whether provided by the Reiki Master or by Reiki first level practitioners, but it did have "limited positive effects on mood and energy levels" as indicated by differing responses to the CES-D item, "I can't get going". Subjects in both Reiki groups showed a significant increase in their ability to "get

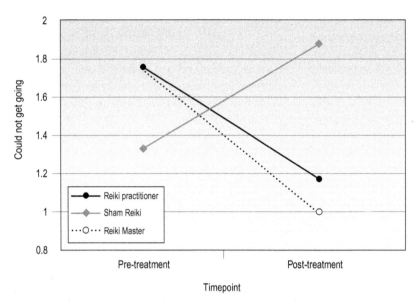

Figure 8.2
Graph showing effects of Reiki on ability to "get going".
(From: Shiflett SC, Nayak S, Bid CB, Miles P and Agostinelli S. Effect of Reiki treatments on functional recovery in patients in poststroke rehabilitation: a pilot study. *Journal of Alternative and Complementary Medicine*, 8(6): 755-563, 2002. Figure 1.)

going" whereas the sham Reiki group became less able to get going (Figure 8.2). When the practitioners were interviewed after the study, neither the Reiki nor the sham Reiki practitioners could identify which category they were in. These two groups did not report any difference in their ability to feel energy flowing through their hands. This is actually not surprising because learning Reiki is rather like learning the piano. The more one practices, the more adept one becomes. Likewise, the more experience one has giving and receiving Reiki, the more sensitive one becomes to feeling the Reiki flow. Using practitioners who do not know whether they have received Reiki attunement raises the question of the effectiveness of a Reiki practitioner who is not confident in their practice. Is Reiki less effective if the practitioner doubts their skill level?

Strengths: This was a randomized, placebo-controlled, double-blinded study, meaning that the participants were not aware of their group assignment and the first level and sham Reiki practitioners were unaware of their grouping.

Weaknesses: The use of historical controls is a major flaw because there is no guarantee that all conditions, such as management and evaluation protocols, would have been identical to those in the experimental case. In addition, the historical controls did not complete the CES-D, but just provided data for their functional independence measure (FIM), another clinical outcome used in this study. In addition, the sample size was small. Another publication (Louw, 2002) criticized this study with regard to the use of the FIM in that this parameter lacks the sensitivity to detect subtle changes in cognition. In addition, the critique makes the point that any potential positive effect of Reiki may have been masked by the heterogeneity of the stroke-induced brain injuries. Different parts of the brain could be affected in different people leading to variation in functional outcomes, some of which might be more conducive to Reiki healing than others. Another confounding variable was that the mean age of the groups differed by 10 years, raising a high likelihood of differences in comorbidities, or the presence of other illnesses. So, overall, although this study indicates that Reiki did not help alleviate depression in stroke victims, there are multiple confounding variables that could be masking any potential positive effect of Reiki.

Future Research: Much more research is needed to determine whether Reiki can successfully alleviate depression in stroke victims. Future studies will require large numbers of subjects, the use of multiple, highly experienced Reiki Masters rather than practitioners who have just received training, as well as sham Reiki and no-treatment control groups.

The purpose of the article by Shore (2004) was to determine the effects of Reiki in 45 people seeking treatment for mild stress or depression. Participants were randomized into one of three groups: Reiki, distance Reiki and sham distance Reiki. Each person in the Reiki or distance Reiki groups received their respective 60–90-minute treatment from a Reiki Master or second level Reiki practitioner once a week for six weeks. The Reiki was hands-on, whereas the distance Reiki was provided by a practitioner who was not present in the room, and in fact could be many miles away. People in the distance Reiki and sham distance Reiki groups entered similar treatment rooms, but those in the sham group did not receive Reiki. The article states that the participants were blinded as to their grouping. This was achieved by deceiving the hands-on Reiki group into thinking they were receiving sham Reiki. The sham distance Reiki and distance Reiki groups were both told that they would receive distance Reiki. At the end of the six-week period, both Reiki groups showed significant reductions in symptoms of psychological stress compared to baseline, as measured by the Perceived Stress Scale (PSS) described in Chapter 7. They also demonstrated reduced depression, as measured by the BDI. In these groups, the PSS and BDI scores continued to decrease throughout the course of one year despite no further treatments. No significant reductions were seen in the sham distance Reiki group, even though they believed they were receiving Reiki. After the experiment was over, the sham distance Reiki group received the full 6-hour Reiki treatment after which they also demonstrated significant decreases in stress and depression.

Strengths: The Reiki practitioners were very carefully selected based on their level of training and the investigators' stipulations that each practitioner must have had at least one year of experience and conducted at least 10 sessions of distance Reiki. In addition, the primary researcher experienced a Reiki session from each potential practitioner to test for quality and effectiveness of treatments. Effectiveness was based on the feeling of subjectively tangibly receiving Reiki energy and of experiencing deep relaxation. This study had the added advantage that it addressed long-term effects of Reiki, monitored over one year.

Weaknesses: The subjects referred themselves and so may have self-selected for their openness to complementary therapies. The sample size was small.

Future Research: Further research is needed with larger groups of participants to determine if these apparently robust effects can be replicated. In addition, it would be interesting to focus on the effects of Reiki on specific psychological disorders.

The purpose of the study by Erdogan and Cinar (2014) was to determine the effect of Reiki on depression of 90 elderly people living in two nursing homes in Turkey. In order to be accepted in the study, the residents had to score at least 14/30 in the Geriatric Depression Scale (GDS), indicating mild depression. The GDS is a 30-item self-report questionnaire designed to identify depression in the elderly. The questions are answered by "yes" or "no" rather than by using a five-point scale. A scoring range of 0–9 is "normal", 10–19 is "mildly depressed", and 20–30 is "severely depressed". Sample questions are: "Are you in good spirits most of the time?"; "Do you frequently get upset over little things?"; "Do you enjoy getting up in the morning?" The accuracy of the GDS is similar to that of the CES-D for evaluating depression and takes about 5–10 minutes to complete. The participants in this study were randomly assigned to one of three groups: Reiki, sham Reiki, and control (no intervention). Reiki was provided by a Reiki Master, and sham Reiki by nurses who just emulated Reiki hand positions but who thought that they were actually providing Reiki. Reiki and sham Reiki sessions lasted 45–60 minutes and were given once a week for eight weeks. The GDS was applied on the first, fourth, and eighth weeks before sessions and on the twelfth week when sessions had stopped. The control group completed the GDS on the same schedule. There was a statistically significant decrease in GDS score in the Reiki group on the fourth, eighth, and twelfth weeks compared to the first week. No significant difference was found in the GDS scores in the sham Reiki and control groups over the period of the study. In addition, the GDS score of the Reiki group was lower than that for the other two groups at the fourth, eighth, and twelfth weeks. During Reiki applications, many of the participants stated that they "felt relaxed, happy, safe, and their ability of coping has increased". In addition, a few participants showed remarkable recoveries from their comorbidities. For example:

. . . an elderly person who was diagnosed with Parkinson disease and who described that they fall often, stated that "before the Reiki application he/she fell four or five times a day", expresses his/her emotions at the end of the seventh week as: "my fallings are now one or two times a week, from now on I feel happy and my crying has decreased, I love life".

Strengths: This study was well designed, using repeated measures over 12 weeks, and participants were randomly assigned to treatment and comparison groups. People in the Reiki and sham Reiki groups were blinded as to their grouping. The Reiki protocol was described in sufficient detail to allow repetition by other investigators. The outcome measure, GDS was appropriate for this population and was adequately described and validated.

Weaknesses: No information was provided regarding the length of time that the Reiki Master had been in practice. The data collectors were aware of the participants' group assignment and so this could introduce bias.

Future Research: Once again, further studies to assess reproducibility would be very useful to confirm evidence for the usefulness of providing Reiki in nursing homes.

The purpose of the study by Baldwin et al. (2017) was to determine the effectiveness of Reiki at reducing the anxiety of 45 patients undergoing knee replacement surgery in hospital. Anxiety was assessed using the STAI. Patients were randomly assigned to one of three groups: Reiki, sham Reiki or rest. Reiki was provided by three Reiki Master hospital employees and sham Reiki by two other hospital employees who had no knowledge of Reiki. All Reiki

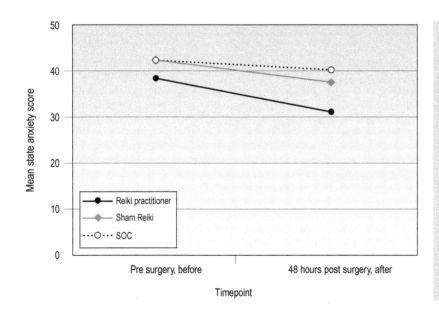

Figure 8.3

Graph showing effects of Reiki on anxiety.

(From: Baldwin AL, Vitale A, Brownell E, Kryak E, Rand W. Effects of Reiki on pain, anxiety, and blood pressure in patients undergoing knee replacement surgery. *Holistic Nursing Practice* 2017; 31(2): 80–89. Figure 2.)

and sham Reiki providers used exactly the same hand positions with the patients. Each patient received three or four
30-minute sessions of either Reiki or sham Reiki from the
same person and were unaware of which "treatment" they
received. The sessions were given 1 hour before surgery and
24, 48, and 72 hours after surgery. Patients in the control
group rested during those periods. The data collectors and
analyzers were blinded as to the grouping or participants
and the group code was not revealed until completion of
the analysis. Only the Reiki group showed significantly
reduced anxiety scores 48 hours after surgery compared to
their anxiety at entry (Figure 8.3). In addition, the Reiki
group had the highest number of hospital discharges at 48
hours versus 72 hours after surgery, implying occurrence
of fewer complications that would otherwise extend their
stay. The Reiki group, but not the sham Reiki or controls,
also showed significantly reduced pain levels, systolic
blood pressure and respiration rates 48 hours after surgery
compared to pre-surgery.

Strengths: This was a randomized, placebo-controlled,
double-blinded pilot study that clearly demonstrated the
feasibility of using Reiki to alleviate anxiety in patients
undergoing knee surgery.

Weaknesses: The patient sample size was small; patients
were recruited from a single hospital center.

Future Research: This feasibility study has paved the
way for a multi-center large scale clinical trial to evaluate
whether Reiki will be a useful addition to routine care of
patients undergoing total knee replacement surgery.

Summary

There is a mix of quality in the published articles related
to the effects of Reiki on anxiety and depression, as can
be seen in Table 8.1. The poorer quality studies, i.e. those
that are not randomized, blinded, placebo-controlled
experiments with enough participants to allow for valid
statistical comparisons between groups, do not contribute greatly to our understanding of the effectiveness of
Reiki in alleviating anxiety and depression. They show

some interesting trends, for example, that Reiki performs as well as other therapies, such as massage, music,
and cognitive behavioral therapy in reducing anxiety or
depression, but they are flawed by problems with experimental design and lack of a valid statistical analysis. For
this reason, there are really only five studies from which
firm conclusions can be drawn. Four of these studies support the use of Reiki as a successful tool for alleviating
anxiety and depression in the following populations: the
elderly; those with chronic medical conditions; patients
undergoing surgery; and otherwise healthy people seeking treatment for depression. The study by Shiflett et al.
(2002) did not support the use of Reiki for reducing overall depression, but the data were difficult to interpret for
reasons already described. Depression comes in different
forms, can have multiple causes and is a very complex
mind-body illness. For those reasons, far more research
is needed in this area to provide the necessary evidence
base for confidently recommending Reiki as a therapy for
depression.

As concluded in the review by Joyce and Herbison
(2015):

*If Reiki is to be regarded as a serious treatment for anxi-
ety or depression then well-designed, well-conducted, and
well-reported studies need to be done. [...]*

*Studies need to be in appropriate patient populations: in
this instance, in people with anxiety or depression, either
clinically diagnosed or by being above cut-offs in anxiety or
depression scores. Reiki should be administered by a trained
Reiki practitioner, and it would be useful to compare it
with something that facilitates blinding of the participants
and different forms of Reiki (e.g. distance Reiki). Outcomes
should include measures of anxiety or depression measured after a reasonable period. These outcomes should be
measured again sometime after the treatment sessions have
stopped to check on the persistence of any effect. Studies
should be large enough to answer questions about whether
such treatments are efficacious. Studies should be reported
in full within a reasonable time of the last outcome being
measured.*

Case Study

CR first came for heart rate variability biofeedback to see if she could learn how to regulate her high blood pressure. She learnt to breathe more slowly and deeply and was soon able to reach a coherent state in which the sympathetic and parasympathetic components of the autonomic nervous system work together in a coordinated fashion. In this way, bodily functions that are regulated by the ANS, such as control of blood pressure, digestion, and blood flow distribution, are optimized for efficiency. CR returned a year later for Reiki because she was anxious about an upcoming court trial. The initial scan indicated that her upper chakras, in the head and throat areas, appeared to be lacking energy. After 30 minutes of Usui Reiki, they felt better balanced. One week later, CR returned for another Reiki session and once again the upper chakras felt weak. Reiki treatment energized the chakras more quickly than before. The practitioner felt guided this time to release tension in the spine. She started with her left-hand middle finger at CR's occiput (back of the skull) and the right-hand middle finger on her coccyx (root of spine) and waited until her pulse was synchronized between both hands. This was repeated with both palms placed flat on CR's spine, fingers of each hand pointing towards each other, one close to CR's head and the other at the base of the spine. After pulse synchronization occurred, the palms were inched closer together and the process was repeated. The practitioner asked CR to make sure that she practiced coherent breathing for at least 5 minutes daily. One week later, CR came for a third session. She said she had been practicing coherent breathing and felt much more in control. On her initial scan, all her chakras felt well-balanced. After 30 minutes of Reiki, CR said she felt strong, stable, and did not feel anxious about the trial. She also said she had decided to maintain a program of healthy exercise and to modify her diet to include less fat and sugar and more protein and vegetables. Receiving Reiki often motivates people to improve their personal habits. It is important to note that CR benefited from a combination of Reiki *and* coherent breathing. Reiki founder, Dr. Usui, always insisted that his students practice coherent breathing while giving and receiving Reiki. This protocol is often neglected by Reiki practitioners even though it places the mind-body into a neutral state that enables the Reiki to work more effectively.

References

Amick HR, Gartlehner G, Gaynes BN, Forneris C, Asher GN, Morgan LC, Coker-Schwimmer E, Boland E, Lux LJ, Gaylord S, Bann C, Pierl CB, Lohr KN. Comparative benefits and harms of second-generation antidepressants and cognitive behavioral therapies in initial treatment of major depressive disorder: systematic review and meta-analysis. *British Medical Journal* 2015; 351: h6019.

Baldwin AL, Vitale A, Brownell, Kryak E, Rand W. Effects of Reiki on pain, anxiety, and blood pressure in patients undergoing knee replacement: a pilot study. *Holistic Nursing Practice* 2017; 31(2), 80–89.

Beard C, Stason WB, Wang Q, Manola J, Dean-Clower E, Dusek JA, Decristofaro S, Webster A, Doherty-Gilman AM, Rosenthal DS, Benson H. Effects of complementary therapies on clinical outcomes in patients being treated with radiation therapy for prostate cancer. *Cancer* 2011; 117(1): 96–102.

Beck AT, Epstein N, Brown G, Steer RA. An inventory for measuring clinical anxiety: Psychometric properties. *Journal of Consulting and Clinical Psychology* 1988; 56: 893–897.

Bowden D., Goddard L, Gruzelier J. A randomized controlled single-blind trial of the efficacy of Reiki at benefitting mood and well-being. *Evidence-Based Complementary and Alternative Medicine* 2011; 2011: 381862.

Bremner MN, Blake BJ, Wagner VD, Pearcy SM. Effects of Reiki with music compared to music only among people living with HIV. *Journal of the Association of Nurses in AIDS Care* 2016; 5: 635–64.

Charkhandeh M, Mansor AT, Hunt CJ. The clinical effectiveness of cognitive behavior therapy and an alternative medicine approach in reducing symptoms of depression in adolescents. *Psychiatry Research* 2016; 239: 325–330.

Dressen LJ, Singg S. Effects of Reiki on pain and selected affective and personality variables of chronically ill patients. *Subtle Energies and Energy Medicine* 1988; 9(1): 51–82.

Ergodan Z, Cinar S. The effect of Reiki on depression in elderly people living in a nursing home. *Indian Journal of Traditional Knowledge* 2014; 15(1): 35–40.

Joyce J, Herbison GP. Reiki for depression and anxiety. *Cochrane Database of Systemic Reviews* 2015; 3(4): CD006833.

Kurebayashi LFS, Turrini RNT, Souza TPB, Takiguchi RS, Kuba G, Nagumo MT. Massage and Reiki used to reduce stress and anxiety: randomized clinical trial. *Revista Latino-Americana de Enfermagem* 2016; 24: 22834.

Louw S. Research in stroke rehabilitation: confounding effects of the heterogeneity of stroke, experimental bias and inappropriate outcome parameters. *Journal of Alternative and Complementary Medicine* 2002; 8(6): 691–693.

Meyer TJ, Miller ML, Metzger RL, Borkovec TD. Development and validation of the Penn State Worry Questionnaire. *Behavior Research and Therapy* 1990; 28: 487–495.

Molina S, Borkovec TD. The Penn State Worry Questionnaire: Psychometric properties and associated characteristics. In: G. C. L. Davey & F. Tallis (Eds.), *Worrying: Perspectives on theory, assessment and treatment* (pp. 265–283). Wiley Series in Clinical Psychology. John Wiley & Sons, Oxford, UK, 1994.

Pariante CM. *Depression, Stress and the Adrenal Axis.* British Society for Neuroendocrinology, UK, 2012. Archived from the original on 11 February 2019.

Richeson NE, Spross JA, Lutz K, Peng C. Effects of Reiki on anxiety, depression, pain and physiological factors in community-dwelling older adults. *Research in Gerontological Nursing* 2010; 3(3): 187–199.

Shiflett SC, Nayak S, Bid C, Miles P, Agostinelli S. Effect of Reiki treatments on functional recovery in patients in post-stroke rehabilitation: a pilot study. *The Journal of Alternative and Complementary Medicine* 2002; 8(6): 755–763.

Shore, AG. Long term effects of energetic healing on symptoms of psychological depression and self-perceived stress. *Alternative Therapies in Health and Medicine* 2004; 10(3): 42–48.

Spielberger CD. *State-Trait Anxiety Inventory: Bibliography* (2nd ed.). Consulting Psychologists Press, Palo Alto, CA, USA, 1989.

Vitale AT, O'Conner PC. The effect of Reiki on pain and anxiety in women with abdominal hysterectomies. *Holistic Nursing Practice* 2006; 20(6): 263–272.

Xing S, Dipaula BA, Lee HY, Cooke CE. Failure to fill electronically prescribed antidepressant medications: a retrospective study. *The Primary Care Companion for CNS Disorders* 2011; 13, p11: PCC.10m00998.

Chapter 9
Reiki for Burnout

What is Burnout?

An excellent definition and description of "burnout" is provided by helpguide.org, a website that was launched by Robert and Jeanne Segal, the parents of Morgan Leslie Segal, who died by suicide in 1996 at the age of 29:

Burnout is a state of emotional, physical, and mental exhaustion caused by excessive and prolonged stress. It occurs when you feel overwhelmed, emotionally drained, and unable to meet constant demands. As the stress continues, you begin to lose the interest and motivation that led you to take on a certain role in the first place.

Burnout reduces productivity and saps your energy, leaving you feeling increasingly helpless, hopeless, cynical, and resentful. Eventually, you may feel like you have nothing more to give.

The negative effects of burnout spill over into every area of life – including your home, work, and social life. Burnout can also cause long-term changes to your body that make you vulnerable to illnesses like colds and flu. Because of its many consequences, it's important to deal with burnout right away.

The above description is consistent with the accepted standard for burnout diagnosis, the Maslach Burnout Inventory (MBI), developed by Christina Maslach and colleagues at the University of San Francisco in the 1970s. According to the MBI, the main symptoms for burnout are:

1. Exhaustion. Emotional energy levels are extremely low.

2. Depersonalization. This is characterized by cynicism and "compassion fatigue".

3. Lack of efficacy. Seeds of doubt are sewn about the meaning and quality of one's work, resulting in reduced care and effort directed to the work.

Physical symptoms of burnout include:

-   Feeling tired and drained most of the time

-   Frequent headaches or muscle pain

-   Lowered immunity

-   Change in appetite or sleep habits

Emotional symptoms of burnout include:

-   Sense of failure and self-doubt

-   Feeling helpless, trapped, and defeated

-   Feeling detached and alone in the world

-   Loss of motivation

-   Increasingly cynical and negative attitude

-   Decreased satisfaction and sense of accomplishment

Behavioral symptoms of burnout include:

-   Withdrawing from responsibilities

-   Isolating oneself from others

-   Procrastinating

-   Using food, drugs, or alcohol to cope

-   Taking out one's frustrations on others

Although the physical symptoms of burnout are similar to those of stress, the emotional responses and behavioral symptoms are quite different. People who are stressed are full beyond capacity; they are over-engaged and possessed by feelings of urgency and hyperactivity.

Chapter 9

Emotionally, they are over-aroused and even small inconveniences can make them angry and frustrated, producing anxiety. All their physical, mental, and emotional overactivity can eventually result in a loss of energy. On the other hand, people suffering from burnout feel empty and lacking in resources. They become less engaged, less motivated, less emotionally responsive, and less hopeful. This leads to detachment and depression. In fact, a recent letter to the editor of Mayo Clinic Proceedings (Bianchi and Schonfeld, 2017), advocated a redefinition of burnout as "job-induced depression" rather than just including the three MBI symptoms. They cited a study involving over 3,000 dentists that showed that the intensity of burnout and depressive symptoms change in parallel over time (Ahola et al., 2014). The authors made the point that if symptoms of depression were included in the definition of burnout, then many more people suffering from this condition would be identified and treated more appropriately.

Burnout and Healthcare Professionals

According to the ECRI Institute, formerly known as the Emergency Care Research Institute, burnout among physicians is alarmingly present and is on the rise (ECRI Institute, 2016): 54.4% of surveyed physicians reported at least one symptom of burnout in 2014, an increase from 45.5% in 2011 (Shanafelt et al., 2015). More recently, the 2018 Survey of America's Physicians, conducted by The Physicians Foundation, stated that:

The number of physicians reporting sometimes, often, or always feeling burned out increased from 74% in 2016 to 77.8% in 2018, suggesting that feelings of burnout are an ongoing condition for many physicians.

These data were based on responses from 8,774 physicians, as well as 2,472 written comments. As seen in Table 9.1, female physicians report the highest rate of burnout, possibly due to their frequent dual roles as professionals and mothers. Employed physicians report higher rates of burnout compared to practice owners; younger physicians, those less than 46 years old, report higher rates of

Table 9.1 Feelings of professional burnout by physician type

	Sometimes/often/always
Aged 45 or younger	81.0%
Aged 46 or older	76.3%
Male	74.1%
Female	84.8%
Employed	80.1%
Owner	76.5%
Primary care physician	78.8%
Specialists	77.2%

(From: "2018 Survey of America's Physicians: Practice Patterns and Perspectives", The Physicians Foundation, p. 32.)

burnout than older physicians. Three factors that cause physicians the most frustration, and may contribute to burnout, are:

1. Poorly designed electronic health record systems that eat into the time physicians could be devoting to their patients.

2. Complicated regulatory and insurance requirements that detract from the physician/patient relationship.

3. Loss of clinical autonomy. According to the report, physicians "often find that their ability to make what they believe are the best decisions for their patients is obstructed or undercut by bureaucratic requirements or third parties who are non-physicians."

In addition, 62.5% of physicians who participated in the report believe they have little input or influence over how the healthcare system is structured and, as a result, they feel powerless. This feeling of powerlessness is one of the key emotional symptoms of burnout.

Burnout in healthcare personnel is not just limited to physicians. Nurses, therapists, medical assistants, and housekeepers are also affected. A publication by the ECRI Institute (2016) states:

Housekeepers are just as vulnerable as the rest of the staff. They're in the room with patients and families for 15 to 20 minutes every day. They develop close relationships and experience deep loss when patients pass away.

In a 2014 analysis of registered nurses and respiratory therapists working in the intensive care unit (ICU), 54% scored "moderate" to "high" for emotional exhaustion on the Maslach Burnout Inventory. Forty percent scored "moderate" to "high" on depersonalization, and 40.6% scored "low" on the personal accomplishment scale. Nurses' overall level of burnout and depersonalization was higher than that of respiratory therapists (Guntupalli et al., 2014).

Nurses in particular are notoriously selfless and many of them are driven by a desire to care for others; this makes them more vulnerable to burnout. In addition, according to Dawn Kettinger, spokeswoman for the Michigan Nurses Association, burnout has probably worsened for nurses in recent times because the workload of the average nurse is greater today than it was 10 or 15 years ago as a result of more technology, documentation, electronic medical records, and added nursing responsibilities. The fast-paced workload can cause nurses to feel overwhelmed and stressed. Over time, this stress can lead to nursing burnout.

In general, the high incidence of burnout in clinical practitioners may be linked to the following factors:

- Healthcare workers often build close relationships with patients and their families and experience deep loss when patients die.

- Physicians and nurses are involved in discussions about adverse events, end-of-life care, and performance of cardiopulmonary resuscitation and medical decisions that, in the end, may not have contributed to patient well-being. All these conversations have the potential to increase stress levels.

- Cost cutting, ever-increasing regulation, and the evolution of the electronic health record (EHR)

have resulted in less control and an abundance of new tasks for providers without any more time to accomplish their work. For example, a quantitative time-and-motion study of outpatient care physicians revealed that they spend 49.2% of their time on EHR and desk work, and 27% of their work day on direct clinical face-to-face time with patients.

- Many healthcare workers are overloaded with numerous, ever-expanding roles and duties.

It is quite clear that the factors leading to burnout are inherent in the environment and the healthcare delivery system and are not merely due to the mental weakness of susceptible individuals. So how can Reiki help? Obviously, the approach must be multi-pronged: first, assess both the measured and perceived effects of receiving Reiki on the symptoms of burnout in healthcare workers; second, if existing research results are promising, extend the research to include larger numbers of participants, a wider range of outcome parameters and all types of clinical personnel; third, determine through further scientific studies whether *self-practice* of Reiki by clinical practitioners is useful as a tool to avoid burnout; fourth, if Reiki self-practice is effective, include a course of practical Reiki education in the career training of all medical personnel; fifth, make organizational changes that will allow time for and encourage Reiki practice by personnel on a daily basis. In order for such dramatic changes to take place in the healthcare system, the evidence for Reiki being an effective tool to eliminate burnout must be solid. At present, the evidence is very sparse but it is promising. In the rest of this chapter, first, the existing research will be reviewed; next, two articles "Enhancing Nursing Practice with Reiki" (https://www.reiki.org/healing/nursingandreiki.html), by registered nurse and Reiki trainer Kathie Lipinski, and "Nurses' Lived Experience for Reiki for Self-Care" by registered nurse, PhD and Reiki Master, Anne Vitale (Vitale, 2009), will be discussed; and, finally, a first attempt to incorporate Reiki training into a nursing degree will be described.

Chapter 9

Current Research on Effects of Reiki on Burnout

There are currently only three published research articles addressing the effects of Reiki on burnout. One refers to female healthcare professionals (Diaz-Rodriguez et al., 2011a), the second to female nurses (Diaz-Rodriguez et al., 2011b), and the third to mental health clinicians (Rosada et al., 2015).

The purpose of the first study was to determine if Reiki treatments have an effect on the symptoms of healthcare professionals diagnosed with Burnout Syndrome (BS). It was hypothesized that a parasympathetic response would occur after Reiki as indicated by changes in heart rate variability (HRV), increases in body temperature and salivary flow rate, and a decrease in salivary cortisol levels. A secondary aim of the study was to analyze the relationships among HRV, body temperature, and salivary changes. Twenty-one self-recruited female healthcare professionals, with a mean age of 44 years, and a psychologist-based diagnosis of BS, attended two treatment sessions held in the morning, one week apart. In the first session, baseline measurements of HRV, body temperature, and stimulated salivary flow rate were collected. Salivary samples were obtained to measure cortisol concentration. Participants were then randomly assigned to a 30-minute Usui Reiki treatment given by a nurse trained to level three Reiki, or placebo non-intentional Reiki (performed by a nurse with no Reiki experience but who mimicked the Reiki hand positions), after which the same measures were repeated. The second session was the same as the first, except that each participant received the alternate treatment compared to the first session. The participants were blinded as to which of their treatments was Reiki and which was placebo. The Reiki treatment, but not the placebo treatment, produced a statistically significant increase in HRV (as measured by SDNN), a decrease in the low frequency component of HRV indicating reduced sympathetic activity, and an elevation of body temperature (Figure 9.1). The high frequency component of HRV, which reflects parasympathetic activity was not affected by either treatment, nor were the salivary flow rate or the salivary cortisol concentrations. These results indicate that

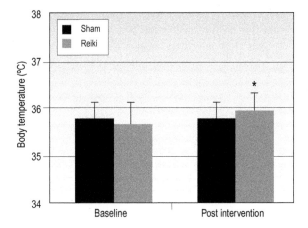

Figure 9.1

Effects of Reiki on body temperature of healthcare professionals with burnout.

(From: Diaz-Rodríguez L, Arroyo-Morales M, Fernández-de-las-Peñas C, García-Lafuente F, García-Royo C and Tomás-Rojas I. Immediate effects of Reiki on heart rate variability, cortisol levels, and body temperature in health care professionals with burnout. *Biological Research for Nursing*, 13(4): 376- 382, 2011a. Figure 2).

Reiki treatment produces a mild but significant relaxation response in nurses with BS symptoms.

Strengths: A very carefully designed placebo-controlled, repeated measures, crossover, single-blinded, randomized trial showing that Reiki promotes relaxation by reducing sympathetic autonomic stimulation, consistent with previous findings in healthy people and in rats. Randomized non-contact Reiki with sham non-contact Reiki control meant that the influence of touch alone or attention alone was eliminated. Confounding variables were minimized by conducting the experiment at the same time of day each time and by asking participants to abstain from caffeine, alcohol, food, and exercise two hours prior to the experiment.

Weaknesses: The effects of respiration rate on HRV were not considered and this may have confounded the low frequency component of the HRV data. The process of respiration contributes to HRV; as one inhales, heart rate increases and, as one exhales, heart rate decreases. When breathing at an average rate of 12–15 breaths per minute, respiration contributes to the high frequency component of HRV, whereas breathing more slowly, at say six breaths per minute, shifts the respiratory component to the low frequency component. Since the respiration rates of participants were not measured, this variation could not be accounted for during the analysis. In addition, HRV measurements were taken immediately after the intervention without any follow-up measures, so that the time duration of any potential benefits was not addressed. Lastly, the sample size was small and restricted to females so the findings may or may not be generalizable.

Future Research: Repeating this study on larger numbers of people, including males, at different sites and performing multiple sessions with follow-up measures is an obvious way to make full use of these promising pilot data.

The purpose of the second study was to investigate the immediate effects of the secretory immunoglobulin A (sIgA), α-amylase activity and blood pressure levels after the application of a Reiki session to 18 female nurses (34–56 years old). The participants had been diagnosed with BS by a psychologist using the Maslach criteria. Secretory IgA is a first-line of defense against pathogenic microorganisms and is found in external secretions that bathe the esophagus and the airways; it is lowered in response to high levels of perceived stress, including burnout. Alpha-amylase is a marker of sympathetic activity and is linked to emotional arousal. Participants were randomly assigned to a Reiki or sham Reiki group, and neither the participants nor the data collectors were aware of the group assignments. Nurses in the Reiki group were treated by a Usui Reiki master with 15 years of clinical experience, who performed Reiki for 30 minutes by holding their hands over various parts of the participant's body without touching. The sham Reiki placebo intervention was administered by a nurse without experience in Reiki who mimicked the Reiki hand positions without touching for 30 minutes. The sham Reiki nurse focused attention on a neutral stimulus with no healing intentions during the session. Blood pressure was recorded, and saliva samples taken before and after the session. One week later, the participants returned, and the experiment was repeated but with each participant in the opposite group from the first session.

The results are presented in Table 9.2. Diastolic blood pressure (DB) was significantly reduced by Reiki but not by sham Reiki. Systolic blood pressure (SB) was reduced more by Reiki than by sham Reiki but the result was not statistically significant. Secretory IgA was significantly increased after Reiki but not after sham Reiki. These results indicate that a single session of Reiki brought immediate and measurable physiological stress relief to the nurses. Although a mechanism for this effect was not defined, it is possible that Reiki reduced sympathetic outflow to the heart and blood vessels, thereby reducing heart rate and relaxing peripheral blood vessels. In addition, it is possible that release of feel-good molecules, such as opiates and serotonin, could have been stimulated by Reiki.

The authors conclude that:

Taken together, these data support the idea that relatively brief but effective relaxation sessions, such as a Reiki treatment, can significantly relieve the negative effects of job stress on specific aspects of the immune system in nurses suffering from BS.

Strengths: This was a randomized, double-blinded, placebo-controlled study which used three different physiological outcome parameters related to stress. All participants had been clinically diagnosed with BS. The crossover design, in which each participant received both Reiki and sham Reiki, can reduce the variability in subject responses. Data were analyzed using robust, reliable, and established statistical tests and the results unambiguously indicated that only the Reiki treatment reduced stress symptoms.

Weaknesses: The sample size was very small and homogeneous and so the results cannot be generalized. Only immediate effects of Reiki were investigated without long-term follow-up.

Future Research: It would be useful to use questionnaires to discover what percentage of nurses and other

Table 9.2 Effects on sIgA, α-amylase activity, and blood pressure levels immediately after the application of a Reiki session in female nurses.

n=18	Placebo session	Reiki session
DB pressure (mm Hg)		
Baseline	70.8 ± 7.6 (95% CI 66.0 – 75.7)	71.1 ± 8.8 (95% CI 65.4 –76.8)
Post-intervention	71.2 ± 9.1 (95% CI 65.4 – 77.1)	66.6 ± 7.9 (95% CI 61.6 –71.7)
Pre-post change	0.4 (95% CI –3.7/4.5)	–4.5 (95% CI –0.6/–9.7)*
SB pressure (mm Hg)		
Baseline	115.4 ± 13.1 (95% CI 107.1 – 123.7)	115.7 ± 12.0 (95% CI 108.1 – 123.4)
Post-intervention	113.6 ± 14.2 (95% CI 104.6 – 122.6)	109.2 ± 12.3 (95% CI 101.4 – 117.1)
Pre-post change	–1.8 (95% CI –0.2/0.3)	–6.5 (95% CI –11.1/–1.8)
sIgA (µg/ml)		
Baseline	21.52 ± 6.67 (95% CI 18.3 – 24.7)	21.56 ± 6.76 (95% CI 18.3 – 24.8)
Post-intervention	19.58 ± 9.97 (95% CI 14.8 – 24.3)	21.51 ± 8.00 (95% CI 21.6 – 29.3)
Pre-post change	–1.94 (95% CI –6.2/2.29)	3.95 (95% CI 1.6/7.3)*
A-amylase activity (U/ml)		
Baseline	149.3 ± 89.4 (95% CI 103.4 – 195.3)	171.0 ± 100.2 (95% CI 119.5 – 222.4)
Post-intervention	171.0 ± 105.0 (95% CI 117.0 – 225.0)	201.4 ± 165.5 (95% CI 16.8 – 287.0)
Pre-post change	21.7 (95% CI –31.4/54.5)	30. 4 (95% CI 1.9/45.2)

Values are expressed as mean ± standard deviation (95% confidence interval) for baseline and post-intervention data as mean (95% confidence interval) for pre-post change. * Statistical significant (P<0.05).

(From: Diaz-Rodriguez et al. The application of Reiki in nurses diagnosed with Burnout Syndrome has beneficial effects on concentration of salivary IgA and blood pressure. *Revista Latino-Americana de Enfermagem* [online], 2011b; 19(5):1132–1138, Table 2.)

clinical practitioners trained in Reiki use self-Reiki on the job to dissipate stressful feelings and, if so, the range of time intervals between their Reiki sessions. Experiments could then be designed to determine whether or not the physiological benefits of Reiki that are related to stress reduction are maintained for those periods. In addition, further studies monitoring opiate and serotoninergic mechanisms could be performed to confirm the importance of these substances in the immediate effects of Reiki.

The purpose of the third study was to determine whether Reiki treatment could reduce the burnout among mental health clinicians, a community at high risk for professional burnout. A convenience sample of 45 volunteer participants (33 women and 12 men) was selected and randomly assigned to either a Reiki or a sham Reiki group in this crossover study. The sample was recruited from community mental health agencies in New England.

All participants were clinicians with at least a Master's degree, who worked 30 or more hours per week and spent at least 50% of their time working directly with clients. Sixteen Reiki practitioners (trained to level two or Master level) with a minimum of five years of practice participated over the duration of the study. Sham practitioners with no Reiki experience were also chosen and taught to mimic the Reiki hand positions so all participants were blinded as to their group assignment. The sham Reiki providers maintained mental arithmetic throughout the sessions to assuage positive feelings and/or healing intentions toward the participant. Each group received a weekly 30-minute hands-on, seated treatment for a period of six weeks. After a minimum rest period of six weeks, the groups were reversed, and the same treatment protocol repeated. Outcomes were measured using the Maslach Burnout Inventory–Human Services Survey, already described, and the Measure Your Medical Outcome Profile Version 2 (MYMOP). This is a well-validated patient-centered outcome questionnaire, developed by the UK Medical Research Council, that asks the participant to select two symptoms to monitor. These symptoms are anything that matters to the individual. The MYMOP also monitors an activity of relevance to the participant, and general sense of well-being. Medications are monitored as well. Data were collected at baseline, after their first six-week treatment, and before and after the second six-week treatment.

The results showed that Reiki treatments given weekly for six weeks significantly reduced burnout symptoms among mental health clinicians. Specifically, Reiki reduced emotional exhaustion significantly more than sham Reiki, was more effective for younger people, and worked better when given during the second six-week treatment. Reiki reduced depersonalization more than sham Reiki and was more effective in single people. Reiki did improve personal accomplishments when given in the first six-week treatment. The MYMOP demonstrated that Reiki was effective for reducing the primary symptom experienced by participants but only if they were single. On the other hand, Reiki improved the ability to perform restricted activities in partnered people. On average, when participants received sham Reiki, they perceived a "worsening quality of life." The authors concluded that their primary hypothesis, that Reiki will reduce a clinician's experience of burnout symptoms, was confirmed. Regarding the more positive effects of Reiki on single people, the authors speculate that partnered people receive positive, gentle touch in their intimate relationships and so the measurable effects of hands-on healing are less dramatic.

Strengths: This randomized, single-blinded, controlled study, using well-validated outcome measures was the first to show that Reiki reduced the experience of burnout in mental health clinicians. It was designed with a washout period of six weeks before the second phase to protect against a carryover effect.

Weaknesses: This study could have benefited from including a third group of either a non-touch therapy or no-treatment as a control to distinguish any benefits derived simply from touch. A no-treatment control group could also help reveal any possible Hawthorne effect which means experiencing ameliorated symptoms simply by knowing one is participating in a study to reduce symptoms.

Edzard Ernst MD, PhD commented negatively on this study in an online blog: https://edzardernst.com/2015/07/a-new-study-of-reiki-healing-with-a-false-positive-result/. According to Wikipedia, Edzard Ernst is an academic physician and researcher specializing in the study of complementary and alternative medicine. He was previously Professor of Complementary Medicine at the University of Exeter, the first such academic position in the world. He retired early from the post due to stopped funding after conflicts with Prince Charles.

Here are his comments concerning the Rosada et al. (2015) study:

Having conducted studies on 'energy healing' myself, I know only too well of the many pitfalls and possibilities of generating false-positive findings with such research. This new study has many flaws, but we need not look far to find the reason for the surprising and implausible finding. Here is my explanation why this study suggests one placebo to be superior to another placebo.

The researchers had to recruit 16 Reiki healers and several non-Reiki volunteers to perform the interventions on the small group of patients. It goes without saying that the Reiki healers were highly motivated to demonstrate the value of their therapy. This means they (unintentionally?) used verbal and non-verbal communication to maximize the placebo effect of their treatment. The sham healers, of course, lacked such motivation. In my view, this seemingly trivial difference alone is capable of producing the false-positive result above.

There are, of course, ways of minimizing the danger of such confounding. In our own study of "energy healing" with sham healers as controls, for instance, we instructed both the healers and the sham healers to abstain from all communication with their patients, we filmed each session to make sure, and we asked each patient to guess which treatment they had received. None of these safeguards were incorporated in the present study – I wonder why!

The claim that the Reiki practitioners used verbal and non-verbal communication to maximize the placebo effect of their treatment is not substantiated. Apparently, Ernst did not contact the authors to ask for further information. Although the authors noted that their sham practitioners practiced mental arithmetic to assuage possible healing intentions towards the participants, they did not make it clear whether the Reiki practitioners practiced in silence. Such a comment would have strengthened the paper. Edzard Ernst notes that an easy way to check whether this problem occurs is to ask each participant to guess which treatment they received. If most of the participants guess correctly, this increases the probability that some other factor, such as the sound of a soothing voice, may have contributed to any beneficial effect of Reiki. Ernst criticizes Rosada et al. for not utilizing such a safeguard. However, his comment just proves that he did not actually read the paper carefully, as shown by the following quote from Rosada et al.:

Multilevel modelling allowed for statistical control of a number of potentially confounding factors, such as people's expectations for which treatment they were receiving . . . their belief about which treatment they had actually received after the treatment was completed. In addition, in the Results section of the paper, it is noted that the participants who thought they did not receive Reiki showed significantly greater improvement in their second worst symptom (MYMOP2). Thus, Edzard Ernst's major critique is untrue.

Future Research: This study lays a strong foundation for larger similar trials. It may also provide future research direction comparing the effectiveness of Reiki on partnered versus non-partnered individuals. Additional positive outcomes in larger studies could lead to Reiki being offered as a regular burnout prevention option for healthcare workers.

Enhancing Nursing Practice with Reiki

According to an article available from the International Center for Reiki Training (https://www.reiki.org/healing/nursingandreiki.html) by Kathie Lipinski, RN, MSN, a Reiki Master teacher, nurse massage therapist, and holistic nurse in private practice:

Working with energy is another way of gathering information on a deeper level. It gives one "subtle clues" as to what is really going on with a person. It helps one to become more aware of the emotional or spiritual component of dis-ease that the nurse can share with the client to gain understanding or insight.

Regarding the use of Reiki to prevent burnout, she says:

The most important benefit of Reiki is the self-care aspect. With all the energies that a nurse has to give in caring for others, a nurse often suffers "burnout." Reiki is an excellent way for nurses to take care of themselves and restore their energy and avoid depletion.

As nurses' roles continue to change and expand, Reiki is there to assist in their professional development. Reiki assists nurses in caring for themselves and restores their energies so they can continue to give of themselves in their role as healthcare advocates. Nurses who practice Reiki are in the unique position to combine both Reiki and their strong medical knowledge to help clients and improve the healthcare system.

She also refers to a book *Reiki and Medicine* by Nancy Eos, MD (Eos, 1995), a practitioner in family and holistic medicine in New York State, in which Dr. Eos says:

Nurses in administrative or management positions use Reiki when doing stressful tasks such as staffing, counselling, and reviewing employees. Reiki calms the situation and creates a more receptive state and clearer thinking. Some managers and staff give themselves Reiki before and during a staff meeting and find the meeting goes smoother.

In 2009, Anne Vitale, PhD, APN, and Reiki Master published a study in which she interviewed 11 female Caucasian nurses who practice Reiki for self-care, to explore their lived experience (Vitale, 2009). Two hundred fifty-two significant statements regarding the nurses' experience with self-Reiki were extracted from the transcripts.

The nurses believed that they practice self-Reiki "by thought," without thinking about it, but self-Reiki practice by touch was also performed periodically:

The nurses discussed using self-Reiki before their workday but used it more often during their workday to keep them centered, balanced, and grounded: a useful strategy for daily workday stress management in healthcare. The nurses reported that it was difficult to find a quiet, private place on a nursing unit to do self-Reiki, frequently practiced in the bathroom or in a bathroom stall, described as a "peaceful sanctuary." Several nurses were in managerial positions and described their offices as "sacred space" to do self-Reiki during their workday. Although these nurses spoke happily about being a nurse, their workday was described as "being in information overload," "feeling frazzled," and these experiences interfere with their preferences to make important patient-care decisions from a "place of calmness." None of the nurses discussed practicing self-Reiki more than once during the workday but described that the calming effects lasted for varying amounts of time. Because of workday time constraints, the nurses reported doing self-Reiki using only one or two hand positions, phrased as "hands over my heart {Heart Chakra}" or "to my solar plexus {Third Chakra}." Self-Reiki practice was described as a routine of daily morning practice to "set intention for the day."

Vitale notes that the use of self-Reiki offered the nurses protection from the ravages of hectic healthcare environments. The fact that the nurses reported that their own personal healing space for Reiki use during the workday was a bathroom or office space indicates that self-Reiki by nurses in hospitals was not seen or valued. Vitale stresses that gathering evidence from practicing nurses about the benefits of caring-healing environments and the creation of reverent, appealing healing environments for all who enter must be a priority of all nurse leaders.

Incorporating Reiki Training in a Nursing Degree

An article by Clark (2013) describes an upper level elective course in Reiki that was included in a bachelor's degree, Science in Nursing (RN-BSN), at the University of Maine, USA. Throughout the course, students were supported to create sustainable caring-healing nursing practices. The course lasted for seven weeks and 14 RN-BSN students enrolled. Students were attuned to Reiki to level two or three and were given the opportunity to give and receive Reiki within the group. They were required to complete all online academic work by answering discussion questions with the use of supporting literature and by replying to other students' postings. Study topics included ethical implications of Reiki utilization in the healthcare setting, exploring how Reiki could be used for one's personal self-care and healing practice, examining the peer-reviewed body of evidence around Reiki and exploring self-care for nurses. Students also experienced mindfulness practices, reflected on their own Reiki practice and attunement experiences, and explored their personal extent of burnout and compassion fatigue. The course outcome was an academic paper in which five peer-reviewed articles on the effectiveness of Reiki were explored, and the ways in which Reiki could be used in the community and in clinical settings were described. In this paper, students also set a path for their future use of Reiki.

All the students agreed that the course outcomes and concepts were met either adequately or in depth. Here are some of the specific comments that were made by the students:

I have used Reiki for self-care. I find myself reaching out to its calmness in times of stress and using the meditation more than I thought I would.

My Reiki is a huge outlet for me, a huge stress reliever, an energy boost, anything I need it to be, whenever I need it to be.

I find myself relying on the time of quiet and peace to try Reiki on myself. I feel a sense of calm. I actually look forward to it. I am spending 15 minutes before my shift in the car to practice Reiki and only a few minutes after shift ends. I do Reiki before bed and I usually fall asleep.

The students also mentioned that they were better prepared to care for others not only in the workplace but also on the home front. While about 40% of the students stated that they initially felt uncomfortable with the apparent dearth of scientific evidence around the effectiveness of Reiki, a realization that Reiki is more of a lived experience than a provable scientific intervention began to emerge from the group. It should be noted that in 2013, when the report was published, there was less published scientific support for Reiki than now. More than half of the students responded to follow-up surveys seven and 10 months after the course ended in which they confirmed that they still used Reiki for themselves and others. They also gave concrete examples of how they were using Reiki in the medical community, supporting patients, families, and fellow nurses in their own healing processes. As a result, an additional component was added to the course in which students provide Reiki in a local hospital's outpatient oncology unit and observe or support cancer patients giving and receiving Reiki.

The Mississippi Nurses Foundation now offers an ongoing 10-hour Reiki self-care training class for nurses with approved continuing education units. Their goal is to encourage professional caregivers to practice self-care by using Reiki as a simple method of stress reduction and relaxation, which also promotes healing.

Summary

Only three research studies on the effects of Reiki on burnout have been published but they are all of high quality, meaning that they were randomized, placebo-controlled experiments, using well-validated outcome parameters, in which the participants were unaware of whether they were in the Reiki or the placebo group.

The results are promising, and the research needs to be extended to include larger numbers of participants. There is now a body of published evidence, obtained from formal and informal interviews with nurses, which nurses are practicing, and benefiting from, self-Reiki to reduce symptoms of burnout. Further scientific studies to quantify the benefits of Reiki self-practice by clinical personnel to reduce burnout would be extremely useful and might motivate healthcare executives to make organizational changes to allow time for, and encourage, Reiki practice by personnel on a daily basis. The one instance in which instruction in Reiki has been included in a nursing degree has been very successful and hopefully Reiki will become a routine elective in the near future.

Case Study

NC was attending a health fair at University of Arizona College of Nursing and came for a sample Reiki session. She was enrolled in a patient advocate course on top of her nursing duties and said she felt overwhelmed. At the start of the session, NC started silently sobbing and said that the Reiki had brought up some emotional issues. I suggested that she come back for a private session the next day. When she returned, she was much more grounded and did not sob. An initial scan of her energy body indicated that she had high energy in her root chakra but low energy elsewhere as if there was some kind of energy blockage. During the session, I asked the Reiki to address emotional issues, to restore emotional and psychological balance, using the Usui symbol for emotion. NC asked how she should receive the Reiki and I asked her to breathe at six breaths per minute, five seconds in and five seconds out, so she would receive the Reiki in a coherent state. Afterwards, her energy body scan felt much more uniform than before. She said that she was very grateful for the Reiki and that she hoped she could reduce the medications she was taking to reduce stress.

References

Ahola K, Hakanen J, Perhoniemi R, Mutanen P. Relationship between burnout and depressive symptoms: a study using the person-centred approach. *Burnout Research* 2014; 1(1): 29–37.

Bianchi R, Schonfeld IS. Defining physician burnout and differentiating between burnout and depression. *Mayo Clinic Proceedings* 2017; 92(9): 1452–1458.

Clark SC. An integral nursing education experience. Outcomes from a BSN Reiki course. *Reiki Holistic Nursing Practice* 2013; 27(1): 13–22.

Diaz-Rodríguez L, Arroyo-Morales M, Fernández-de-las-Peñas C, García-Lafuente F, García-Royo C, Tomás-Rojas I. Immediate effects of Reiki on heart rate variability, cortisol levels, and body temperature in healthcare professionals with burnout. *Biological Research for Nursing* 2011a; 13(4): 376–382.

Diaz-Rodriguez L, Arroyo-Morales M, Cantarero-Villanueva I, Férnandez-Lao C, Polley M, Fernández-de-las-Peñas C. The application of Reiki in nurses diagnosed with Burnout Syndrome has beneficial effects on concentration of salivary IgA and blood pressure. *Revista Latino-Americana de Enfermagem* [online], 2011b; 19(5):1132–1138.

ECRI Institute. Burnout in healthcare: The elephant in the room. *Risk Management Reporter* 2016 Dec 14. https://www.ecri.org/components/HRC/Pages/RMRep1216.aspx.

Eos, N. Reiki and Medicine. Published by Nancy Eos, 1995.

Guntupalli KK, Wachtel S, Mallampalli A, Surani S. Burnout in the intensive care unit professionals. *Indian Journal of Critical Care Medicine* 2014; 18(3):139–143.

Rosada RM, Rubik B, Mainguy B, Plummer J, Mehl-Madrona L. Reiki Reduces Burnout Among Community Mental Health Clinicians. *The Journal of Alternative and Complementary Medicine* 2015; 21(8): 489–495.

Shanafelt TD, Hasan O, Dyrbye LN, Sinsky C, Satele D, Sloan J, Colin P, West CP. Changes in burnout and satisfaction with work-life balance in physicians and the general US working population between 2011 and 2014. *Mayo Clinic Proceedings* 2015; 90(12):1600–1613.

Vitale A. Nurses' lived experience of Reiki for self-care. *Holistic Nursing Practice* 2009; 23(3): 129–145.

Chapter 10
Reiki for Improving Range of Motion

What is Range of Motion?

Range of motion (ROM) is a measurement of movement around a joint. The four types of joint movement (not including rotation) are flexion, extension, abduction, and adduction. Flexion refers to a movement that decreases the angle between two body parts. For example, flexion at the elbow refers to decreasing the angle between the ulna (lower arm) and the humerus (upper arm), whereas extension is the opposite, as illustrated in Figure 10.1. *Adduction* is the movement of a body part toward the body's midline. So, if a person has their arms straight out at the shoulders and brings them down to their sides, it is adduction. *Abduction* is any motion of the limbs or other body parts that pulls away from the midline of the body. For example, swinging the hands from the side of the body up to the shoulder or higher is abduction. Examples of adduction and abduction of the shoulder joint are shown in Figure 10.2.

Measuring Range of Motion

The instrument used to measure ROM is a goniometer. The word goniometer is derived from the Greek terms *gonia* and *metron*, which mean angle and measure, respectively. There are two "arms" of the goniometer: the stationary arm and the moveable arm. The arms are connected at one end by a rotating axis that is centered on a measuring scale similar to a protractor, as seen in Figure 10.3. Each arm is positioned at specific landmark points on the body and the center of the goniometer is aligned at the joint to be measured. The stationary arm is positioned along the longitudinal axis of the *stabilized* joint segment and the moveable arm parallel to the longitudinal axis of the *moving* joint segment. Positioning the goniometer correctly is crucial; if the arms of the goniometer are not aligned properly, the measure will be inaccurate. Similarly, moving the axis of the goniometer off the joint line will yield an incorrect measurement.

According to Mayo Clinic Hope & Healing (Quinn, 2019), generally accepted normal ranges of motion of several different joints are as follows:

Hip

- Flexion: 0 to 125 degrees

- Extension: 115 to 0 degrees

- Hyperextension (straightening beyond normal range): 0 to 15 degrees

- Abduction (moving away from the central axis of the body): 0 to 45 degrees

- Adduction (moving towards the central axis of the body): 45 to 0 degrees

- Lateral rotation (rotation away from the center of the body): 0 to 45 degrees

- Medial rotation (rotation towards the center of the body): 0 to 45 degrees

Knee

- Flexion: 0 to 130 degrees

- Extension: 120 to 0 degrees

Ankle

- Plantar flexion (movement downward): 0 to 50 degrees

- Dorsiflexion (movement upward): 0 to 20 degrees

Chapter 10

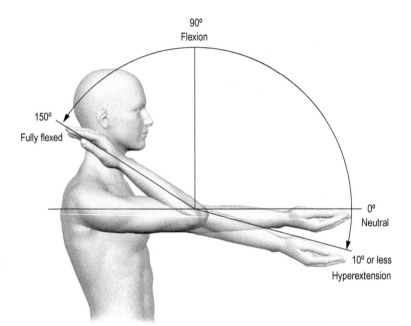

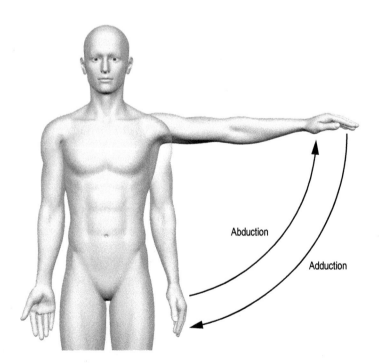

Figure 10.1
Diagram depicting range of motion at elbow joint.
(From: American Academy of Orthopedic Surgeons.)

Figure 10.2
Diagram showing abduction and adduction of shoulder joint.
(From: Mraz S. What's the Difference Between Abduction and Adduction? (Biomechanics) *Machine Design*, 22 July 2014.)

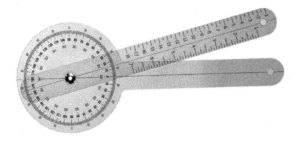

Figure 10.3

Example of a goniometer used to measure range of motion. (From: Manchester-Bedford Myoskeletal, "Range of Motion". http://www. mbmyoskeletal.com/learning/range-of-motion/)

Shoulder

- Flexion: 0 to 180 degrees
- Extension: 0 to 50 degrees
- Abduction: 0 to 90 degrees
- Adduction: 90 to 0 degrees
- Lateral rotation: 0 to 90 degrees
- Medial rotation: 0 to 90 degrees

Elbow

- Flexion: 0 to 160 degrees
- Extension: 145 to 0 degrees
- Pronation (rotation inward): 0 to 90 degrees
- Supination (rotation outward): 0 to 90 degrees

Wrist

- Flexion: 0 to 90 degrees
- Extension: 0 to 70 degrees
- Abduction: 0 to 25 degrees
- Adduction: 0 to 65 degrees

Issues that Impede Range of Motion

Limited ROM is a term used when a joint has a reduction in its ability to move. There are numerous intrinsic factors that can affect ROM of a specific type of joint, some of which can be modified and some which cannot. Examples of factors that cannot be controlled include the internal resistance within the joint and bony structures that limit movement. Age and gender also affect ROM. Older people generally have lower ROM than younger people and require more time to reach their full ROM. On average, men have smaller ROMs to women in some areas, with the greatest difference, 29.7%, occurring in the hand. Factors that can be modified to some extent are the elasticity of muscle tissue and the muscle's ability to relax and contract.

Apart from the intrinsic properties of the joint, extrinsic factors such as injury and disease can limit ROM. ROM can be limited by injuries to the soft tissues surrounding a joint, such as skin, muscle, tendon, and ligament. Such injuries may be acute, such as when a joint is hit by a strong, external force, or chronic. Most chronic injuries arise from repetitive overuse and are inflammatory in nature. Examples are tendinitis (inflammation of a tendon), bursitis (inflammation of the bursa, fluid-filled cushion pads in the joints), and epicondylitis (irritation of the epicondyle, which surrounds the rounded parts of the bones in a joint). Muscle strains or tears are also included in this category. With regard to disease, rheumatoid arthritis and osteoarthritis are the main diseases that limit ROM.

Characteristics of Osteoarthritis

Osteoarthritis is the most prevalent type of arthritis and is commonly referred to as the wear-and-tear type of arthritis. In the United States, about 27 million people live with the condition. Osteoarthritis is most common among adults over 65 years old, and women are more likely to develop osteoarthritis than men, especially after age 50. The main risk factors for developing arthritis are:

- Overweight or obesity—Excess body weight adds burden to weight-bearing joints but, in addition,

Chapter 10

there may be metabolic effects associated with extra weight and obesity that increase the risk of osteoarthritis.

- Genetic predisposition—Studies have associated certain gene variations with an increased risk of developing osteoarthritis.

- Occupations that require intense joint loading, especially repetitively, increase the risk of developing osteoarthritis. This is true of jobs that require lifting, kneeling, squatting, or climbing.

Osteoarthritis has long been thought to arise from the breakdown of cartilage in one or more joints. Cartilage is a hard, slippery tissue which provides a cushion between the bones of joints, allowing the bones to glide over one another. It also absorbs shock from physical movements. When cartilage degradation occurs, joints can deteriorate to the point of rubbing bone against bone which may alter the structures, such as muscles and tendons, that surround joints. These changes can lead to severe chronic pain and loss of mobility. More recently it has been discovered that many other factors play a role in the development of osteoarthritis including production of pro-inflammatory mediators and destructive enzymes. For example, wear and tear from joint loading stimulates the production of pro-inflammatory factors and proteases which contribute to joint deterioration.

Characteristics of Rheumatoid Arthritis

Rheumatoid arthritis differs from osteoarthritis in that it is an autoimmune disorder in which the immune system mistakenly attacks its own cells and tissues, primarily those of the joints. While rheumatoid arthritis can occur at any age, symptoms usually start between the ages of 40 and 60 and the risk increases with age. Overall, the chances of developing rheumatic arthritis will more than triple between the ages of 35 and 75, increasing from 29 cases per 100,000 people to 99 cases per 100,000, according to research from the Mayo Clinic. Women are three times as likely to be afflicted as men, so gender-dependent hormonal differences may play a role in development of the disease. Smoking, obesity, infections, and physical and emotional stress can increase both the chances of getting the disease and the severity of symptoms. More details of the risk factors are listed below:

- Genetic predisposition—People born with specific genes, called human leukocyte antigen (HLA) class II genotypes are more likely to develop rheumatoid arthritis. Environmental factors, such as obesity or smoking, may increase the chances that these genes will be activated.

- Smoking—Multiple studies show that cigarette smoking can increase the risk of developing rheumatoid arthritis and can make the disease symptoms worse.

- Overweight or obesity—Being obese can increase the risk of developing rheumatoid arthritis and studies indicate that there is a correlation between degree of obesity and chances of developing rheumatoid arthritis. Being overweight or obese triggers inflammation because the release of inflammatory proteins, called cytokines, from fat cells aggravate the symptoms of rheumatoid arthritis.

- Infection—There is evidence to suggest that infections such as flu may trigger rheumatoid arthritis.

- Physical and emotional stress—Physical overexertion and emotional stress may cause rheumatoid arthritis symptoms to flare up, possibly due to the release of stress hormones such as cortisol and adrenaline that intensify the immune response.

Since both types of arthritis affect multiple joints and increase inflammation, pain, and stiffness there is a high probability that ROM will be impaired in one or more joints.

Therapies to Improve Range of Motion

The most usual non-surgical treatment for impaired ROM caused by injury and/or inflammation is **physical therapy**. A physical therapist works with patients to create an individualized program to strengthen the muscles around the joint, increase ROM and reduce pain. The program may include several types of interventions such as manual manipulation, therapeutic exercise, functional training, and electrotherapeutic modalities in which sensory nerves are stimulated by frequency-modulated electric current or by lasers or ultrasound. A recent review of non-operative treatment for rotator cuff tears (Edwards et al., 2016) showed support for the use of physical therapy:

Recent studies have suggested that patients opting for physical therapy have demonstrated high satisfaction, an improvement in function, and success in avoiding surgery.

Anti-inflammatory drugs are sometimes used in conjunction with physical therapy to reduce the pain and swelling that contributes to decreased ROM, but it is important that physical therapists are judicious in their use. According to Duchesne et al. (2017):

In summary, anti-inflammatory drugs could have beneficial and adverse effects on muscle regeneration depending on the chronic inflammatory state (local or systemic) and on the type of injury or disease. Thus, anti-inflammatory modalities could be part of a therapeutic strategy along with physical therapy in order to treat chronic disorders, but their use should be carefully selected based on scientific evidence.

Acupuncture is another therapy that is claimed to improve ROM in patients suffering from various forms of arthritis. However, the scientific evidence is not convincing. Only the abstract portions of the few existing publications are readily available, and they are of poor quality, lacking in important information and details. For that reason, they are not discussed in this chapter. The only systematic review of the topic (Green et al., 2005) is limited to the effects of acupuncture on shoulder ROM. Nine research studies were analyzed and only one small study

showed that acupuncture plus exercise was better than just exercise for improving pain, range of motion, and function for up to five months. Overall, the authors concluded:

Due to a small number of clinical and methodologically diverse trials, little can be concluded from this review. There is little evidence to support or refute the use of acupuncture for shoulder pain although there may be short-term benefit with respect to pain and function. There is a need for further well-designed clinical trials.

Massage therapy is also often sought by people with rheumatoid arthritis because it is believed that massage can induce relaxation and encourage gentle joint movement, both of which translate into less pain and improved mood. These claims are supported by scientific evidence, at least with respect to massage for shoulder injuries. A systematic review of the effectiveness of massage on the ROM of the shoulder (Yeun, 2017) based on seven studies and including 237 participants, concluded that massage is effective in improving shoulder flexion and abduction, especially when delivered as sports massage:

Sports massage showed the largest significant effect in all the outcome variables. It includes techniques like effleurage, petrissage, and friction. Effleurage is rubbing the skin lightly from the distal site to the proximal site using the extremities. It reduces edema and promotes muscle relaxation by facilitating the flow of the lymph nodes. Petrissage is performed for the purpose of increasing the movability of the muscle, by twisting the area between the muscle and the skin after holding the soft tissue. Friction is pressing the skin soft tissue deeply using a thumb, by putting it on the bone or on the fascia of the muscle.

However, the authors do mention some limitations of the papers included in their review:

First, as there have not been many randomized controlled trials (RCT), the quality of the studies that were included in the analysis was not high. Later, if more papers that conducted RCT are collected, meta-analysis will need to be performed. Second, the homogeneity of the papers that were included in the analysis was low, and the papers that were included in the analysis were not many; thus, subgroup analysis for the intervention moderators could not be performed.

Usually, if a person's impaired ROM is a result of an injury, their goal is 100% recovery, but in the case of arthritis or the presence of a genetic abnormality, the process cannot be reversed. The aim, then, is to slow down the degenerative joint damage, maintain mobility, minimize pain, and increase overall quality of life. Since emotional stress can cause flare-ups in inflammatory processes that may be contributing to impair ROM, it is a good idea to include **stress reduction therapies** in any treatment plan. Any therapy that induces relaxation will probably also decrease the inflammatory response. As described in Chapter 7, the process of relaxation stimulates the vagus nerve, which inhibits production of inflammatory cytokines that damage the tissue. **Reiki,** especially when practiced in conjunction with deep, slow breathing, as taught by Reiki founder, Mikao Usui, has been shown to stimulate the vagus nerve. So, Reiki is an obvious choice for a stress reduction therapy to help increase ROM. In fact, similar to massage, people often seek out Reiki as a way to reduce the pain related to joint problems and to increase ROM. There is currently just one published scientific study on the topic of the effectiveness of Reiki in increasing the

ROM of impaired joints (Baldwin et al., 2013). This paper is summarized below.

How Reiki, Compared to Other Therapies, Affects Range of Motion

This study (Baldwin et al., 2013) investigates the effect of Reiki compared to sham healing, Reconnective Healing (RH), physical therapy (PT) or rest on 78 people with reduced ROM of arm elevation in the scapular plane resulting from shoulder injuries (structural damage) and/or inflammation. A photograph of a person with limited ROM in the scapular plane is shown in Figure 10.4. The ROM of each arm is described by the angle of the arm to the horizontal. To be included in the study, each participant had to have the ROM of at least one of their arms limited to somewhere between 30° below the horizontal plane and 60° above the horizontal plane. Only people without any experience of energy healing were invited to participate in the trial. Shoulder pain is a common musculoskeletal symptom, accounting for 16% of all musculoskeletal complaints and lifetime prevalence of shoulder pain can range from 7% to 36% of the population.

The participants were randomly assigned to one of the five groups and they received a single 10-minute session

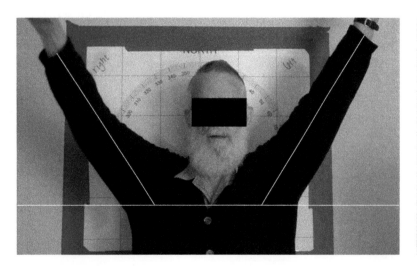

Figure 10.4
Measuring range of motion from a video still. This person has limited ROM in the scapular plane.

(From: Baldwin AL, Fullmer K, Schwartz GE. Comparison of physical therapy with energy healing for improving range of motion in subjects with restricted shoulder mobility. *Evidence-Based Complementary and Alternative Medicine.* 2013; 2013:329731. Figure 2).

of their assigned treatment or control procedure. The mean age for each group was 61.3 ± 53.2(SD) (control), 58.5 ± 59.4 (sham), 64.4 ± 56.6 (PT), 66.6 ± 58.3 (Reiki), and 59.8 ± 52.2 (RH). Each person in the RH group received treatment from one of three Reconnective healers. Reconnective healers work with their hands to sense and manipulate the biofield, or energy field surrounding the patient (Rubik, 2002), and they purportedly tune into the healing energy frequencies needed by each recipient. Unlike Reiki, there is no specific process involved in which practitioners focus on the present moment through concentrating on their breathing. All Reconnective healers receive training from instructors who have followed a prescribed syllabus (see: www.thereconnection.com). People who have received RH anecdotally report a range of sensations including warmth, tingling, cold, and throbbing, as well as physiological responses such as rapid eye movements, deepening breath, stomach gurgling and muscle twitching. The three Reconnective healers selected for this study were experienced instructors from The Reconnection LLC Teaching Team, who train students worldwide. The three chosen Reiki practitioners were Reiki Masters who had been practicing Usui Reiki professionally for a minimum of four years. The three selected licensed physical therapists did not include energy work in their repertoire, had practiced PT for over 10 years, and were experienced in treating complex medical and physical conditions in a range of traditional PT settings. Three people who had absolutely no experience with any form of energy healing were chosen to be sham healers.

All practitioners were instructed not to reveal what type of therapist they were so that the participants would be blinded regarding their treatment type. They were all told that the participants had ROM limitations resulting from shoulder injuries or arthritis. Reconnective healers used mainly hands-off treatment, whereas Reiki practitioners used mainly hands-on treatment for each participant. Physical therapists gave their normal basic manipulation of the shoulder joints and surrounding deep tissue in an attempt to increase shoulder abduction and flexion. Sham healers were asked to wave their hands slowly over the par-

ticipant's shoulder area and upper body, 6–12 inches away from their body and to occasionally draw their hands back away from them, similar to the actions of Reconnective healers. People in the "rest" group lay on a massage table in a quiet room accompanied by a student who sat reading silently.

Pre- and post-measures of ROM were made by asking each participant to stand close in front of a wall, without touching it, with their arms at their sides. They were then video-recorded as they moved their arms out to the sides and then up towards their head, in a scapular plane (not bringing their arms forward) as far as they could go, while keeping their arms straight. Range of motion was measured by video analysis rather than using a goniometer because it is less invasive and because there was no need for the 0.1° accuracy of the goniometer. Participants were asked to rate their degree of pain (by marking their pain level on a horizontal 100 mm scale on which 0 was no pain and 100 was extreme pain), after they had raised their arms to the maximum possible height.

The pre- and post-treatment ROM values for each treatment are shown in Figure 10.5. On average, ROM increased by 3°, 0.6°, 12°, 20° and 26° for control, sham, PT, Reiki, and RH groups, respectively. Statistical analysis showed that sham treatment was no better than the no-treatment control and that *PT, Reiki and RH were all significantly more effective than sham*. The asterisks in Figure 10.5 indicate that the pre/post difference is greater than for sham healing. Reconnective healing was significantly more effective than PT but there was no significant difference between Reiki and PT. The pre- and post-treatment values for self-reported pain for each treatment can be seen in Figure 10.6. On average, the pain score decreased by 0%, 15.4%, 11.5%, 10.1%, and 23.9% for control, sham, PT, Reiki, and RH groups, respectively. Unlike the ROM results, the sham treatment was significantly more effective in reducing pain than the no-treatment control; in fact, none of the other treatments were any more effective than the sham treatment for reducing pain. The asterisks in Figure 10.6 indicate that the pre/post difference is greater than for control. For that reason, the reduction in pain experienced by

Chapter 10

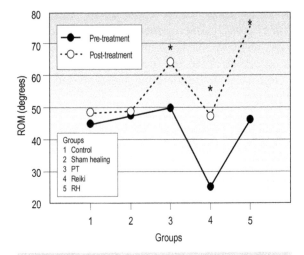

Figure 10.5

Graph showing how Reiki and other modalities affect ROM.

(From: Baldwin AL, Fullmer K, Schwartz GE. Comparison of physical therapy with energy healing for improving range of motion in subjects with restricted shoulder mobility. Evidence-Based Complementary and Alternative Medicine. 2013; 2013:329731. Figure 3).

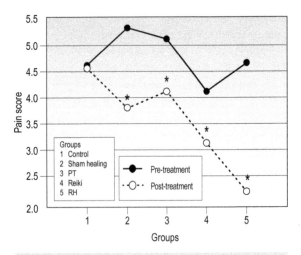

Figure 10.6

Graph showing how Reiki and other modalities affect perceived pain.

(From: Baldwin AL, Fullmer K, Schwartz GE. Comparison of physical therapy with energy healing for improving range of motion in subjects with restricted shoulder mobility. Evidence-Based Complementary and Alternative Medicine. 2013; 2013:329731. Figure 4).

participants apart from those in the no-treatment group can be attributed to the placebo effect. The success of the sham healing in reducing pain was probably stimulated by the expectation of healing arising from the appearance and actions of the sham healer that may have then triggered a release of endogenous opiates or activated the dopaminergic system.

This study shows that Reiki and RH are just as effective as PT at improving ROM and decreasing pain in people with shoulder injuries. These energy healing therapies only involve light or no touch, so if they are as effective as manual manipulation (PT) in improving ROM, this would imply that manual manipulation is not essential for alleviating this particular impairment. However, one limitation of this study is that the results are confined to those seen in a single 10-minute treatment session with no follow-up. Therefore, there is no way of telling whether the beneficial effects of one of the therapies (Reiki, PT, or RH) would last longer than the others. Nevertheless, the results suggest that it would be beneficial for physical therapists to be trained in energy healing as well as PT so that they could reduce the need for manual work on patients, at least in cases of shoulder limitations. In a study addressing job strain in physical therapists (Campo et al., 2009), 58% of the 882 physical therapists interviewed experienced a work-related ache or pain, during the year prior to the survey, that resulted from treating and handling patients. Training physical therapists in Reiki would provide them with another effective tool to benefit their patients and to reduce their own physical workload.

<u>Strengths</u>: This is a randomized, placebo-controlled, double-blinded study in which high-level practitioners were selected for all disciplines. The study is a proof of concept that the use of Reiki or RH is equally as effective as manual manipulation PT in improving ROM in patients with painful shoulder limitation when evaluated immediately after a 10-minute treatment.

<u>Weaknesses</u>: One limitation is that the results are confined to those seen in a single 10-minute treatment session with no follow-up.

Future Research: Further research is needed to determine whether the healing effect of a 10-minute Reiki or RH session is sustained over a time any longer than for a 10-minute PT session. Also, future research into the possible physiological mechanisms to explain the beneficial effects of Reiki in this case would be useful. Once a mechanism can be defined, there is potential for improving the efficacy of Reiki.

Case Study

KC came with immobility in her left arm and osteoarthritis in her fingers; she could not reach very far up her back. She had a 1-hour Reiki session in which she lay supine on the Reiki table for all except for the last 10 minutes, during which time she lay on her stomach. I instructed her to breathe deeper and slower than usual so that she would enter a more receptive state. I gave KC Usui Reiki and sensed a lot of energy entering KC's heart, arms, and hands. KC said she felt very relaxed and she also experienced some tinging sensations. For the last 10 minutes, I placed my hands in contact with KC's shoulders and I felt tingling in my hands, indicating that the Reiki energy was flowing. The session ended with a spinal tension release, in which I placed both palms on KC's spine so that they were aligned with the spine and pointing towards each other. One hand was close to KC's head and the other was at her waist level. With my hands in this position, I waited until my middle-finger pulses were synchronized. After pulse synchronization occurred, I inched my palms closer together and repeated the process.

KC returned 10 days later and reported that her mobility was much improved and that she had been practicing breathing more deeply and slower than she usually did. I gave her a 1-hour session, very similar to before, in which she lay supine most of the time, except for the last 10 minutes when I performed the spinal tension release. Once again, KC said she felt very relaxed and then she left. I did not see KC again for several months. By chance, we met at a social gathering and she mentioned how well she felt, how her mobility had improved, and how useful she found the deep, slow breathing for improving her relaxation.

References

Baldwin AL, Fullmer K, Schwartz GE. Comparison of physical therapy with energy healing for improving range of motion in subjects with restricted shoulder mobility. *Evidence-Based Complementary and Alternative Medicine* 2013; 2013:329731.

Campo MA, Weiser S, Koenig KL. Job strain in physical therapists. *Physical Therapy* 2009; 89(9): 946–956.

Duchesne E, Dufresne SS, Dumont NA. Impact of inflammation and anti-inflammatory modalities on skeletal muscle healing: from fundamental research to the clinic. *Physical Therapy* 2017; 97(8): 807–817.

Edwards P, Ebert J, Joss B, Bhabra G, Ackland T, Wang A. Exercise rehabilitation in the non-operative management of rotator cuff tears: a review of the literature. *International Journal of Sports Physical Therapy* 2016; 11(2): 279–301.

Green S, Buchbinder R, Hetrick SE. Acupuncture for shoulder pain. *Cochrane Database of Systematic Reviews* 2005, Issue 2. Art. No.: CD005319.

Quinn E. Generally accepted values for normal range of motion in joints. Verywell health, Mayo Clinic Hope & Healing. Updated 15 March 2019 (https://www.verywell health.com/what-is-normal-range-of-motion-in-a-joint -3120361).

Rubik B. The biofield hypothesis: its biophysical basis and role in medicine. *Journal of Alternative and Complementary Medicine* 2002; 8(6): 703–718.

Yeun YR. Effectiveness of massage therapy on the range of motion of the shoulder: a systematic review and meta-analysis. *Journal of Physical Therapy Science* 2017; 29(2): 365–369.

Chapter 11
Reiki and Surgery

Pre-Surgery Anxiety

It is natural to feel anxious about surgery and anesthesia because people, in general, fear the unknown and do not like to pass control of their well-being to other people, even if those people are medical experts. Severe anxiety can put one into the fight-or-flight mode and cause unpleasant symptoms, such a pounding and racing heart, irregular heartbeat, nausea, stomach tightness or diarrhea, shortness of breath, and insomnia. In addition, when one is anxious, it is difficult to think clearly and remember instructions that might be important prior to surgery. The sympathetic, arousal-promoting component of the autonomic nervous system is overstimulated at the expense of the parasympathetic, relaxing component. As described in Chapter 5, breathing more deeply and slower than usual rebalances the autonomic nervous system, increasing the activity of the parasympathetic system. This shift promotes a feeling of calm and enhances cognitive skills (Lehrer et al., 2003). Receiving Reiki, in combination with breathing more slowly, adds to one's ability to control anxiety. Several research papers already discussed in Chapter 5 (Friedman et al., 2010; Diaz-Rodriguez et al., 2011) and Chapter 8 (Dressen and Singg, 1998; Baldwin et al., 2017) provide quantitative evidence that receiving Reiki reduces anxiety. Therefore, a Reiki session prior to surgery is likely to be very beneficial for most people who are anticipating surgery. The John Harvey Gray Center for Reiki Healing recommends receiving Reiki prior to surgery for the following reasons:

Since Reiki is a balancing and harmonizing energy, it helps to release stress and tension and places the body in its optimal state for healing. Reiki is not just for physical healing. Reiki works at all levels . . . physical, emotional, mental, and spiritual.

If the person's energy level is in the average or good range, you may give a complete Reiki session the same day or on the eve of the surgery, doing all three Reiki patterns (front of the torso; head, neck and shoulders; back of the torso, back of the knees and the plantar surface of the feet). Administer Reiki in each of the positions for 2–3 minutes each. However, if the person's energy level is low, then it would be more beneficial to them to receive a series of Reiki sessions prior to surgery. Start at least one week prior to surgery, giving daily sessions (same three patterns, 5 minutes per position).

What Problems are Experienced by Patients after Surgery?

After surgery, patients may experience uncomfortable short-term effects from anesthesia, physical trauma, limited mobility, and possible infection. According to the Mayo Clinic (https://www.mayoclinic.org/tests-proce dures/anesthesia/about/pac-20384568), **short-term effects of anesthesia** post-surgery include:

- Nausea

- Vomiting

- Dry mouth

- Sore throat

- Muscle aches

- Itching

- Shivering

- Sleepiness

- Mild hoarseness

Major surgery also imposes **severe trauma** on the body, causing a stress response that stimulates various metabolic and hormonal changes (Burton et al., 2004). The hormonal

Chapter 11

Table 11.1 Table of hormonal changes associated with surgery.				
	Pituitary	**Adrenal**	**Pancreatic**	**Others**
Increased secretion	Growth hormone (GH)	Catecholamines	Glucagon	Renin
	Adrenocorticotropic hormone (ACTH)	Cortisol		
	β-Endorphin	Aldosterone		
	Prolactin			
	Arginine vasopressin (posterior pituitary) (AVP)			
Unchanged secretion	Thyroid stimulating hormone (TSH)			
	Luteinizing hormone (LH)			
	Follicle stimulating hormone (FSH)			
Decreased secretion			Insulin	Testosterone
				Oestrogen
				Tri-iodothyronine (T_3)

(From: Burton D, Nicholson G and Hall G. Endocrine and metabolic responses to surgery. *Continuing Education in Anaesthesia, Critical Care & Pain*, 2004; 4(5): 144-147, Table 2).

changes associated with surgery are summarized in Table 11.1. Note in particular the increased secretion of catecholamines, such as adrenaline and noradrenaline, that increase heart rate; the stress hormone cortisol, that makes the body more sensitive to the effects of catecholamines; and the stress hormone aldosterone, that increases sodium reabsorption into the blood, leading to osmotically-induced water retention in the bloodstream and consequential increases in blood pressure above the normal values.

Pain is very common after surgery and, if the pain is severe, it may slow down the healing process by preventing the person from participating in the gentle, stretching exercises or walking that are necessary to promote recovery. Walking increases the circulation and promotes the flow of oxygen throughout the body, which is essential for wound healing. It also strengthens muscle tone and improves gastrointestinal and urinary tract function. An absence of physical activity leads to sluggish circulation and increases the chances of formation of stroke-inducing blood clots.

Depending on the type of operation that has been performed, individuals, post-surgery, are sometimes instructed to **restrict their movement** or avoid certain activities, such as aerobics, jogging, or swimming, until the bone or tissue heals. This situation can have a significant negative impact on patients' lives, especially when it prevents an individual from driving their car or from attending social activities, and it may lead to **depression**. Individuals who are suffering from depression are less likely to follow a doctor's orders which may impair the healing process and lead to complications.

According to the International Association for Reiki Practitioners:

Every surgical procedure takes a toll on the body, whether it is a minor laparoscopic procedure or a minor surgery. After the procedure is complete, it will take time for the individual to heal. Until healing is complete, the individual cannot return to his or her normal life. In order to speed the recovery, surgical patients often spend time resting, taking medication or participating in various types of therapy. Some people may also schedule Reiki sessions with the goal of encouraging the body to heal more quickly.

How is Post-Surgical Pain Usually Treated?

Post-surgical pain is usually managed with various pain-reducing medicines (analgesics). The type, delivery method, and dose of medication for each individual depends on the type of surgery performed, the expected extent of recovery, and the patient's own needs.

Pain medications, as indicated by the Mayo Clinic (https://www.mayoclinic.org/pain-medications/art-2004 6452) include the following:

- **Opioids:** These are powerful pain medications that diminish the perception of pain. They trigger release of the body's own endorphins which muffle pain and boost feelings of well-being. Examples of opioids are fentanyl, hydromorphone, morphine, oxycodone, oxymorphone, and tramadol.

- **Local anesthetics:** These drugs cause a short-term loss of sensation at a particular area of the body. Examples are lidocaine and bupivacaine.

- **Nonsteroidal anti-inflammatory drugs (NSAIDs):** These are drugs that lessen the inflammatory response which exacerbates pain and swelling. Examples are ibuprofen, naproxen, and celecoxib.

- **Other non-opioid pain relievers** include acetaminophen and ketamine. Side effects include a sedative effect, ranging from mild (feeling sleepy) to severe (not breathing), and nausea or vomiting. They may also cause itching and constipation.

When used as prescribed, most of these pain-relieving medications make surgical procedures more tolerable and speed up recovery. However, if opioids are taken for longer than five consecutive days, they can be addictive. The Centers for Disease Control, USA, guidelines suggest limiting initial opioid prescriptions to three days, stating that opioids for more than seven days "will rarely be needed," except for active cancer, palliative, or end-of-life care. Unfortunately, patients often take their prescribed opioids for longer than this period. According to a recent survey (Kennedy-Hendricks et al., 2016), more than 60% of Americans who are prescribed opioids keep any pills that are left over for future use. The National Institute of Drug Abuse, USA, refers to the current situation as an "Opioid Overdose Crisis":

Every day, more than 130 people in the United States die after overdosing on opioids. The misuse of and addiction to opioids—including prescription pain relievers, heroin, and synthetic opioids such as fentanyl—is a serious national crisis that affects public health as well as social and economic welfare. The Centers for Disease Control and Prevention estimates that the total "economic burden" of prescription opioid misuse alone in the United States is $78.5 billion a year, including the costs of healthcare, lost productivity, addiction treatment, and criminal justice involvement. Since drug use may involve side effects and/or addiction, it is wise to offer patients other therapies to use in conjunction with the prescribed drugs with the aim of reducing drug dosage and length of application. Hospitalized patients who practice mindfulness techniques, such as deep breathing, and change the pain sensations through imagery, report less pain than those who do not (Garland et al., 2017). In fact, about a third of the 244 patients in this study were able to relieve pain by 30%, which is equivalent to taking 5 mg of the opioid oxycodone.

With regard to Reiki, according to the International Association of Reiki Professionals (IARP):

Research studies have shown that Reiki offers a number of different benefits, some of which may be beneficial to people who are recovering from a surgical procedure.

They list the benefits as follows:

1. Reiki may reduce anxiety before and after surgery. "Because anxiety may inhibit the healing process, it stands to reason that reducing anxiety through Reiki sessions may be beneficial to the healing process."

2. Reiki may help or reduce depression after surgery.

3. Reiki may reduce stress levels. "Stress causes inflammation to build up in the body, which may delay healing."

4. Reiki may improve quality of sleep. "When the body is trying to heal from an injury, trauma, or surgi-

Chapter 11

cal procedure, good quality sleep is essential. Reiki produces feelings of relaxation for many clients, and people often report that they experience improved sleep quality after beginning Reiki therapy."

5. Reiki reduces sensations of pain.

The following section reviews the existing research studies related to the effects of Reiki on patients undergoing surgery and presents evidence that supports many of the claims made by IARP.

Studies of Effects of Reiki on Symptoms Post-Surgery

There are currently seven peer-reviewed, published research studies addressing the effects of Reiki on symptoms experienced by patients after surgery. The types of surgery involved are:

- Abdominal hysterectomy (Vitale and O'Connor, 2006)

- Dental surgery in children (Kundu et al., 2014)

- Knee replacement (two papers) (Notte et al., 2016; Baldwin et al., 2017)

- Caesarean (two papers) (Midilli and Eser, 2015; Midilli and Gunduzoglu, 2016)

- Breast cancer (pre-surgery) (Chirico, 2017).

Abdominal Hysterectomy

The purpose of this pilot study was to compare reports of pain and levels of state anxiety in two groups of women (with and without Reiki treatment) after abdominal hysterectomy. The hypothesis of this study was that there would be a greater decrease in pain in subjects adjunctively treated with Reiki touch therapy.

Twenty-two women, ranging in age from 40 to 73 years and scheduled to undergo hysterectomies for non-cancer diagnoses, who were consented for the study, were ran-

domly assigned to one of two groups. Demographic information and medical records were obtained for each participant by the principal investigator. This information was used to check for pre-test differences between individuals in the control and treatment groups. There were no differences between groups on the variables of age, duration of diagnosis, previous hospitalizations, or previous surgeries. Patients in the control group (n=12) received traditional nursing care throughout their length of stay. Patients in the treatment group (n=10) were given three 30-minute Reiki treatments per the study regimen. Reiki treatment was given: 1) In the surgery center after an intravenous drip for surgery had been started; 2) 24 hours postoperatively; and 3) 48 hours postoperatively. Treatments two and three were performed in the patient's room.

Reiki treatments were performed by medical center-employed, registered nurses with a minimum level three certification as a Reiki practitioner and were supervised by a Reiki Master-level registered nurse (RN). For consistency, a standard Reiki hand position protocol was followed with each of 10 hand positions held for 3 minutes each. All participants followed a standard pain medication protocol. Data were collected using the State component of the State-Trait Anxiety Inventory (STAI) and a visual analog 0–10 scale for pain measurement, where 0 represented no pain, and 10 the worst possible pain.

Self-reported pain levels differed in the first 24 hours post-operatively (3.8 for the treatment group versus 5.4 for the control group on a 10-point scale) but not at 48 and 72 hours. Use of pain analgesics by patients was mixed but there was a general lessening of need in the treatment group. Anxiety on the day of discharge was positively affected in the treatment group (a score of 27.00 ± 7.05 (SD) vs 38 ± 9.64 (SD) for control). The length of surgery was longer for the control group than for the treatment group (mean=72 minutes for control group versus mean=59 minutes for treatment group) using the same anesthesia protocol.

<u>Strengths</u>: This was a well-designed, randomized pilot study with suitable control and treatment groups. The

Reiki treatments were standardized with the same Reiki practitioner administering treatment for a given patient. Data collectors were blinded as to the group assignment of patients. The results clearly indicate that Reiki induces a desirable relaxation effect pre-operatively and at 24 hours post-operatively, and also exerts a positive effect on pain levels.

Weaknesses: There was a small number of participants and it was unclear whether the participants had previous experience with Reiki. There was no sham Reiki control group, and so the effects cannot be distinguished from touch therapy alone. As a result, the patients were aware of their group assignment, and so the Reiki group may have had a higher expectation for a positive result.

Future Research: This pilot study supports the need for further and more extensive research on the effects of Reiki in a health care setting. The indication of shorter surgical procedures for patients receiving pre-operative Reiki therapy could have an especially profound impact.

Dental Surgery in Children

The purpose of this study was to examine the effects of Reiki as a complementary therapy, in addition to prescription drugs, for post-operative pain control in pediatric patients undergoing dental surgery. The hypothesis was that a single session of pre-operative Reiki, compared to sham Reiki, would reduce post-operative pain intensity, analgesic requirements of the patients, and the incidence of side effects, as well as improving parent satisfaction. This study was approved by an institutional bioethics committee and signed parental consent was required for each child to participate. Thirty-eight children (aged 9 months to 4 years) were randomly assigned to receive one session, lasting 20–30 minutes, of either Reiki or sham Reiki before surgery. The Reiki practitioners were Reiki Masters and the sham Reiki providers were members of the research team who were not trained in Reiki. All practitioners and providers used the same standardized script to communicate with participants and families, and the same hand positions. After surgery, post-operative pain scores (using

a scale appropriate for pre-verbal children), drug requirements, side effects, and parental satisfaction were assessed by an observer and by the child's assigned nurse. Neither the families nor the data collectors knew the group assignment of each child. The data were analyzed statistically to determine any differences between the two groups.

The blinding process (not telling each participant their group assignment) was successful. Only one quarter of the parents correctly guessed which treatment (Reiki or sham Reiki) their child was receiving. Pain scores and opioid requirement decreased after 30 minutes post-operatively for both groups, and the number of participants also decreased after 30 minutes due to early discharge. The authors state that no statistically significant difference was observed between groups on any outcome measure. However, the results section clearly shows that the dose of pain medication used during the surgery was significantly lower for the Reiki group than for the sham group; this finding was not discussed. The authors concluded that this experiment does not support the effectiveness of Reiki as a complementary therapy for post-operative pain control in pediatric patients.

Strengths: This is one of the few double-blind, randomized controlled studies investigating the effect of Reiki as an addition to opioid therapy for pain control in children. This strong study supports the feasibility of conducting rigorous Reiki research studies with children.

Weaknesses: This was a pilot study and so the sample size is small. Although the authors employed a sham Reiki group, they did not include a control group (i.e. no intervention). This makes it difficult to interpret the results; although there was no statistically significant difference between the Reiki and sham groups, it is possible that both groups would have had significantly lower pain scores and analgesic usage than a control group, but the study design did not allow for this to be tested.

Future Research: Larger studies with both sham Reiki and no-intervention groups are needed to gain useful information about the role of Reiki in reducing post-operative pain. This particular experiment indicated that sham Reiki was just as effective as real Reiki at reducing perceived pain. It would be interesting to design research studies to determine whether touch alone is more effective at reducing pain in young children than in adults. In addition, the use of more objective outcome parameters, such as neuroendocrine and biochemical changes experienced by patients, before and after surgery, with and without Reiki, would strengthen this field of research.

Knee Replacement

Two published studies are available. The study by Notte et al. (2016) will be discussed first. The purpose of this pilot study was to determine the impact of Reiki therapy on patients undergoing total knee arthroplasty (TKA). Specific goals were to investigate whether Reiki treatments reduce perceived pain, decrease the use of pain medication following surgery and improve overall satisfaction with the hospital experience. This study was approved by an Institutional Review Board and subjects gave their consent for participation. The subjects were 43 patients undergoing TKA, who were randomized into either a Reiki (n=23) or a non-Reiki (n=20) group. The Reiki group received one 20-minute session before surgery, one 30-minute session after surgery, and one 20-minute session each on three post-operative days. The non-Reiki group received care as usual. Reiki sessions were given by nurses certified in Reiki. Each patient received their Reiki when they were lying in their hospital bed or sitting in a chair by the bedside. Reiki practitioners placed their hands lightly on, or just above, the subject while the subject was listening to music through headphones. Pain was assessed, using the numeric rating scale, before and after Reiki sessions for the Reiki group, and during normal check-ins for the control group. A questionnaire was distributed on the day of discharge to assess satisfaction with the Reiki and with the hospital experience.

Reiki therapy sessions significantly reduced pain, except during the sessions in the Post-Anesthesia Care Unit (PACU) immediately following surgery. No statistically significant differences were found in pain medica-

tion use between the Reiki and the non-Reiki groups. Participants in both groups rated their hospital experience as good, very good, or excellent.

Strengths: This study suggests that Reiki reduces TKA post-operative pain in a hospital setting, but the evidence is not strong, as described below. On a more encouraging note, as a result of positive feedback and decreased pain ratings following Reiki sessions from this research project, a Reiki program was established at the hospital.

Weaknesses: The same sample size was small; the authors attribute the small number of participants to difficulty with the recruitment process. Unfortunately, although it was stated that pain was assessed in the non-Reiki group using the numerical scale, no data were presented. Another weakness was that the Reiki practitioners who participated in the study were trained to different levels and there was no standardization of the hand positions. In addition, the subjects receiving Reiki also listened to music, whereas the control group did not, and so it is possible that it was the music that caused the reduction in pain intensity rather than the Reiki. The study would have been more valuable if a sham Reiki group had been included. As it was, there was no blinding of the participants regarding knowledge of their group assignment.

Future Research: Larger studies with Reiki, sham Reiki and no intervention groups are essential in order to obtain robust data regarding the effectiveness of Reiki at reducing pain and anxiety before and after surgery. The amount of time for which the benefits are sustained following a Reiki session of given length should also be explored.

The second study of the effects of Reiki on patients undergoing TKA (Baldwin et al., 2017) has already been discussed in Chapter 8 in terms of the resulting alleviation of anxiety. In brief, the purpose was to determine the effectiveness of Reiki at reducing the anxiety of 45 patients undergoing TKA in hospital. The results regarding pain intensity, blood pressure, pain medication, and length of hospital stay are added here. This study is much stronger than the study by Notte et al., for the following reasons. Patients were randomly assigned to one of three groups: Reiki, sham Reiki, or rest. Reiki was provided by three Reiki Master hospital employees and sham Reiki by two other hospital employees who had no knowledge of Reiki. All Reiki and sham Reiki providers used exactly the same hand positions with the patients. Each patient received three or four 30-minute sessions of either Reiki or sham Reiki from the same person and were unaware of which "treatment" they received. The sessions were given 1 hour before surgery and 24, 48 and 72 hours after surgery. Patients in the control group rested during those periods. The data collectors and analyzers were blinded as to the grouping or participants and the group code was not revealed until completion of the analysis.

The following data were collected from patients prior to and after all Reiki sessions or corresponding rest periods: pain level (using the 0–10 visual analog numeric pain rating assessment scale) and blood pressure (BP) (using inpatient data monitors). Anxiety was assessed using the STAI before treatment on the day of surgery and again after the last treatment. As described in Chapter 8, only the Reiki group showed significantly reduced anxiety scores 48 hours after surgery compared to their anxiety level at entry (see Figure 8.3). The Reiki group, but not the sham Reiki or controls, showed significantly decreased pain levels 48 hours after surgery compared to pre-surgery (Figure 11.1). With regard to BP, only the Reiki group showed systolic BP and diastolic BP values that were statistically significantly reduced 48 hours after surgery compared to pre-surgery (Figures 11.2A,B). The decrease in systolic BP was a desirable response in the patients because mean systolic BP was bordering onto hypertension before surgery. The sham Reiki group showed significantly reduced systolic BP, but diastolic BP was not significantly changed. The standard of care group (controls) group showed a trend for reduction of systolic BP but little change for diastolic BP. On the basis of observed trends, it is possible that if the sample sizes for the groups had been larger, there may have been significant reductions in BP for all three groups, suggesting that this effect may not be mediated by Reiki treatment per se. The Reiki group used the lowest number of doses of as-needed pain medication (22 doses or 2.4 doses per

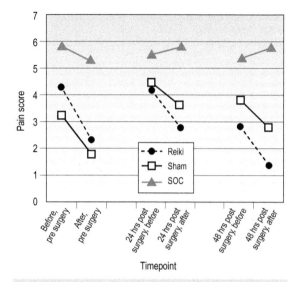

Figure 11.1

Results of pain intensity of patients before and after Reiki, sham Reiki or rest during their hospital stay for knee surgery.

(From: Baldwin AL, Vitale A, Brownel, E, Kryak E, Rand W. Effects of reiki on pain, anxiety, and blood pressure in patients undergoing knee replacement surgery. *Holistic Nursing Practice* 2017; 31(2): 80–89. Figure 1).

patient) compared to the sham Reiki group (36 doses or 6 doses per patient) and the control group (29 doses or 5.5 doses per patient). As shown in Figure 11.3, the Reiki group had the highest number of hospital discharges at 48 hours versus 72 hours after surgery, implying occurrence of fewer complications that would otherwise extend their stay.

Strengths: This was a scientifically rigorous IRB-approved study with randomized, blinded protocols, that included a sham Reiki control group as well as a normal standard of care control. All Reiki practitioners were experienced Reiki Masters who used standardized hand positions that were mimicked by the sham Reiki providers.

Weaknesses: The patient sample size was small; patients were recruited from a single hospital center.

Future Research: This feasibility study supports the pursuit of a multi-center, large-scale clinical trial to evalu-

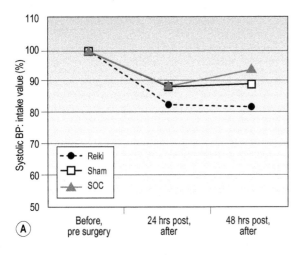

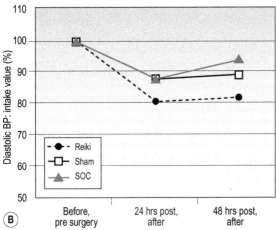

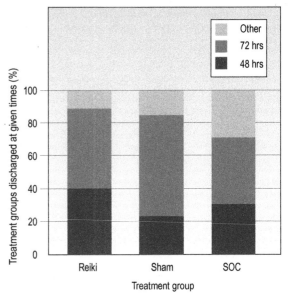

Figure 11.3

Histogram showing percentage of patients discharged at different times after knee surgery as a function of their treatment group.

(From: Baldwin AL, Vitale A, Brownel, E, Kryak E, & Rand W. Effects of reiki on pain, anxiety, and blood pressure in patients undergoing knee replacement surgery. *Holistic Nursing Practice* 2017; 31(2): 80–89. Figure 4.)

Figure 11.2

Results of (**A**) systolic and (**B**) diastolic blood pressure of patients before and after Reiki, sham Reiki or rest during their hospital stay for knee surgery.

(From: Baldwin AL, Vitale A, Brownel, E, Kryak E, Rand W. Effects of reiki on pain, anxiety, and blood pressure in patients undergoing knee replacement surgery. *Holistic Nursing Practice* 2017; 31(2): 80–89.)

ate whether Reiki will be a useful addition to routine care of patients undergoing total knee replacement surgery.

Caesarean Section Surgery

Tulay Sagkal Midilli, RN, PhD is lead author on two studies to determine whether Reiki can reduce the pain and anxiety experienced by women undergoing planned or unplanned Caesarean section surgery (Midilli and Eser, 2015; Midilli and Gunduzoglu, 2016). In both cases, the protocols were approved by an institutional bioethics committee and all participating subjects gave their written consent. The first experiment was performed on 90 women, 18–45 years old who were hospitalized for Caesarean section. They were randomly assigned to Reiki or control (rest only) groups. Reiki or rest period were administered to the patients, in their rooms, within the first 24 and 48 hours post-surgery. Patients in the Reiki group received treatment to each of 10 identified regions of the body for 3 minutes, resulting in a total of 30 minutes of Reiki for each session. The exact hand positions used were based on the study by Vitale and O'Connor (2006) and are listed in Table 11.2. The rest periods for the control group also lasted for 30 minutes. The

Table 11.2 Table listing Reiki hand positions used with patients post-surgery for Caesarean section.

Positions	Place of Reiki application on patient
Approach patient on left side of body	
1. First hand position	Place left hand on patient's Power Chakra*
	Place right hand on patient's Crown Chakra
2. Second hand position	Place right hand on patient's third eye
	Place left hand directly under patient's head
3. Third hand position	Place left hand on patient's Throat Chakra
	Place right hand under patient's neck
4. Fourth hand position	Place left hand on patient's Power Chakra
	Place right hand on patient's Heart Chakra
5. Fifth hand position	Place left hand on patient's lower abdomen
	Place right hand under patient's back (lumbar)
6. Sixth hand position	Place left hand holding patient's left hand
	Place right hand on patient's left shoulder
7. Seventh hand position	Place left hand under patient's left foot (ball of)
	Place right hand under patient's left hip bone
Approach patient on right side of body	
8. Eighth hand position	Place left hand on patient's right shoulder
	Place right hand holding patient's right hand
9. Ninth hand position	Place right hand under patient's right foot (ball)
	Place left hand on patient's right hip bone
10. Tenth hand position	Place right and left palms of hands under patient's feet

*Power Chakra: energy center for self-esteem, self-worth and identity; Crown Chakra: spiritual connection to a higher power; Third Eye: mental processes and intuition; Throat Chakra: energy center for expression, communication and will; Heart Chakra: center for love and relationships. These centers store thoughts, emotions, beliefs, and attitudes regarding the above, and are only 5 of the 7 main midline Chakras, or energy centers, connecting the physical, emotional, mental, and spiritual body.

From: Midilli TS, Eser I. Effects of Reiki on post-Caesarean delivery pain, anxiety, and hemodynamic parameters: a randomized, controlled clinical trial. *Pain Management Nursing*, 16(3):388-399, 2015. Figures 3–5).

researchers were careful to administer the Reiki or rest periods within 4–8 hours of application of postoperative analgesia, to minimize extraneous variables. Pain intensity (visual analog scale), anxiety (state anxiety scale), blood pressure, heart rate, and respiration rate were measured before and after each Reiki or rest treatment. After both treatments, analgesics were provided as needed and the number and dosage recorded.

Patients in the Reiki group showed significantly less pain (76.60% reduction) and anxiety (29.61% reduction) between the first pre-treatment and second post-treatment measurement, as well as a reduced respiration rate. No differences were seen in the control group. The results for pain intensity and anxiety are shown in Figures 11.4 and 11.5. Patients in the Reiki group needed significantly fewer analgesics than those in the control group. Blood pressure and pulse rate were not affected by either treatment.

Strengths: This is a randomized, controlled study that utilizes established outcome parameters and robust statistical methods to provide evidence supporting the use

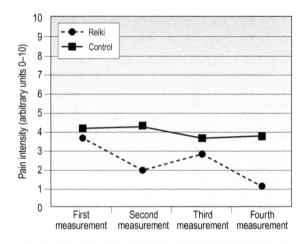

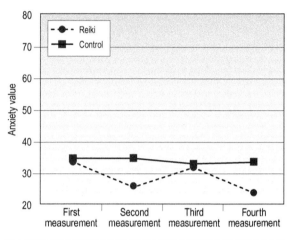

Figure 11.4

Graph showing pain intensity of patients before and after Reiki or rest (control) given 24 hours (first and second measurements) or 48 hours (third and fourth measurements) post-surgery.

(From: Midilli TS, Eser I. Effects of Reiki on post-Caesarean delivery pain, anxiety, and hemodynamic parameters: a randomized, controlled clinical trial. *Pain Management Nursing* 2015; 16(3): 388–399. Figures 3–5.)

Figure 11.5

Graph showing anxiety levels of patients before and after Reiki or rest (control) given 24 hours (first and second measurements) or 48 hours (third and fourth measurements) post-surgery.

(From: Midilli TS, Eser I. Effects of Reiki on post-Caesarean delivery pain, anxiety, and hemodynamic parameters: a randomized, controlled clinical trial. *Pain Management Nursing* 2015; 16(3): 388–399. Figures 3–5.)

of Reiki as a pain and anxiety-relieving method in women after Caesarean delivery.

<u>Weaknesses</u>: Although the Reiki protocol was clearly described, no information was provided about the qualifications and experience of the Reiki practitioners. In addition, the Reiki practitioner also collected the data and so was not blinded as to the group assignment of participants, introducing the possibility of bias. There was no sham Reiki group included to account for the effects of touch alone on patient pain and anxiety; thus, the patients were not blinded as to their treatment type.

The second experiment was performed on 45 women, 18–45 years old who were hospitalized for Caesarean section. This time the study was single-blinded, randomized, and double-controlled. Patients were randomly assigned to Reiki, sham Reiki, and control groups and were unaware of their group assignment (blinded). The term "double-

controlled" refers to the fact that there were two control groups: sham Reiki to control for the touch aspect of Reiki and the no-intervention group. For these reasons, this study was scientifically far more robust than the previous attempt. In this study, instead of administering Reiki to the whole body, Reiki or sham Reiki was only applied for 15 minutes to the incision area within the first 24 and 48 hours after the operation and within 4 to 8 hours of the application of standard analgesics. The control group rested for 15 minutes during these times. Pain severity and vital signs were evaluated immediately before and after the Reiki, sham Reiki, or rest periods. Afterward, the number of hours after each application when patients needed analgesics and the number of doses taken were recorded.

Data analysis revealed that the Reiki group had significantly less pain and less need for analgesics than the sham Reiki and control groups. A reduction in pain of 76.06% was determined in the Reiki group patients between the first pre-treatment and second post-treatment measurement. There was no difference in vital signs; all vital signs of all patients both before and after treatment had normal values. With regard to analgesic use, it was determined that on the first and the second days, patients in the Reiki group felt the need for analgesics later than those in the other two groups. In addition, the Reiki group required a lower number of analgesic doses on the third day than the other two groups.

Strengths: This study is important and moves the field forward since it is a scientifically strong study with methodological excellence, being a single-blinded, randomized, double-controlled study. The results are consistent with other studies suggesting that Reiki reduces pain and contributes relevant empirical data on reduced analgesic usage.

Weaknesses: This was a small study with only 15 patients in each arm of the study. There was no explanation about the specific level of Reiki training by personnel treating patients, and similar to the previous study, the person administering Reiki also collected the data.

Future Research: More studies with larger numbers of participants are needed, in which the frequency and duration of Reiki application are compared, before it can be concluded that applying 15 minutes of Reiki to the incision area after a Caesarean section operation is effective for reducing pain and the number of analgesics requested by each patient.

Breast Cancer (Pre-surgery)

The purpose of this study (Chirico, 2017) was to evaluate Reiki as an intervention in reducing anxiety and improving mood in breast cancer patients pre-surgery and to evaluate the role that self-efficacy for coping with cancer plays in the process. It was hypothesized that: (i) patients in the group receiving Reiki would have a reduced perceived anxiety and an improvement in mood; (ii) patients with high self-efficacy, or coping skills, would have lower

levels of perceived anxiety and more positive mood states; and (iii) those with high self-efficacy would draw more benefit from the Reiki treatment. Women, ages 23–65 and newly diagnosed with breast cancer, were recruited for the study during their pre-surgery hospitalization. All patients were approached by a psychologist who described the research project and presented the informed consent form, together with a document with written information. Fifty-five patients in the intervention group were given 1 hour of Reiki treatment by a Reiki Master on the day prior to surgery. The 55 patients in the standard care group received no Reiki treatments. Both groups completed questionnaires administered by a psychologist trained in diagnostic interviews. The interviews/questionnaires were given to the Reiki group patients on the day prior to surgery just before the Reiki session and just after the session, before sleep. The control group patients participated in their interviews at equivalent times. Mood state was measured by the Profile of Mood States (POMS) inventory. Anxiety was measured by the state form of the STAI.

Study results confirmed all three hypotheses, showing that Reiki therapy as an intervention the day before surgery is effective at improving patients' general well-being and that patients with greater coping skills were better able to manage anxiety regardless of group. Also, patients with greater coping skills demonstrated a more powerful effect of the Reiki intervention on both anxiety and mood than the patients with low coping skills, confirming that a patient's self-efficacy for coping with cancer can influence the effect of a Reiki treatment. The results regarding effects of Reiki on anxiety are shown in Figure 11.6, split between "high coping" and "low coping" individuals. Reiki was associated with reduced anxiety for both coping levels but was more effective for the high-level copers. For people in the control group, there was no change in anxiety for high-level copers, and an increase in anxiety score for low-level copers. The results for mood states are presented in Figure 11.7, in terms of tension, depression, and vigor. Reiki helped reduce tension for both coping levels, but only reduced depression and increased vigor for the

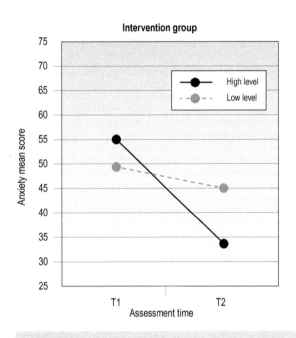
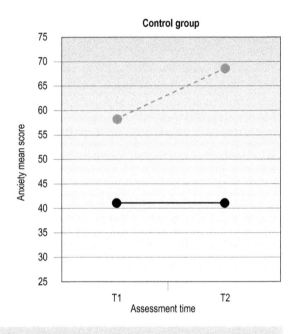

Figure 11.6

Mean anxiety scores of patients before (T1) and after (T2) receiving Reiki one day before surgery for breast cancer compared to those of control group not receiving Reiki. Results are separated according to whether patients have a high or low self-efficacy level, as judged by questionnaire.

(From: Chirico A. Self-efficacy for coping with cancer enhances the effect of Reiki treatments during the pre-surgery phase of breast cancer patients. *Anticancer Research* 2017; 37(7): 3657–3665. Figure 1.)

high-level copers. For individuals in the control group, the high copers showed little change and the low copers showed a slight increase in tension, a marked increase in depression and a small increase in vigor. It is surprising to see increased vigor in the low-level copers of the control group, but in the text, it is actually stated:

The analysis of the simple effects showed that patients of the control group with high levels of self-efficacy showed an increment in their vigor across the time while these levels remain substantially the same in patients with low self-efficacy.

This statement makes more sense and suggests that there was a typing error in the figure. Overall, the authors conclude:

A cancer patient more confident in their ability to cope with the disease-related stressors drew better benefits coming from the Reiki intervention than the patients with lower confidence in coping with the disease stressors.

Strengths: This is a well-designed study that confirms previous findings that Reiki decreases pre-operative anxiety. It also reveals new findings about the importance of a patient's self-efficacy for coping with cancer in optimizing the beneficial effects of Reiki treatment.

Weaknesses: There is no sham Reiki group and so the effects of touch are not separated from those of Reiki, per se.

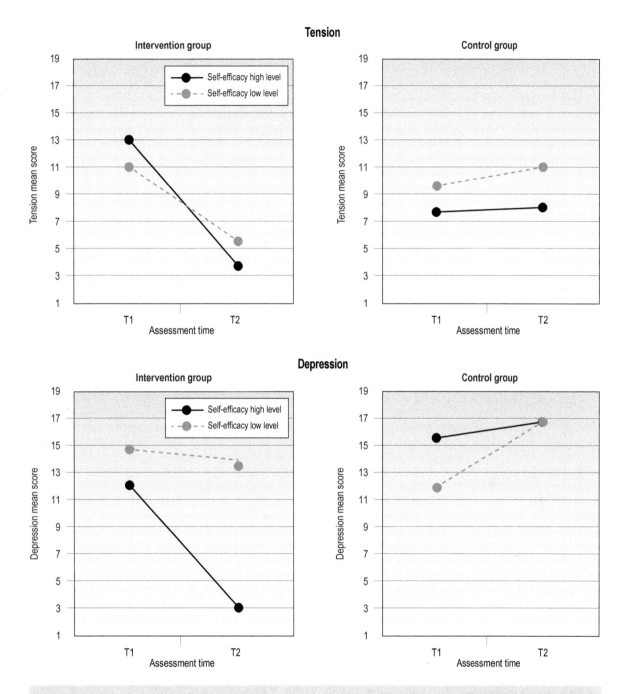

Figure 11.7

Mean scores for tension, depression and vigor (overleaf) of patients before (T1) and after (T2) receiving Reiki one day before surgery for breast cancer compared to those of control group not receiving Reiki. Results are separated according to whether patients have a high or low self-efficacy level, as judged by questionnaire. *(Continued)*

(From: Chirico A. Self-Efficacy for coping with cancer enhances the effect of Reiki treatments during the pre-surgery phase of breast cancer patients. *Anticancer Research* 2017; 37(7): 3657–3665. Figure 2.)

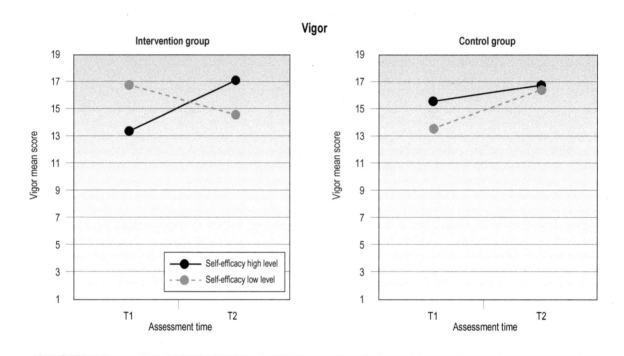

Figure 11.7
(continued)

<u>Future Research</u>: The authors recommend additional larger studies to investigate the effects of Reiki treatment in longitudinal studies with different timing, applied at different points in the cancer trajectories, and taking into consideration the role of self-efficacy in coping with cancer.

Summary

There is strong scientific evidence to recommend the use of Reiki as an adjunct to analgesics in order to reduce pain and anxiety in patients undergoing surgery. Of the six studies in which the effects of Reiki on surgery-related pain were assessed, five of them were positive. All four studies in which the effects of Reiki on anxiety were monitored showed a statistically significant decrease in patients' anxiety following Reiki treatment. All five studies in which levels of analgesic medication requested by the patients were compared between groups showed that Reiki significantly reduced that need. These results are particularly relevant for the fields of Reiki in post-partum care, nursing, and in-patient hospital settings. Given the safety of Reiki and the recent Centers for Disease Control and Prevention and US Food and Drug Administration warnings on Tylenol, NSAIDs, and opioids, an inexpensive method with no known side effects that has statistically meaningful results in strong methodological studies deserves further consideration. Interestingly, comparing these results with those for general anxiety that is not associated with surgery, as described in Chapter 8, Reiki appears to be far more effective in reducing surgery-related anxiety. One possibility for this difference could be that surgery-related anxiety is an acute phenomenon rather than a chronic issue that is perhaps easier to alleviate.

Case Study

LV had early stage cancer in her left breast. She was already trained to first level in Usui Reiki. LV requested a Reiki session to prepare her for a pre-surgery intervention to precisely locate the tumor. The practitioner gave her a 1-hour Karuna Reiki session. The initial scan, with palms moving slowly over LK's body, a few inches away, did not reveal any intense "hot spots". Not much energy flow was felt by the practitioner during the first 5 minutes, but after that, the energy felt much stronger, as indicated by pulsing sensations in the practitioner's hands. The practitioner placed her hands a few inches above LK's breasts and concentrated more on the left breast. Sometimes she felt guided to place one hand on LK's crown or solar plexus. After the session, LK said that she felt the energy flooding through her whole body.

LK returned for another session after she had had the breast surgery. She said that the radiologist had asked whether she was a runner because her heart rate remained low throughout the procedure, and normally the radiologist only sees that in runners. LK was not a runner but practiced Reiki daily. Fortunately, the tumor was only 5 mm in diameter and the lymph nodes were clear. The initial Reiki scan revealed a hot patch over the left breast that had not been detected previously. It is possible that this was due to the surgery. After 30 minutes of Karuna Reiki, the final scan showed a much more uniform energy field. LK said she felt "much more together" and had a positive attitude about the six weeks of radiotherapy she was about to undergo. LK agreed to self-treat herself daily with Reiki. Six years later, LK is cancer-free.

References

Baldwin AL, Vitale A, Brownel, E, Kryak E, Rand W. Effects of reiki on pain, anxiety, and blood pressure in patients undergoing knee replacement surgery. *Holistic Nursing Practice* 2017; 31(2): 80–89.

Burton D, Nicholson G, Hall G. Endocrine and metabolic response to surgery. *Continuing Education in Anaesthesia, Critical Care & Pain* 2004; 4(5): 144–147.

Chirico A. Self-Efficacy for Coping with Cancer Enhances the Effect of Reiki Treatments During the Pre-Surgery Phase of Breast Cancer Patients. *Anticancer Research* 2017; 37(7): 3657–3665.

Diaz-Rodriguez L, Arroyo-Morales M, Fernandez-de-las-Penas C, Garcia-Lafuente F, Garcia-Royo C, Tomas-Rojas I. Immediate effects of Reiki on heart rate variability, cortisol levels, and body temperature in health care professionals with burnout. *Biological Research for Nursing* 2011; 13: 376–382.

Dressen LJ, Singg S. Effects of Reiki on pain and selected affective and personality variables of chronically ill patients. *Subtle Energies and Energy Medicine* 1998; 9(1): 51–82.

Friedman RSC, Burg MM, Miles P, Lee F, Lampert R. Effects of Reiki on autonomic activity early after acute coronary syndrome. *Journal of the American College of Cardiology* 2010; 56: 995–996.

Garland EL, Baker AK, Larsen P, Riquino MR, Priddy SE, Thomas E, Hanley AW, Galbraith P, Wanner N, Nakamura Y. Randomized Controlled Trial of Brief Mindfulness Training and Hypnotic Suggestion for Acute Pain Relief in the Hospital Setting. *Journal of General Internal Medicine* 2017; 32(10): 1106–1113.

Kennedy-Hendricks A, Gielen A, McDonald E, McGinty EE, Shields W, Barry CL. Medication Sharing, Storage, and Disposal Practices for Opioid Medications Among US Adults. *JAMA Internal Medicine* 2016; 176(7):1027–1029.

Kundu A, Lin Y, Oron AP, Doorenboz AZ. Reiki therapy for postoperative oral pain in pediatric patients: Pilot data from a double-blind, randomized clinical trial. *Complementary Therapies in Clinical Practice* 2014; 20: 21–25.

Chapter 11

Lehrer PM, Vaschillo E, Vaschillo B, Lu SE, Eckberg DL, Edelberg R, Shih WJ, Lin Y, Kuusela TA, Tahvanainen KU, Hamer RM. Heart rate variability biofeedback increases baroreflex gain and peak expiratory flow. *Psychosomatic Medicine* 2003; 65(5): 796–805.

Midilli TS, Eser I. Effects of Reiki on post-Caesarean delivery pain, anxiety, and hemodynamic parameters: a randomized, controlled clinical trial. *Pain Management Nursing* 2015; 16(3): 388–399.

Midilli TS, Gunduzoglu NC. Effects of Reiki on pain and vital signs when applied to the incision area of the body after Caesarean section surgery. *Holistic Nursing Practice* 2016; 30 (6), 368–378.

Notte BB, Fazzini C, Mooney RA. Reiki's effect on patients with total knee arthroplasty: a pilot study. *Nursing* 2016; 46 (2): 17–23.

Vitale AT, O'Conner PC. The effect of Reiki on pain and anxiety in women with abdominal hysterectomies. *Holistic Nursing Practice* 2006; 20(6): 263–272.

Chapter 12
Reiki for Pain

Frequent Sources of Pain

There are two major categories of pain: short term (acute) or long term (chronic).

- *Acute pain* is a severe or sudden pain, such as resulting from an injury or a surgery, which resolves within a certain amount of time.

- *Chronic pain* is persistent, lasting for months or even longer, and may be considered a health condition in itself.

Pain occurs when nerve endings become extra sensitive to stimulation, or are damaged by an accident, surgery, infection, or disease. A common form of pain resulting from disease-mediated nerve damage occurs in diabetes in the form of a painful burning sensation in the hands and feet. Some of the most frequent forms of pain are back and neck pain, joint pain (such as arthritis), headaches, pain from an injury, cancer pain, pain from inflammation (such as inflammatory bowel disease), and pain-related conditions such as fibromyalgia (a disorder that causes widespread musculoskeletal pain).

Pain is not just a physical entity, however. An injury or disease that is extremely painful for one person may not bother another. According to the Mayo Clinic (www.mayoclinic.org/understanding-pain/art-20208632):

A person's experience of pain is shaped by the complex emotional and cognitive processing that accompanies the physical damage or sensation. So pain really is in your head as well as your body.

Factors that influence a person's pain perception include:

i.   Genetic factors

ii. Gender – women report more frequent and severe pain than men.

iii. Psychological factors – pain is more prevalent in people with depression, anxiety, or low self-esteem.

iv. Social factors such as stress and social isolation.

v.   Past experiences of painful episodes – such memories make one more sensitive to pain in the present moment.

This psychological aspect of pain makes the study of pain relief particularly susceptible to the placebo effect in which a person's perceived pain is decreased after a fake "treatment" but no active therapy is given. This favorable response is due purely to the patient's belief that they are being given a special treatment that will help them, even if, in reality, they are not. With regard to Reiki, the most common way to distinguish between real and placebo responses is to compare the effects of Reiki to those of sham Reiki, in which a person who is untrained in Reiki performs the same hand positions as the Reiki practitioner. However, although this means of discernment is quite effective, it is not 100% reliable because it is possible that even a person who is untrained in Reiki might have some natural healing ability. Even so, if pain relief occurs through the placebo effect, it is still pain relief, and so the placebo response in itself is valuable, even though it is commonly disparaged.

According to Professor Ted Kaptchuk of Harvard-affiliated Beth Israel Deaconess Medical Center in Boston:

The placebo effect is more than positive thinking – believing a treatment or procedure will work. It's about creating a stronger connection between the brain and body and how they work together.

Placebos may make you feel better, but they will not cure you. They have been shown to be most effective for conditions like pain management, stress-related insomnia, and cancer treatment side effects like fatigue and nausea.

One possible reason why experiencing placebos may reduce symptoms is that the placebo could trigger a release of endorphins. Endorphins have a similar structure to morphine and other opiate painkillers and act as natural painkillers. Pain is a very common problem that interferes with people's ability to take part in their daily activities. In addition, pain can negatively affect relationships and interactions with others especially since it can sap an individual's energy and make one feel less healthy overall. For these reasons it is important to thoroughly explore possible therapies for reducing pain.

Studies of the Results of Reiki on Pain Perception

There are currently 13 peer-reviewed, published papers reporting on Reiki as a pain-relieving therapy. Five of the studies involve pain related to surgery (Vitale and O'Conner, 2006; Midilli and Gunduzoglu, 2016; Notte et al., 2016; Baldwin et al; 2017; Shaybak, 2017). Two studies describe the effects of Reiki on pain that is associated with cancer (Olson et al., 2003; Tsang et al., 2007). The remaining studies relate to back pain (Jahantiqh et al., 2018) and to pain associated with: a variety of chronic illnesses (Dressen and Singg, 1998), age-related disorders (Richeson et al., 2010), diabetic neuropathy (Gillespie et al., 2007) and movement of the arms in people with shoulder issues (Baldwin et al., 2013). One other study mentioned in Chapter 8 (Bremner et al., 2016) that investigates the effect of simultaneous Reiki *and* music on various outcomes, including pain, is not included in this chapter because there was no Reiki alone group. Another study mentioned in Chapter 11 (Kundu et al., 2010) that explored the effect of Reiki on post-surgical pain and anxiety in children undergoing dental surgery is also not included because it only included Reiki and sham Reiki groups and therefore had no standard of care control group with which to compare.

Effects of Reiki on Pain Related to Surgery

All of the papers that fit this category, except for Shaybak, 2017, were described in Chapter 11. The previously reported papers all demonstrated that Reiki was significantly more effective than the control procedures at reducing surgery-related pain. Surgeries included were hysterectomy (Vitale and O'Connor, 2006), Caesarean section (Midilli and Gunduzoglu, 2016) and knee replacement surgery (Notte et al., 2016; Baldwin et al., 2017).

The purpose of the Shaybak study was to determine the effect of Reiki on pain associated with the incision site in the saphenous vein (superficial vein in the leg) after coronary artery bypass grafting (CABG). Current methods used for non-narcotic and narcotic pain management, as well as unrelieved pain, can cause dangerous states for patients after heart surgery, and may lead to potentially longer hospital stays. Forty patients were randomly assigned to Reiki and sham Reiki groups for four days, on average, after their CABG operation. These patients had provided verbal and written consent to be included in the study. The mean age of the control and intervention groups were 59.05 ± 6.16(SD) and 61.55 ± 7.01(SD) years, respectively. Sixty percent of patients in both the intervention and control groups were male. The patients received Reiki from a Reiki Master, and sham Reiki from a nurse untrained in Reiki, from a distance of two feet, towards the whole body for 6 minutes and towards the root chakra for 3 minutes. The intensity of pain was assessed before and after the Reiki or sham Reiki using the Visual Analog Scale. The *sensory* (how the pain feels) and *affective* (how pain affects emotions) qualities of pain were also assessed at the same times using the short and modified version of the McGill Pain Questionnaire (MPQ). Typical items describing the sensory aspects are "throbbing", "shooting", and "stabbing". The four words used to assess the affective quality are: "tiring/exhausting", "sickening", "fearful", and "punishing/cruel". All these items were scored by the patient on a four-point scale from "none" to "severe". The post-intervention score for pain sensory quality was significantly lower for the Reiki group than for the sham Reiki group (1.31 vs 2.13; $p = 0.019$) after controlling for confounding variables, indicating that the Reiki produced some relief. However, no statistically significant difference was found between the two groups in the mean scores of pain severity and affective quality of pain in the legs.

Strengths: This study confirms previously published research that Reiki is an effective non-pharmacological option for pain relief. Another strength is the use of non-touch Reiki treatment eliminating the possibility of pain relief through light touch.

Weaknesses: The weaknesses are as follows: no standard of care group was included; Reiki and sham Reiki sessions were not offered until the fourth day after surgery; the sessions only lasted 9 minutes and that very brief amount of time was, on occasion, interrupted by nursing and medical care; the patients may have been more focused on chest pain rather than leg pain.

Future Research: It is significant to note that these positive results were achieved with so brief a Reiki session, under such conditions. This study validates the need for a larger scale study (adjusting for the above weaknesses) on non-touch Reiki for pain relief after surgery.

Effects of Reiki on Pain Associated with Cancer

The purpose of the study by Olson et al., 2003 was to determine whether Reiki has beneficial effects on pain, quality of life, and analgesic use in cancer patients undergoing palliative treatment. The participants were cancer patients receiving palliative care for pain (nine males, average age 59.5 and 15 females, average age 56). The experimental protocol was approved by an institutional ethics committee and written consent was obtained from the patients included in the study. One group (n=13) received pain medications (opioids) with rest and the other group (n=11) received pain medications (opioids) with Reiki therapy. Participants either rested or received Reiki for 90 minutes on days 1 and 4 according to group assignment. In both cases, these interventions occurred 1 hour after the patients' first afternoon analgesic dose. Reiki was given hands-on by a Usui Reiki master to 18 specific areas of the body for 90 minutes. Quality of life (QOL) was assessed using a multi-dimensional questionnaire on days 1 and 7.

The following measures were performed before and after Reiki or rest: self-reported pain evaluation using the Visual Analog Scale (10-point); blood pressure; heart rate; respiration rate; analgesic use. Statistical comparisons were applied to data from both groups.

Reiki therapy intervention used with cancer patients resulted in a significant decrease in pain compared to the control group on days 1 and 4 (Tables 12.1 and 12.2). Diastolic blood pressure and heart rate also decreased significantly in the Reiki group, but not the control group, on day 1, but the differences were not statistically significant on

Table 12.1 Pain, blood pressure, heart rate, and pulse for Arm A and Arm B on day 1					
	Arm A (Opioid plus rest)		Arm B (Opioid plus Reiki)		
Variable	Before	After	Before	After	Kruskal-Wallis Comparing Change in Arm A and Change in Arm B
Pain (10 cm VAS)	4.5	4.2	4.5	3.3	$P = 0.035$
Systolic blood pressure (mm Hg)	109	108	121	117	ns
Diastolic blood pressure (mm Hg)	64	65	72	68	$P = 0.005$
Heart rate (beats/minute)	80	80	78	71	$P = 0.019$
Respirations (breaths/minute)	18	18	17	17	ns

(From: Olson K, Hanson J, Michaud M. A phase II trial of Reiki for the management of pain in advanced cancer patients. *Journal of Pain Symptom Management* 2003; 26(5): 990–997. Figures 2–4).

day 4. The psychological component of QOL was significantly improved on day 7 compared to day 1 for the Reiki group only (Table 12.3).

Strengths: Overall, the study design was good in that a control group was included and some statistically significant findings were obtained. Only one Reiki practitioner was used for all patients, providing consistency in the study. In addition, the Reiki sessions lasted as long, or even longer than, a normal Reiki session. Physiological and psychological measures were obtained from the participants and the data were analyzed using standard statistical analysis.

Weaknesses: There was no sham Reiki group and so it is not possible to separate the effects of Reiki from the effects of touch. Only a small number of patients participated in the study and they all knew their group assignment, so the Reiki group may have had an inherent expectation of a positive result.

Additional Note: There was difficulty in recruiting a larger number of participants because of reluctance by eligible patients to be placed in the non-Reiki treatment group. As a result of this study, Reiki is now offered by volunteers, free of charge, on the inpatient palliative unit that was the primary recruitment site.

Future Studies: The results of this study justify spending resources on further research with larger numbers of participants and inclusion of a sham Reiki group.

Table 12.2 Pain, blood pressure, heart rate, and pulse for Arm A and Arm B on day 4					
	Arm A (Opioid plus rest)		**Arm B (Opioid plus Reiki)**		
Variable	**Before**	**After**	**Before**	**After**	**Kruskal-Wallis Comparing Change in Arm A and Change in Arm B**
Pain (10 cm VAS)	3.8	3.7	3.9	2.4	*P* = 0.002
Systolic blood pressure (mm Hg)	113	112	119	116	*ns*
Diastolic blood pressure (mm Hg)	65	65	71	67	*ns*
Heart rate (beats/minute)	78	77	78	76	*ns*
Respirations (breaths/minute)	18	17	17	16	*ns*

(From: Olson K, Hanson J, Michaud M. A phase II trial of Reiki for the management of pain in advanced cancer patients. *Journal of Pain Symptom Management* 2003; 26(5): 990–997. Figures 2–4).

Table 12.3 Quality of Life data for day 1 and day 7					
	Arm A (Opioid plus rest)		**Arm B (Opioid plus Reiki)**		
Subscale	**Day 1**	**Day 7**	**Day 1**	**Day 7**	**Kruskal-Wallis Comparing Change in Arm A and Change in Arm B**
Psychological (10 cm VAS)	5.1	5.1	5.4	6.2	*P* = 0.002
Social (10 cm VAS)	2.8	2.9	3.0	3.0	*ns*
Physical (10 cm VAS)	6.7	6.7	7.0	7.5	*ns*

(From: Olson K, Hanson J, Michaud M. A phase II trial of Reiki for the management of pain in advanced cancer patients. *Journal of Pain Symptom Management* 2003; 26(5): 990–997. Figures 2–4).

The study by Tsang et al. (2007) examined the effects of Reiki on fatigue, pain, anxiety, and overall QOL in 16 patients (13 female, median age 59) experiencing cancer-related fatigue, an extremely common side effect in patients undergoing cancer treatment and recovery. All patients consented for this trial, which was approved by a university research ethics committee. These patients had recently completed chemotherapy treatment and scored 3 or higher on the Edmonton Symptom Assessment System (ESAS) tiredness questionnaire item. A unique aspect of this study compared to others was that the longevity of the effects of Reiki on patient symptoms was also assessed. This was a two-arm, randomized, counterbalanced, crossover study as depicted in Figure 12.1. Group A (n=8) received five consecutive daily Reiki treatments followed by a one-week "washout" period, two additional Reiki treatments, and then two weeks of no treatments. The "washout" period was included to determine to what degree the measured effects of the first five Reiki treatments were sustained over the week. Patients then switched over and participated in the "rest" protocol. Group B (n=8) began with resting for approximately 1 hour per day for five consecutive days followed by a one-week washout period of no scheduled rest and then an additional week of no treatments. Patients then crossed over and participated in the Reiki protocol described above. The Reiki practitioner was an Usui Reiki master with over 10 years of experience, including working with cancer patients. On average, each Reiki or rest session lasted 45 minutes. Before and after each Reiki session or rest period, participants completed ESAS questionnaires to monitor daily tiredness, pain, and anxiety. Before and after each treatment arm, participants completed Functional Assessment of Cancer Therapy Fatigue subscale (FACT-F) and Functional Assessment of Cancer Therapy, General Version (FACT-G) questionnaires to assess overall fatigue levels and general QOL. All are considered reliable instruments for collecting this kind of data in clinical trials. Patients mailed in their questionnaires at the end of each phase of the study.

Regarding incremental, day-to-day effects of Reiki or rest on fatigue, pain, or anxiety, there was a significant reduction in all areas in the Reiki condition and no statistically significant changes in the resting group. Pain scores

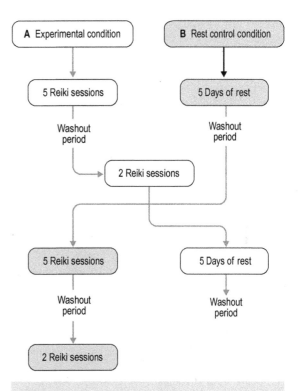

Figure 12.1

Flow chart showing Reiki and rest protocol for patients experiencing cancer-related fatigue.

(From: Tsang K, Carlson L, Olson K. Pilot crossover trial of Reiki versus rest for treating cancer-related fatigue. *Integrated Cancer Therapy* 2007; 6 (1): 25–35. Figure 1).

for the Reiki condition, pre-five-day treatment vs post were 2.44 ± 2.45 (SD) vs 0.88 ± 1.50. Corresponding scores for the rest condition were 2.20 ± 2.60 (SD) vs 1.67 ± 2.29, which did not constitute a significant change. There was a significant difference in change scores between the Reiki and rest conditions in the pre- and post-treatment general cancer assessment tests indicating that the Reiki condition resulted in overall improved quality of life over and above that associated with rest alone. The beneficial effects of Reiki on fatigue, pain, and anxiety lasted longer than the monitored washout period of seven days.

<u>Strengths:</u> This pilot project adds valuable information about the time course of potential benefits of Reiki to

the body of research on cancer-related pain, fatigue, and anxiety.

Weaknesses: Problematic aspects of this study include the absence of a sham Reiki arm. Participants were not blinded regarding their treatment type, and there was little or no oversight of participants when at home during a rest period. Also, the treatments were somewhat variable in length, and the research endpoints consisted of written questionnaires as opposed to objective physiologic measurements. In addition, it is not clear that the effect size was clinically relevant due to the small number of participants. Finally, the day-to-day pre and post scores for pain over each of the five Reiki days were not included in the results, and so it is not known whether all the benefit occurred on the first day and then stabilized, or if the benefit accrued gradually.

Future Research: A finding of interest is the sustained effects of the Reiki treatments suggesting that future studies should allow for a longer washout period than seven days to test for longer duration of benefits.

Effects of Reiki on Pain from Other Sources

Back Pain (Jahantigh et al., 2018)

The purpose of this study was to determine the effectiveness of Reiki, compared to physiotherapy or to standard of care (SOC), in relieving lower back pain and improving the activities of daily living (ADL) in 60 patients who had intervertebral disc hernia (IVDH). The patients were randomly assigned to one of the three groups. Patients in the Reiki group received a 15-minute distant Reiki session by a Reiki master on three consecutive days. Participants in the physiotherapy group underwent 7 to 10 sessions of physiotherapy for 60–90 minutes. Patients in the SOC group received 75mg indomethacin and 50mg methocarbamol every 8 hours, as did the patients in the other two groups. Data were collected using a demographics survey, the Visual Analog Scale for pain, and the Instrumental ADL (ADL-IADL) questionnaire.

There were no significant differences in the demographic data among the study groups. Pain was significantly reduced (p<0.002), and ADL significantly improved (p<0.011) in the Reiki group compared to the SOC group. There was no significant difference in the participants' average pain level or ADL score post-treatment between physiotherapy and Reiki groups. The authors concluded that Reiki and physiotherapy are both effective methods in managing pain and improving ADL in patients with IVDH. However, Reiki is a more cost-effective and faster treatment method than physiotherapy.

Strengths: The sample size was adequate for pilot data and reliable scales were used for measuring pain and ADL.

Weaknesses: The Reiki group only received three 15-minute distant Reiki sessions whereas the physiotherapy group received 7-10 sessions each lasting 60-90 minutes. It was not stated whether the data analyst was blinded with respect to the data grouping and there was no mention of the experience level of the Reiki Master.

Various Chronic Diseases (Dressen and Singg, 1998)

As described in Chapter 8, the purpose of the study by Dressen and Singg (1998) was to test the effects of Reiki on pain, depression, and anxiety in 120 self-selected patients who were chronically ill with a variety of medical conditions including headaches, coronary heart disease, and cancer. Patients were randomly assigned to one of four groups: Reiki, sham Reiki, Progressive Muscle Relaxation (PMR) and control (no therapy). All groups except the control group received 10 bi-weekly, 30-minute sessions of their treatment. Three months after the post-testing, the Reiki group participants were contacted for the follow-up testing to examine the differences in mean scores between the post-test and follow-up measures. The overall pain intensity was measured using the five-point rating scale, Present Pain Intensity (PPI) included in the MPQ. This scale provides pain ratings ranging from 1 to 5 as follows: 1– mild, 2 – discomforting, 3 – distressing, 4 – horrible, and 5 – excruciating. Three other dimensions measuring the quality of pain were also included from the MPQ: sensory, affective, and evaluative. Sensory relates to the feeling of the pain (throbbing, sharp), affective to the emotional impact (cruel, vicious), and evaluative to the cognitive

McGill Pain Questionnaire

Patient's name _____ Date _____ Time _____ am/pm

PRI S _____ A _____ E _____ M _____ PRI(T) _____ PPI _____

(1–10) (11–15) (16) (17–20) (1–20)

Flickering ☐	Tiring ☐
Quivering ☐	Exhausting ☐
Pulsing ☐	
Throbbing ☐	Sickening ☐
Beating ☐	Suffocating ☐
Pounding ☐	
	Fearful ☐
Jumping ☐	Frightful ☐
Flashing ☐	Terrifying ☐
Shooting ☐	
	Punishing ☐
Pricking ☐	Gruelling ☐
Boring ☐	Cruel ☐
Drilling ☐	Vicious ☐
Stabbing ☐	Killing ☐
Lancinating ☐	
	Wretched ☐
Sharp ☐	Blinding ☐
Cutting ☐	
Lacerating ☐	Annoying ☐
	Troublesome ☐
Pinching ☐	Miserable ☐
Pressing ☐	Intense ☐
Gnawing ☐	Unbearable ☐
Cramping ☐	
Crushing ☐	Spreading ☐
	Radiating ☐
Tugging ☐	Penetrating ☐
Pulling ☐	Piercing ☐
Wrenching ☐	
	Tight ☐
Hot ☐	Numb ☐
Burning ☐	Drawing ☐
Scalding ☐	Squeezing ☐
Searing ☐	Tearing ☐
Tingling ☐	Cool ☐
Itchy ☐	Cold ☐
Smarting ☐	Freezing ☐
Stinging ☐	
	Nagging ☐
Dull ☐	Nauseating ☐
Sore ☐	Agonizing ☐
Hurting ☐	Dreadful ☐
Aching ☐	Torturing ☐
Heavy ☐	
	PPI
Tender ☐	0 No Pain ☐
Taut ☐	1 Mild ☐
Rasping ☐	2 Discomforting ☐
Splitting ☐	3 Distressing ☐
	4 Horrible ☐
	5 Excruciating ☐

Brief ☐	Rhythmic ☐	Continuous ☐
Momentary ☐	Periodic ☐	Steady ☐
Transient ☐	Intermittent ☐	Constant ☐

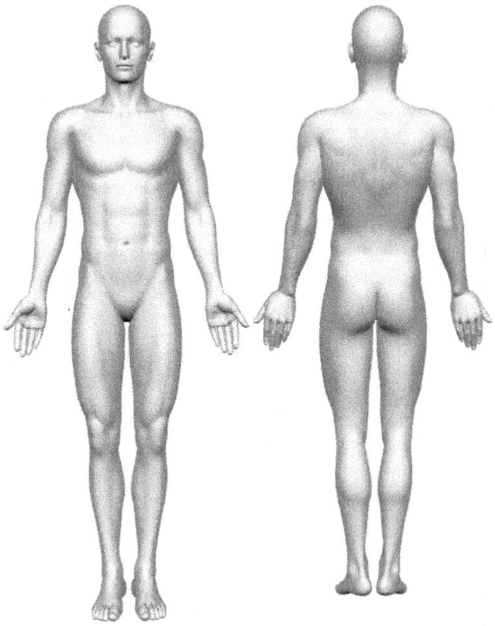

E = External
I = Internal

Comments

Figure 12.2

The McGill Pain Questionnaire.

(From: NIH/Warren Grant Magnusen Clinical Center).

Chapter 12

aspect (annoying, unbearable). A copy of the full MPQ is shown in Figure 12.2. There is strong support for the reliability, validity and consistency of the MPQ.

The Reiki group showed the largest decrease in pain intensity (2.26 to 0.86), pain sensory quality (13.08 to 8.80), and pain evaluative aspect (2.71 to 1.11), but not in pain affective quality or pain total scale. However, after three months there were further significant decreases in all pain measures. According to the authors:

These findings showed two things: first, that gains made by the recipients of Reiki were maintained over longer period of time, and second, that in case of two pain variables (PRI R: affective and PRI-R: total scale) that did not show significant pre-test to post-test change, significant reduction in pain did take place at three-month follow-up testing.

In addition, as indicated by their "Post-Research Comments", the authors appeared to be surprised about the effectiveness of Reiki in improving the pain perception and mood of their chronically ill patients:

We were amazed with several things while completing this study. First, the willingness on the part of medical and mental health professionals to refer patients for this research project was most encouraging. Second, the subjective accounts of benefits of Reiki from most participants coincided with the subjective accounts presented by others in Reiki literature. One of the most astonishing reports came from an HIV-positive patient whose lab work following only two of the 10 Reiki treatments indicated a dramatic rise in CD4 cell count. Third, in all her academic career of over 20 years, present co-author Singg had never experienced such a low dropout rate in any other experiment as was the case in the present study. Participants in all groups were most motivated to receive Reiki. One reason might be the need to reduce chronic pain associated with their medical conditions.

Pain, Depression and Anxiety in the Elderly (Richeson et al., 2010)

This pilot study evaluated the effects of Reiki on pain, depression, and anxiety in older adults living in a com-

munity setting. Twenty volunteers (age 55 or older, with medical diagnosis of pain, depression, and/or anxiety) were randomized into an experimental or wait-list control group. All participants read and signed an informed consent form approved by the university's Institutional Review Board prior to participating in the study. The experimental group received Reiki for 30 minutes once per week for eight weeks; the control group was offered Reiki only after the study had concluded. Both Reiki practitioners were Reiki Masters with eight to 10 years of experience. The researchers' goal was to study the effect of Reiki on pain, depression, anxiety, heart rate (HR), and blood pressure (BP) in older adults. Before and after the eight-week period, the following outcome parameters were measured: Faces Pain Scale (FPS); HR; BP; Geriatric Depression Scale (GDS-15); Hamilton Anxiety Scale (HAM-A). In addition, those receiving Reiki were asked five interview questions to obtain descriptions of their experiences; one of the authors analyzed the content and created categories for recurring phrases.

As shown in Table 12.4, the Reiki group showed significant improvement on measures of pain, depression, and anxiety, but no statistically significant changes in blood pressure or heart rate. The most common experiential description was "relaxation" following Reiki treatments. Selected participant quotes were:

- "Very relaxed after Week 1; felt peace of mind... relaxed and joyful after Week 3."
- "Best hour of the week."
- "Peaceful and relaxing."
- "Effects of relaxed feeling lasted longer after the second treatment."
- "Complete relaxation after Week 1."
- "Relaxed, like a pink cloud surrounds me all day after treatment."

Strengths: This trial explored a different sample population (community-based older adults). Multiple Reiki ses-

Table 12.4 Results related to pain, depression, anxiety, heart rate, and blood pressure (n=20)

Measure	Experimental Group (n = 12)			Control Group (n = 8)		
	Pretest	Post-test	p Value[a]	Pre-test	Post-test	p Value[a]
	Median (IQR) Mean (SD)	Median (IQR) Mean (SD)		Median (IQR) Mean (SD)	Median (IQR) Mean (SD)	
GDS-15	7.5 (4.0) 7.8 (3.7)	3.5 (5.5) 5.0 (4.4)	0.0005*	4.0 (4.0) 4.3 (3.4)	5.0 (7.0) 6.1 (4.5)	0.0313*
HAM-A	21 (23.5) 25.2 (14.4)	10 (19.5) 17.5 (15.5)	0.0005*	18.0 (17.0) 21.2 (12.9)	28.0 (21.5) 28.5 (13.5)	0.0313*
FPS	3 (2.5) 4.8 (1.3)	1 (2.0) 2.2 (1.2)	0.0078*	2.5 (1.5) 5.0 (1.3)	4.0 (2.0) 7.6 (1.2)	0.0156*
HR	65 (14.5) 65.0 (8.4)	62 (7.0) 64.1(4.2)	0.7793	62.0 (11.0) 64.0 (6.5)	62.0 (8.0) 63.2 (6.1)	1.00
	n (%)	n (%)	p Value[b]	n (%)	n (%)	p Value[b]
BP						
Good	5 (41.67)	6 (50)	0.3679	6 (75)	2 (25)	0.3679
At risk	6 (50)	6 (50)		4 (25)	4 (50)	
High risk	1 (8.33)	0 (0)		0 (0)	0 (0)	

[a] p values based on the one-sample (Fisher's exact) rank test.
[b] p values based on the generalized McNemar's test (Stuart-Maxwell test).
* Significant at p < 0.05.

(From: Richeson NE, Spross JA, Lutz K, Peng C. Effects of Reiki on anxiety, depression, pain and physiological factors in community-dwelling older adults. *Research in Gerontological Nursing* 2010; 3(3): 187–199. Table 1).

sions were provided to each participant. Both quantitative and qualitative outcome parameters were used, resulting in both precise, objective data as well as information about the participants' subjective experiences.

Weaknesses: The sample size was small and there was no sham Reiki group so the positive effects could have been due to touch. There was no blinding of subjects or data collectors regarding the group assignment of participants. The Reiki treatment was not standardized with each participant but given according to "participant need". One of the two Reiki practitioners was part of the research team. Most disappointing was the lack of data collection before and after each of the eight sessions which would have given a timeline of Reiki's effects on the participants. For that reason, it is not possible to tell whether the whole of each beneficial effect of Reiki was manifested after the first week and then plateaued, or whether the improve-

ment was additive and took several weeks. Another possibility could be that the benefits occurred after a single session but were temporary and restored after each subsequent session.

Diabetic Neuropathy (Gillespie et al., 2007)

The purpose of this study was to determine whether Reiki would alleviate pain and improve mobility and QOL in subjects with type 2 diabetes and painful diabetic neuropathy (PDN). Two hundred and seven subjects with these disorders were recruited and randomly assigned to one of three treatment groups: Reiki (93 subjects), sham Reiki (88 subjects) or usual care (26 subjects). The groups were well-matched with respect to age, gender, years with diabetes and hemoglobin A1c concentration (which evaluates the amount of glucose in the blood). Participants in the Reiki and sham Reiki groups were blinded as to their group assignments and had two 25-minute sessions the first week followed by weekly treatments for the rest of the 12-week period. The sham Reiki practitioners were actors trained to mimic the Reiki practitioners. Patients in the usual care group were just assessed at the start and end of the 12-week period. The primary outcome was the MPQ. Secondary end points were a 6-minute walk test, the Epidemiology Diabetes Intervention and Complications QOL Questionnaire, the Well-Being Questionnaire, and the Diabetes Treatment Satisfaction Questionnaire. Compared to the baseline results, the total score for pain descriptors improved significantly for both the Reiki and sham Reiki groups but not for the usual care group. Global pain scores and walking distance improved from baseline in both Reiki and sham Reiki groups, but there was no significant difference between Reiki and sham Reiki. Reiki was no more effective than sham Reiki at decreasing pain perception and improving walking distance in subjects with PDN. However, the authors did recognize that these results highlighted the importance of the partnership between the healthcare provider and the patient in optimizing their well-being:

However, the reduction of pain symptoms observed in both treatment groups is consistent with the concept that the formation of a "sustained partnership" between the healthcare provider and the patient can have direct therapeutic benefits.

Strengths: This was a randomized, blinded, placebo-controlled study with sham Reiki and no-intervention groups which included a fairly large number of participants. The reduction of symptoms observed in both the Reiki and sham Reiki groups is consistent with some other studies relating to pain alleviation, and with the concept that a sustained partnership between the healthcare provider and the patient can have direct, therapeutic benefits.

Weaknesses: Possible limitations include relatively low pain scores at baseline in all the groups and the inability to retain the subjects in the usual care group. Another weakness was the lack of information about the credentials of the Reiki practitioners.

Shoulder Issues (Baldwin et al., 2013)

As described in Chapter 10, the purpose of this research was to compare the efficacies of Reiki, sham Reiki, Reconnective Healing (RH) and physical therapy (PT) in improving limited range of motion (ROM) of arm elevation in the scapular plane, and in reducing the pain experienced during this movement. All the participants were diagnosed with shoulder injuries (structural damage) and/or inflammation. Treatments were only given for 10 minutes in a single session. The pre- and post-treatment values for self-reported pain for each treatment can be seen in Figure 10.6. On average, the pain score decreased by 0%, 15.4%, 11.5%, 10.1%, and 23.9% for control, sham, PT, Reiki, and RH groups, respectively. Similar to the study on pain related to diabetic neuropathy (Gillespie et al., 2007), the sham Reiki treatment was just as effective as Reiki in reducing the pain experienced by participants, who had shoulder injuries or inflammation, as they raised their arms.

Summary

Every one of the 13 studies investigating the effects of Reiki on pain perception showed that the subjects who received Reiki experienced statistically significant lower self-reported levels of pain than those who received standard care. Seven of the studies included a sham Reiki group for comparison, and of those seven, three (Gillespie et al., 2007; Baldwin et al., 2013; Jahantiqh et al., 2018) demonstrated that Reiki was not significantly better than sham Reiki and, in two cases, not significantly more effective than physical therapy. These results demonstrate for sure that there is a placebo component to Reiki's ability to control pain perception. People in pain are usually comforted by the presence of a person who appears to be trying to help them by offering light touch. A scientific study (Goldstein et al., 2016) highlighted the powerful analgesic effect of social touch and also suggested that empathy between partners may explain the pain-alleviating effects of social touch. A more recent paper (Hein et al., 2018) confirmed that if a person in pain is physically touched by another person, their perceived pain is lessened. Interestingly, in this experiment, if the person touching them was a stranger, the beneficial effect was greater than if they were a friend. Not only did the people being touched report lower levels of pain, but brain imaging indicated less activation of the regions of the brain corresponding to the actual pain response. The authors hypothesized that the people in pain did not expect to receive help from a stranger, were pleasantly surprised, and so the pain-relieving effect of touch was boosted.

On the other hand, four studies (Dressen and Singg, 1998; Midilli and Gunduzoglu, 2016; Shaybak et al., 2017; Baldwin et al., 2017) showed that Reiki was significantly *more* effective than sham Reiki. These results cannot be explained by touch and indicate that Reiki can act above and beyond the placebo effect in provid-

ing pain relief. While the number of studies is limited, there is scientific evidence to suggest that Reiki may be effective for reducing pain and that it can act beyond the placebo effect.

How Much Reiki is Needed to Reduce Pain?

Even though the studies described above are varied regarding the type of pain addressed and the number and duration of Reiki sessions given, they do provide some useful information about the number and duration of Reiki sessions needed to provide significant pain relief for various conditions. This information is tabulated in Table 12.5. It must be stressed that all the conclusions drawn from this table are preliminary because they are based on a small number of investigations. Bearing in mind this limitation, the following conclusions are listed below:

Table 12.5 Number and duration of Reiki sessions needed to provide significant pain relief

Study	Issue	# Sessions	Session length (min)	Time between sessions	Percent pain relief
Baldwin et al., 2013	Shoulder injury/ inflammation	1	10	NA	11.5%
Shaybak et al., 2017	Leg incision	1	9	NA	NS 62% for sensory
Midilli & Gunduzoglu, 2016	Caesarean surgery	2	15	24 hr	76.6%
Olson et al., 2003	Cancer	2	90	3 days	51% 27% session 1; 43% session 2
Vitale & O'Connor, 2006	Hysterectomy surgery	3	30	24 hr	No baseline values. All relief in first 24 hrs
Baldwin et al., 2017	Knee surgery	3	30	24 hr	66% 38% after session 2
Jahantigh et al., 2018	Back pain	3	15	24 hr	54%
Notte et al., 2016	Knee surgery	5	30	24 hr	66%
Tsang et al., 2007	Cancer	5	45	24 hr	68%
Richeson et al., 2010	General age-related	8	30	1 week	54%
Dressen & Singg, 1998	Chronic illnesses	10	30	3.5 days	62% (15% more after 3-month follow-up) 33% for sensory (77% more after follow-up)
Gillespie et al., 2007	Diabetic neuropathy	13	25	1 week	18% (no better than sham Reiki)

- A single 9- or 10-minute Reiki session can provide a small but significant relief from pain.

- Even two Reiki sessions can provide a large degree of pain relief for an acute or a chronic condition.

- Between three and five 30-minute Reiki sessions, given 24 hours apart, consistently provide a large degree of pain relief from both acute and chronic issues.

- The small number of studies involving more than five Reiki sessions do not indicate that more than five sessions give more protection than three sessions.

- Two studies show that pain relief is further enhanced after the second Reiki session compared to after the first session.

- One study indicates that pain relief is sustained and even enhanced up to three months after completion of a set of Reiki sessions with no further Reiki.

- The sensory aspect of pain may respond differently to Reiki than does pain in its totality.

- Reiki sessions spaced one week apart do not appear to provide much pain relief from diabetic neuropathy. Perhaps more frequent Reiki sessions would be more effective in alleviating pain from this debilitating condition.

Overall, it seems that giving at least two or three 30-minute Reiki sessions to patients with a variety of acute and chronic conditions will substantially alleviate their pain. As indicated by the papers reviewed in Chapter 8, it is not just the physical aspect of pain that is relieved by Reiki but the mental and emotional aspects as well. This conclusion, based on a limited number of scientific studies, is consistent with the following comment by the International Association of Reiki Practitioners (IARP):

Unlike most other treatments, Reiki is a multi-purposed method that can heal both physical and emotional ailments. Through Reiki, some patients suffering from pain due to cancer, injury, or psychological or emotional distress have found relief where other methods were not successful.

Future Research

As stated in a review of the effect of Reiki on pain and anxiety in adults (Thrane and Cohen, 2014):

Continued research using Reiki therapy with larger sample sizes, consistently randomized groups, and standardized treatment protocols is recommended.

It is essential that future research studies on this topic include Reiki, sham Reiki, and standard of care (SOC) groups, that participants are unaware of their group assignment (except for SOC), that data collectors and analyzers are blind as to data grouping, that at least three 30-minute Reiki sessions are provided to each subject, and that there are follow up measurements for at least several months after the end of the treatment.

Case Study

CG had suffered from migraines since childhood. The migraines had worsened over the last few months. On top of that, she was going through a divorce. She was taking medication for migraine, but it made her feel drowsy. For that reason, she was searching for an alternative, so she came for a Reiki session. CG began her Reiki session lying face down so that the practitioner could easily access the base of her head and her neck region (as indicated in *Reiki for Common Ailments* by Mari Hall, 1999). The practitioner did Karuna Reiki, using the first four symbols on those areas, for about 10 minutes and then did a spinal tension release. Next, CG lay supine and the practitioner continued Karuna Reiki, focusing on CG's throat, upper chest and solar plexus. The practitioner felt an intense energy that seemed to be flowing into the throat. When she was working on CG's chest, she noticed a complicated pattern of energy movement in her hands which eventually settled down to a slow pulsing. After the 40-minute session was over, the practitioner mentioned to CG about the energy at the throat and asked her if she had problems speaking her mind, since the throat chakra is linked to communication. CG said that it takes a while for her to speak her mind even with relatives and close friends. The practitioner recommended two more sessions.

One week later, CG returned for her second session. She said that she had just had one headache since the last session and that it was not a migraine. The practitioner worked on the back of CG's head and neck while CG sat in a chair. Then CG lay supine on the Reiki table while the practitioner worked on her heart and solar plexus. The practitioner felt a lot of energy that seemed to be flowing into the heart area. She ended the session by placing her hands on the soles of CG's feet. Afterwards, CG said that she felt very relaxed and she noticed a tingly sensation in her fingers. CG asked what she should expect during the next few days, and the practitioner said that she might expect fewer headaches and a stronger emotional energy to help her cope with her difficult time. The session lasted 30 minutes.

One week later, CG came for her third session. She said that she had not had any headaches since the last session. The practitioner asked CG to lie supine and then did Karuna Reiki, using the first four symbols, on CG's head, throat, heart, solar plexus, hands and root chakra. This time the practitioner did not feel any intense energy flows as she had during the first two sessions; the energy flow felt gentle and even. After the session, CG said that she felt very relaxed and that she was glad that the migraines had not reoccurred. The practitioner recommended that in the future CG might consider learning Reiki for herself.

References

Baldwin AL, Fullmer K, Schwartz GE. Comparison of Physical Therapy with Energy Healing for Improving Range of Motion in Subjects with Restricted Shoulder Mobility. *Evidence-Based Complementary and Alternative Medicine* 2013; 2013: 329731.

Baldwin AL, Vitale A, Brownel E, Kryak E, Rand W. Effects of Reiki on pain, anxiety, and blood pressure in patients undergoing knee replacement surgery. *Holistic Nursing Practice* 2017; 31(2): 80–89.

Dressen LJ, Singg S. Effects of Reiki on pain and selected affective and personality variables of chronically ill patients. *Subtle Energies and Energy Medicine* 1998; 9(1): 51–82.

Gillespie E, Gillespie B, Stevens M. Painful diabetic neuropathy: Impact of an alternative approach. *Diabetes Care* 2007; 30(4): 999–1001.

Goldstein P, Shamay-Tsoory SG, Yellinek S, Weissman-Fogelz I. Empathy Predicts an Experimental Pain Reduction During Touch. *The Journal of Pain* 2016; 17(10): 1049–1057.

Hall M. *Reiki for Common Ailments*. Piatkus, London, 1999.

Hein G, Engelmann JB, Tobler PN. Pain relief provided by an outgroup member enhances analgesia. *Proceedings of the Royal Society B. Biological Sciences* 26 September 2018; 285 (1887).

Jahantiqh F, Abdollahimohammad A, Firouzkouhi M, Ebrahiminejad V. Effects of Reiki versus physiotherapy on relieving lower back pain and improving activities daily living of patients with intervertebral disc hernia. *Journal of Evidence-Based Integrative Medicine* 2018; 23, 1–5.

Midilli TS, Gunduzoglu NC. Effects of Reiki on pain and vital signs when applied to the incision area of the body after Cesarean section surgery. *Holistic Nursing Practice* 2016; 30 (6), 368–378.

Notte BB, Fazzini C, Mooney RA. Reiki's effect on patients with total knee arthroplasty: a pilot study. *Nursing* 2016; 46 (2): 17–23.

Olson K, Hanson J, Michaud M. A phase II trial of Reiki for the management of pain in advanced cancer patients. *Journal of Pain Symptom Management* 2003; 26(5): 990–997.

Richeson NE, Spross JA, Lutz K, Peng C. Effects of Reiki on anxiety, depression, pain, and physiological factors in community-dwelling older adults. *Research in Gerontological Nursing* 2010; 3(3): 187–199.

Shaybak E. Effects of Reiki energy therapy on saphenous vein incision pain: A randomized clinical trial structure. *Der Pharmacy Lettre* 2017; 9 (1): 100–109.

Thrane S, Cohen SM. Effect of Reiki therapy on pain and anxiety in adults: an in- depth literature review of randomized trials with effect size calculations. *Pain Management Nursing* 2014; 15(4): 897–908.

Tsang K, Carlson L, Olson K. Pilot crossover trial of Reiki versus rest for treating cancer-related fatigue. *Integrated Cancer Therapy* 2007; 6(1): 25–35.

Vitale AT, O'Conner PC. The effect of Reiki on pain and anxiety in women with abdominal hysterectomies. *Holistic Nursing Practice* 2006; 20(6): 263–272.

Chapter 13
Reiki for Chemotherapy

Problems Experienced by Patients Undergoing Chemotherapy

Chemotherapy is often given to patients to reduce the chances of the cancer spreading or returning. Cancer cells grow fast and so chemotherapy drugs are designed to preferentially kill fast-growing cells. Unfortunately, these drugs do not just kill the cancer cells; they also destroy some healthy tissue, too. As illustrated by Figure 13.1, possible side effects include mouth sores, easy bruising, hair loss, nausea and vomiting, neuropathy (painful nerve damage), and digestive problems. Other side effects include a weakened immune system, anemia, and fatigue. In fact, cancer-related fatigue is one of the most common side effects of chemotherapy. According to the American Cancer Society:

People describe it as feeling weak, listless, drained, or "washed out." Some may feel too tired to eat, walk to the bathroom, or even use the TV remote. It can be hard to think or move. Rest does not make it go away, and just a little activity can be exhausting. For some people, this kind of fatigue causes more distress than pain, nausea, vomiting, or depression.

The causes of cancer-related fatigue are not fully understood. It may be the cancer and/or the cancer treatment. Here are some possible causes:

- Cancer and cancer treatment can change normal protein and hormone levels that are linked to inflammatory processes which can cause or worsen fatigue.

- Treatments kill normal cells and cancer cells, which leads to a build-up of cell waste. Your body uses extra energy to clean up and repair damaged tissue.

- Cancer forms toxic substances in the body that change the way normal cells work.

Overall, the number and severity of side effects varies greatly from person to person. According to *Medical News Today* (Villines, 2018):

Side effects are unpredictable and depend on the type of chemotherapy drug a person is using.

The combination of fatigue, pain, and other side effects that a person may experience during chemotherapy often leads to emotional distress, fear, anxiety and depression. Therefore, the side effects of chemotherapy are multimodal, meaning that they affect not only a person's physical condition and function, but also their mental and emotional stability. More importantly, these side effects may also prevent doctors from delivering the prescribed dose of chemotherapy at the specific time and the schedule of the treatment plan. If the time schedule of the therapy is compromised, this may limit a patient's ability to achieve the best outcome from treatment. As described in previous chapters, Reiki acts on all levels of the human condition and so would be a good candidate for use in cancer patients to decrease the physical and psychological side effects of chemotherapy. This may explain the increased number of published studies in recent years investigating the use of Reiki in cancer patients to control the side effects of chemotherapy. Most of the existing published scientific studies do support Reiki's effectiveness in alleviating pain, improving mood states, reducing fatigue, and decreasing anxiety and depression in most people, whether or not they have cancer.

Current Methods for Alleviating Symptoms

A comprehensive description of allopathic methods for alleviating symptoms arising from chemotherapy is provided by Texas Oncology which is: "an independent, physician-led practice that offers treatments and conducts research to enable more cancer patients to receive high-quality care while staying close to the critical support of

Chapter 13

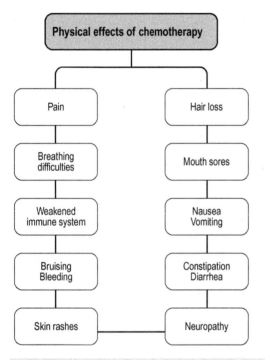

Figure 13.1
Possible side effects of chemotherapy on the body.
(From: Villines Z. What are the side-effects of chemotherapy? *Medical News Today.* www.medicalnewstoday.com/articles/323485.php.)

the brain (Harris, 2010). This production of serotonin is one of the most sensitive signals to cause nausea and vomiting during the first 24 hours after chemotherapy. Blocking this signal is one way to prevent acute symptoms that are relatively short-lived. The newest serotonin inhibitor, Alloxi®, also prevents delayed nausea and vomiting, which occurs two to five days after treatment.

Pain

Pain is one of the most common and feared symptoms of cancer and is usually treated with various pain medications, the type being dependent on the severity of the pain. Pain is rated on a scale of 1–10, with 0 being no pain and 10 the worst pain imaginable. The World Health Organization recommends the following approach for relief of cancer pain:

For mild to moderate pain (1–3 on the scale) pain, over-the-counter medications, such as acetaminophen (Tylenol®) or non-steroidal anti-inflammatory drugs, such as ibuprofen, are prescribed. For moderate to severe pain (4–6), opioids, such as tramadol or dihydrocodeine are used, sometimes in conjunction with Tylenol®. For severe pain (7–10), stronger opioids are prescribed, such as morphine or oxycodone.

However, as described in Chapter 11, opioids can be addictive. In addition, pain medications have other side effects of their own, such as drowsiness, constipation, nausea, and vomiting. In addition to taking pain killers, patients are sometimes encouraged to use acupuncture, biofeedback, massage, and imagery to reduce their pain levels.

Anemia

Anemia refers to a reduced red blood cell count, which in this case arises because chemotherapy drugs kill the fast-growing cells in the bone marrow that produce red blood cells. A low red blood cell count results in insufficient hemoglobin; since hemoglobin carries and delivers oxygen to the all the cells of the body, this means that the body's cells do not receive sufficient oxygen for optimal function. The cells have insufficient oxygen to

family and friends." A brief summary of their methods to reduce the main side effects of chemotherapy, derived from their website (www.texasoncology.com/cancer -treatment/chemotherapy/managing-chemotherapy-side -effects) is presented below.

Nausea and Vomiting

Modern anti-vomiting drugs, called antiemetics, have reduced the severity of nausea and vomiting with chemotherapy. Serotonin inhibitors are currently the most effective antiemetics for patients with cancer. Chemotherapy triggers a massive release of serotonin from enterochromaffin cells in the inner wall of the intestine and the serotonin stimulates nerves leading to the vomiting center in break down the sugars to release energy. In fact, paucity of red blood cells is a major cause of the fatigue that is almost always experienced by cancer patients undergoing chemotherapy. It is not only the red blood cells that are killed; white blood cells and platelets are also affected. White cells mediate the immune response, and so a deficiency in white cells increases the chances of infection. A low platelet count can lead to the bruising often associated with chemotherapy. Common symptoms of the different types of low blood cell counts are listed in Table 13.1. Anemia is treated by injecting blood cell growth factors, such as erythropoietin, that stimulate the cells in the bone marrow to produce more red blood cells, white blood cells, or platelets. These factors can be produced in laboratories and are approved by the Food and Drug Administration (FDA) for the treatment of cancer patients with low blood counts. Unfortunately, treatment with the blood cell growth factors currently available results in side effects including edema, nausea, vomiting, and diarrhea.

Fatigue

The fatigue experienced by chemotherapy patients is often caused by anemia, so is treated by injecting blood cell growth factors as described previously. In addition, patients are advised to maintain good nutrition, but this is difficult because the chemotherapy often produces a loss of appetite. Interestingly, moderate exercise is encouraged because inactivity can actually decrease the body's ability to produce energy.

Depression

Depression is most often treated with a combination of counseling and anti-depressant drugs. The drugs usually take three to six weeks to start working and may be associated with some side effects. Patients are often recommended to continue to take the medication for six to nine months. Currently, the most common antidepressant drugs are called **selective serotonin reuptake inhibitors (SSRIs)** that increase the concentration of the "feel good" molecule, serotonin. Although that sounds like a desirable outcome, it is not a good remedy if the patient is suffering from nausea and vomiting, which are other symptoms of chemotherapy. As described earlier in this chapter, production of serotonin is one of the most sensitive signals to cause nausea and vomiting. In addition, SSRIs do cause some other side effects, such as agitation, nervousness, decreased sex drive, insomnia, and headaches. In addition to counseling and taking antidepressants, patients with depression are sometimes recommended to practice meditation, yoga, and deep breathing.

How Reiki Affects Patients Undergoing Chemotherapy

As described in the previous section, the current methods for alleviating symptoms caused by receiving chemotherapy can be effective. However, the drugs used to treat the side effects of chemotherapy have side effects themselves. For example, drugs used to treat the nausea of chemotherapy may cause the patient to feel depressed, and vice

Table 13.1 Common symptoms of low blood counts		
Low red blood cells	**Low white blood cells**	**Low platelets**
Fatigue or tiredness	Infection	Excessive bruising
Trouble breathing	Fever	Excessive bleeding
Rapid heart rate		Nosebleeds
Difficulty staying warm		
Pale skin		
Dizziness or light headedness		

(From: https://www.texasoncology.com/cancer-treatment/side-effects-of-cancer-treatment/common-side-effects/low-blood-counts.)

versa. One huge benefit of Reiki is that it has no side effects. Thus, including Reiki in a patient's treatment plan will do no harm, and as indicated by the scientific research summarized in this section, there is a good chance that it will significantly improve outcomes. There are several major advantages that Reiki has over the current treatments used to alleviate the symptoms of chemotherapy:

- Reiki is a multi-purpose method that can alleviate both physical and emotional discomfort.

- Reiki is non-invasive and does not add to, or compete with, the cocktail of powerful chemotherapeutic agents already circulating in the patient's body.

- Reiki is very low cost.

There are currently five published studies reporting on clinical trials using Reiki to reduce the symptoms of chemotherapy, three of which appeared within the last five years. These publications will be described and critically reviewed in chronological order. The articles by Olson et al. (2003) and Orsak et al. (2015) were already discussed in detail in Chapters 12 and 7, respectively, and will just be summarized here.

The purpose of the study by Olson et al. (2003) was to determine whether Reiki has beneficial effects on pain, quality of life and analgesic use in cancer patients undergoing palliative treatment. The 24 participants, who were cancer patients receiving palliative care for pain, all received either Reiki and opioids or opioids alone. Participants either rested or received Reiki for 90 minutes on days 1 and 4, according to group assignment. Reiki resulted in a significant decrease in pain compared to the control group on days 1 and 4 (see Tables 12.1 and 12.2). Diastolic blood pressure and heart rate also decreased significantly in the Reiki group, but not the control group, on day 1. There was no quantitative decrease in the use of pain medications in the Reiki group compared to the control. However, the psychological component of QOL was significantly improved on day 7 compared to day 1 for the Reiki group only (Table

12.3). Although no sham Reiki group was included and the number of participants was small, these results are promising and justify spending resources on further research.

The study by Catlin et al. (2011) was designed to determine whether provision of Reiki therapy during outpatient chemotherapy infusion is associated with increased comfort and well-being of patients. Another goal was to support the Oncology Nursing Society's research agenda to improve the quality of life of patients with cancer. Chemotherapy patients who were receiving treatment at a single chemotherapy center and who agreed to participate were consented for the study. Sixty-three participants per group were randomly assigned to one of three additional treatments during the infusion: 1) standard care, 2) 20 minutes of sham Reiki, or 3) 20 minutes of actual Reiki. Patients and infusion center nurses were blinded as to whether sham or actual Reiki therapy was being administered. The sham Reiki therapist was chosen specifically for her disbelief in the efficacy of Reiki and was asked to perform mental arithmetic or create mental shopping lists to distract her while executing sham Reiki. Patients completed two different well-being assessment questionnaires (Healing Touch Comfort Questionnaire and Well-Being Analog Scale), both before and after the infusion. The questionnaires were then collected and statistically examined based on the patient numerical responses.

Both the actual Reiki and the sham Reiki raised the comfort and well-being levels of the participants; the standard care group had the same results in pre- and post-infusion assessments. There was no statistically significant difference between the sham Reiki and the actual Reiki. It is postulated in the paper that the positive effect on well-being may be due to the physical presence of a therapist, sham or actual.

<u>Strengths</u>: This is a randomized, blinded study with a good sample size and a sham Reiki arm as part of the protocol.

<u>Weaknesses</u>: The treatment was a one-time, 20-minute session for each of the participants in the sham and actual

Reiki groups; assessment of multiple treatments was not undertaken. The Reiki practitioner was said to be "trained and experienced", but no details were given regarding the Reiki level and years of experience. In addition, only self-report evaluations were used to assess the efficacy of the Reiki.

Fleisher et al. (2014) designed a study to evaluate the outcomes of an integrative Reiki volunteer program on patients in a large, urban, academic cancer center over a nine-month period. This experiment was approved by the University of Pennsylvania Review Board. The main objective was to assess the effectiveness of the Reiki program by collecting subjective distress scores from 162 participants before and after Reiki sessions and by analyzing patients' answers to open-ended questions asked after each Reiki session, in terms of the presence of key words and recurring themes. Reiki treatments (10–30 minutes) were provided by Reiki Masters or practitioners training to be Reiki Masters, to outpatients on a voluntary basis during chemotherapy or radiation treatment, to inpatients during hospital stays and to a small number of caregivers and staff. A total of 305 Reiki treatments were provided to the participants. There were highly statistically significant decreases in distress, anxiety, depression, pain, and fatigue. Over 80% of participants liked the Reiki session, found it helpful, and would recommend Reiki to others. Individuals reported that Reiki induced relaxation and enhanced spiritual well-being.

Strengths: This study, while not a randomized controlled trial demonstrating cause and effect, informs readers of the acceptability, feasibility, and outcomes of Reiki for management of distress and symptoms during cancer treatments. This work was performed by a very strong study team at the University of Pennsylvania, well-versed in integrative oncology. The authors describe the competency assessment of Reiki practitioners, describe techniques and tools in enough detail for other investigators to repeat the experiment, and self-assess the study's limits.

Weaknesses: Only one-time treatments were included in the protocol and only subjective evaluations were used

to determine the effectiveness of each Reiki treatment. Most importantly, there is no comparison with patients from the same population who did not receive Reiki.

The study by Orsak et al. (2015) investigated whether Reiki treatment would improve the quality of life, mood state and symptom distress of 36 women undergoing four sessions of chemotherapy for breast cancer. The clinical outcomes used in the research to assess well-being were "Quality of Life", "Symptom Distress" and "Mood States". This was a two-phase study. The first established the base levels for the outcome parameters by obtaining data from 10 patients undergoing chemotherapy. In the second phase, patients were randomly assigned to one of two groups. One group (15 patients) received 30 minutes of Reiki during chemotherapy and the other group (11 patients) had a companion who conversed with them and was present for 30 minutes. It was hypothesized that both Reiki and companionship would make the side effects of chemotherapy more bearable, but that the effects of Reiki would be more marked. Results showed that neither Reiki nor companionship decreased symptom distress compared to standard care, but all patients found Reiki to be relaxing. Patients in both the Reiki and companion groups showed improvements regarding quality of life and mood and reduced fatigue, but the standard care group did not.

Strengths: This study is unique in that it compares Reiki with the presence of a companion and with standard care during the chemotherapy of women with breast cancer. The outcome scales are well-defined and the statistical analysis is thorough. The study is significant in demonstrating that complementary modalities such as Reiki and companionship can assist in the tolerance of conventional chemotherapy treatments.

Weaknesses: The number of patients involved was small and the patients were not blinded as to their grouping. Although the companion was allowed to speak with the patient throughout the 30-minute session, conversation with the Reiki practitioner was limited to a few explanatory words at the start of the session. In addition, since the companions were also Reiki practitioners, it is possible that they were unconsciously sending Reiki to the patients. Only self-report evaluations were used to assess the efficacy of the Reiki.

Finally, the study by Demir et al. (2015) attempted to determine the effect of distant Reiki on pain, anxiety, and fatigue in cancer patients receiving chemotherapy. In distant Reiki, the practitioner first states the name of the patient and then sends the healing energy to the patient remotely. In this case, the practitioner was over 8 km from the patients. The protocol was approved by the research committee of the University of Istanbul Institute of Oncology. Participants were 18 cancer patients receiving chemotherapy in a hospital in Turkey. The patients were randomly divided into two groups, Reiki or non-Reiki (control), but were blinded as to grouping. One advantage of using distant Reiki is that since the Reiki practitioner is not in the room with the patient, it is not possible for the patient to know whether they are in the Reiki group or the control group. A second degree Usui Reiki practitioner, who had been practicing for more than four years, sent distant Reiki to individuals in the Reiki group for 30 minutes each day for five days. Patients assessed their levels of pain, stress, and fatigue using a numeric rating scale (0–10) before the study and after its completion. Patients in the Reiki group showed significantly less pain (45% reduction), stress (68% reduction), and fatigue (39% reduction) after treatment compared to before the session whereas, in the control patients, those values increased.

Strengths: This study is well conceived in terms of blinding of patients to treatment received and the statistical processes used. It is significant to note that these positive results were achieved with as few as five 30-minute distance-only Reiki sessions for each of the participants. No in-person treatments were used in this study. This is one of the few published scientific studies of distance Reiki.

Weaknesses: The main weakness is the small sample size. In addition, only self-reported evaluations were used to assess the efficacy of the Reiki.

Summary of Research Results and Future Direction

All five published research studies on the effects of Reiki on cancer patients undergoing chemotherapy gave positive results with regard to reducing pain, fatigue, anxiety, depression, and distress, and to increasing quality of life, comfort, and well-being. Two of the studies involved large numbers of participants (Catlin et al., 2011; Fleisher et al., 2014). In the three cases in which Reiki was compared to standard of care (Olson et al., 2003, Catlin et al., 2011, Demir et al., 2015), Reiki was significantly better at improving patients' outcomes. When Reiki was compared with sham Reiki (Catlin et al., 2011), or with the presence of a companion (Orsak et al., 2015), both pairs of treatments resulted in similar improvements. These results might appear to indicate that Reiki's beneficial effects are totally derived from human contact, rather than from some additional mechanism specific to energy healing. However, neither of the studies is really a fair comparison. In one case, the "companions" were also Reiki practitioners and were allowed to converse with the patient whereas the "Reiki practitioners" were not. In the other case, patients only received one 20-minute session of Reiki or sham Reiki, which may not have been of adequate duration for Reiki to exert effects beyond those associated with simple touch. It is essential that, in future experiments, Reiki "dosage" is explored in the context of its effectiveness in reducing symptoms of chemotherapy. What is the optimal number of sessions, length of sessions, and frequency of sessions necessary to alleviate symptoms? All future studies should be double blinded and randomized and include two control groups: sham Reiki and standard of care. In this way, the effects of touch alone can be calibrated over multiple treatments and separated from the total effect of Reiki. In addition, hands-on Reiki could be compared to Reiki given with the hands hovering over the patient to determine whether actual touch contributes to the beneficial effects of Reiki. Two corresponding sham Reiki groups (hands-on and hands-off) would separate out the effects of "touch alone" from the effects of a person being present with the patient but not touching them. All of these groups could be compared to standard of care. In this way, the importance of the roles that presence and touch play in the Reiki experience could be determined. Despite the little that is known about how Reiki actually works, and the small number of studies that address the effects of Reiki on cancer patients receiving chemotherapy, the results obtained so far look promising.

Case Study

DB was a nurse who had had a colonoscopy two months previously and had been diagnosed with stage 3a cancer. She had had surgery and was now on chemotherapy. DB had had two chemotherapy treatments and was scheduled for 10 more over the next six months. In addition, she had experienced uterine cancer (stage 1) three years before, and had had a hysterectomy. DB thought there "must be something going on with my body". She had not had Reiki before. The practitioner gave DB a 1-hour session of Karuna Reiki, starting with a scan. During the scan, she felt an area of heat over the center of DB's lower abdomen. During the session, the practitioner noticed that she became very hot herself as she placed her hands on DB's cheeks (see Figure 4.6B). The practitioner also sensed, in her hands, a lot of movement of energy as she worked on DB's abdominal area. Just before the end of the session, DB asked for a bathroom break. On returning, and when the session was completed, DB said that she felt very relaxed and that during the session very often she could still sense the practitioner's hands in a particular area, even though she knew that the practitioner had moved on to another region of her body. The practitioner recommended that DB return for a 30-minute session just before her next chemotherapy treatment the following week.

For the next session, the practitioner started Karuna Reiki but it took about 15 minutes, working through chakras 7, 6, and 5 before she started to feel the energy. She felt it at the fourth chakra. From the fourth to the first chakra, the energy felt very strong. After the session, DB said that she felt very relaxed: a quiet relaxation. She usually feels anxious before her chemotherapy appointments but this time she felt no anxiety, even though her appointment was within the next hour. DB did not return for more Reiki sessions. Seven years later, DB is healthy and is working as a coordinator for home health.

References

Catlin A, Taylor-Ford RL. Investigation of standard care versus sham Reiki placebo versus actual Reiki therapy to enhance comfort and well-being in a chemotherapy infusion center. *Oncology Nursing Forum* 2011; 38(3): E212–E220.

Demir M, Gulbeyaz C, Kelam A, Aydmer A. Effects of distant Reiki on pain, anxiety and fatigue in oncology patients in Turkey: a pilot study. *Asian Pacific Journal of Cancer Prevention* 2015; 16:4859–4862.

Fleisher KA, Mackenzie ER, Frankel ES, Seluzicki C, Casarett D, Mao JJ. Integrative Reiki for cancer patients: A program evaluation. *Integrative Cancer Therapies* 2014; 13(1): 62–67.

Harris DG. Nausea and vomiting in advanced cancer. *British Medical Bulletin* 2010; 96: 175–185.

Olson K, Hanson J, Michaud M. A phase II trial of Reiki for the management of pain in advanced cancer patients. *Journal of Pain Symptom Management* 2003; 26(5): 990–997.

Orsak G, Stevens A, Brufsky A, Kajumba M, Dougall AL. The effect of Reiki therapy and companionship on quality of life, mood, and symptom distress during chemotherapy. *Journal of Evidence-based Complementary and Alternative Medicine* 2015; 20(1): 20–27.

Villines Z. What are the side-effects of chemotherapy? *Medical News Today* 2018. www.medicalnewstoday.com/articles/323485.php.

Chapter 14

Providing Reiki in Hospitals – Practicalities

Reasons for Establishing Reiki Programs in Hospitals

Giving Reiki to a person in hospital can be a very rewarding and affirming experience, for both the receiver and the provider. Based on the published scientific research pertaining to the effects of Reiki on physical and psychological health, it is not difficult to justify spending time and money on providing Reiki in hospitals. Almost all of the research studies described in the previous chapters support the use of Reiki as a tool to improve health. Although the number of articles is small, they consistently show that Reiki can:

- Reduce pain (14 articles)

- Assist with pain and anxiety reduction in patients pre- and post-surgery (six articles)

- Reduce symptoms associated with chemotherapy (five articles)

- Reduce emotional stress (six articles)

- Improve relaxation and well-being (eight articles)

- Reduce anxiety and depression to some extent (four articles).

In addition, three studies show that Reiki reduces burnout in nurses, physicians and other hospital workers.

Pain, anxiety, and stress accompany almost any disease or disorder being treated, and most surgeries being performed, in hospitals. Reiki ameliorates pain, stress, and in some cases, anxiety. Since Reiki is safe, has no side effects, and is low cost there is absolutely no reason not to make it available to all patients and hospital workers who request it. In the latest American Hospital Association survey in 2010, approximately 42% of the 714 responding hospitals were incorporating integrative medicine therapies into the hospital setting. The top modalities offered included pet therapy, massage, music/art, guided imagery/relaxation training, and Reiki/Healing Touch (HT).

Benefits for Patients and Caregivers

Reiki is, by its nature, complementary to allopathic medicine, and the reduction of anxiety and sense of calm that it brings to patients can increase their speed of recovery and improve the outcomes of traditional therapy. Greater fear or distress prior to surgery has been associated with poorer outcomes including longer hospital stays, more postoperative complications, and higher rates of rehospitalization (Kiecolt-Glaser et al., 1998). In addition, psychological stress leads to clinically relevant delays in wound healing and can increase susceptibility to wound infection (Walburn et al., 2009). Emotional stress can also impair the efficacy of some drug treatments. For example, when a person is under a lot of stress, the body produces more of the stress hormone, cortisol. Excess cortisol increases the concentration of glucose in the bloodstream and reduces the effectiveness of insulin, used to treat type 1 diabetes. As another example, mental stress reduces the ability of levodopa to suppress tremor intensity in Parkinson's disease patients (Zach et al., 2017). However, the stress response can be controlled. A gentle, non-invasive therapy such as Reiki reduces stress and promotes relaxation. Reiki will work in conjunction with allopathic medicine and surgery to significantly improve patient outcomes.

As described in Chapter 9, Reiki also benefits caregivers. There is now a body of published evidence showing that nurses are practicing and benefiting from self-Reiki to reduce symptoms of burnout. Burnout reduces productivity, saps one's energy, and leaves one emotionally drained and unable to meet constant demands. It is obvious that if Reiki reduces these symptoms, the caregivers, the patients, the hospital administrators, and the financial advisors will all benefit and recover their equilibrium.

Chapter 14

The benefits of Reiki for patients and caregivers are summarized as follows:

For patients:

1. Reduces stress, anxiety.

2. Promotes feelings of control and engagement with respect to own well-being.

3. Promotes trust between patient and caregiver(s).

4. Additive benefit to conventional drug therapies potentially allowing reduced medication, fewer side effects and toxicities.

5. Possible shorter recovery times.

For caregivers:

1. Reduces stress/burnout.

2. Promotes positive well-being, sense of competence.

Potential Business Value for Reiki in Hospitals

There are three main reasons why offering Reiki may benefit hospitals financially. One is because hospital patients are increasingly asking for complementary therapies, including Reiki, in addition to standard care, and so they are more likely to choose hospitals that offer these services. In an online article from *STAT News* (Ross et al., 2017), it is stated that there is "a booming market for 'natural' therapies" and "There's no question that patients want alternative medicine. It's a $37 billion-a-year business". In addition:

"A national consortium to promote integrative health now counts more than 70 academic centers and health systems as members, up from eight in 1999. Each year, four or five new programs join," said Dr. Leslie Mendoza Temple, the chair of the consortium's policy working group.

Shelley Adler, who runs the Osher Center for Integrative Medicine at the University of California, San Francisco, reported:

"The center is on pace to get more than 10,300 patient visits this fiscal year, up 37% from 2012. It's expanding its clinical staff by a third."

Duke University's integrative medicine clinic has also seen strong growth: total visits jumped 50% in 2015 to more than 14,000, Dr. Adam Perlman, the executive director, told IntegrativePractitioner.com.

Interestingly, the point of the *STAT News* article from which the above quotes were obtained is that hospitals are willing to provide services in complementary and integrative medicine because they benefit financially and because *that is what the patients want, regardless of whether or not there is supportive scientific evidence.* However, for Reiki, there is scientific evidence for potential business value in hospitals, as shown by reasons two and three.

The second reason is there is evidence that patients who receive Reiki before and after surgery require less pain medication and are discharged from hospital faster on average than those who do not. Both of these results were seen in patients undergoing knee replacement surgery (Baldwin et al., 2017) and in more than 8,000 patients enrolled in the Reiki program at Columbia/HCA Portsmouth Regional Hospital, Portsmouth, New Hampshire, USA. Thirdly, based on the measurements of the physical and psychological benefits of Reiki to hospital nurses and other healthcare workers (Vitale, 2009; Diaz-Rodriguez et al., 2011a, 2011b; Clark, 2013; Rosada et al., 2015), there is likely to be a reduction in hospital staff turnover. For all these reasons, Reiki, as a caring-healing approach to patient care, should be of significant financial impact to insurers, patients, and providers.

Some Reiki Programs Currently Offered at Healthcare Institutions

USA

1. New York-Presbyterian Hospital/Columbia University Medical Center, New York, NY

2. Duke Integrative Medicine, Durham, NC

3. Yale-New Haven Hospital, New Haven, CT

4. Cleveland Clinic Wellness Institute, Lyndhurst, OH

5. Memorial Sloan-Kettering Cancer Center, New York, NY

6. Banner University Medical Center, Tucson, AZ

7. Tucson Medical Center, Tucson, AZ

8. Children's Hospital Boston, Boston, MA

9. Dana Farber/Harvard Cancer Institute, Boston, MA

10. Hartford Hospital Integrative Medicine, Hartford, CT

11. Abramson Cancer Center of the University of Pennsylvania, West Chester, PA

12. Johns Hopkins Integrative Medicine and Digestive Center, Lutherville-Timonium, MD

13. Portsmouth Regional Hospital, Portsmouth, NH

14. Mayo Clinic, Rochester, MN

UK

1. University College Hospital Macmillan Cancer Centre, London

2. Southampton General Hospital, Southampton

3. Welcome Treatment Centre, Sherwood Forest Hospitals, Sutton-in-Ashfield, Nottinghamshire

4. Trinity Holistic Centre, South Tees Hospital, Middlesbrough

Australia

1. Solaris Cancer Care Centres, Western Australia

2. Footprints Day Centre, Perth, Western Australia

Types of Reiki Programs

1. Grouped by type of practice:

- Run by hospital staff only – Dana Farber Cancer Institute, MA, USA

- Staff and lay practitioners – New York Presbyterian Hospital, NY, USA

- Mostly lay practitioners – Hartford Hospital Integrated Medicine, CT, USA

- Managed by external company – University Medical Center, AZ, USA

- Fee charged for Reiki – Cleveland Clinic, OH; Dana Farber Cancer Institute, MA, USA

- No fee for Reiki – most facilities

- Staff integrates Reiki into practice

- Boston Children's Hospital, MA, USA (125 staff members)

- Yale-New Haven Children's Hospital, CT, USA (25 staff members)

2. Grouped by type of clients:

- Treats both inpatients and outpatients – Memorial Sloan-Kettering Cancer Center, NY, USA

- Treats specific inpatients only – New York Presbyterian Hospital, NY

- Reiki for all inpatients – Hartford Hospital, CT, USA

- Reiki for out-patients only – Duke University, NC, USA

- Reiki for both patients and family members – Columbia University Medical Center, NY, USA

- Staff receive Reiki – most facilities

Examples of Patient and Employee Outcomes

A few hospitals that offer Reiki have monitored patient, and sometimes employee, outcomes before and after receiving Reiki and have made these data available to the public. As mentioned in Chapter 2, Hartford Hospital, Hartford, Connecticut, USA, obtained patient outcome measurements during program development, and both employee and patient outcomes after the program was expanded. These outcomes show that patients and employees responded very positively to Reiki. Pain, anxiety, and nausea were reduced, their ability to sleep improved, and the likelihood of patients choosing Hartford Hospital for future admissions increased. These data are shown in Figures 2.3–2.7. Figure 2.4 demonstrates measurements of patient relaxation and pain before and after Reiki, that were taken during development of the program. The number of patients involved is not listed. Figure 2.6 shows the effects of Reiki or massage on sleep and nausea in patients. The results are very positive, but the relative contributions of Reiki and massage are not defined, nor is the number of patients involved. Figure 2.7 demonstrates the effects of Reiki, acupuncture, and massage on pain and anxiety of 189 patients (36 receiving Reiki, 76 receiving acupuncture, 84 receiving massage). Once again, the effects are positive but the relative contributions of the various therapies are not presented. Figure 2.5 shows measurements of the effects of Reiki on relaxation, pain and fatigue of 44 employees that were taken during development of the program. A statistical analysis is included, demonstrating highly significant positive results for all parameters. Figure 2.3 indicates that after expansion of the Reiki program at Hartford Hospital, over 84% of patients tested indicated they were more likely to choose Hartford Hospital for future admissions because of the Integrative Medicine Program.

An example of changes in outcome measurements of 79 patients receiving Reiki at St. Charles Cancer Center, Bend, Oregon, USA, is shown in Table 14.1. The overall average change in the pain scale was a 1.5-point decrease (range 0–8).

When the 103 Reiki sessions with patients who rated their pain as a zero before and after the session (experiencing no pain) were adjusted for, the "corrected" average decrease in the pain level improved to 2.26 points. The overall average change in the anxiety level was a 2.7-point decrease (range 0–9). When the 48 Reiki sessions with patients who rated their anxiety as a zero before and after the session (experiencing no anxiety) were eliminated from these data, the average decrease improved to 3.2 points. Finally, the well-being scores also improved after a Reiki session compared to baseline. The well-being scale is the "opposite" of the pain and anxiety scales, with a rating of zero meaning the patient felt miserable, and 10 meaning they felt excellent. The overall average change in the well-being scale was a 1.9 increase (range 0–10). When the 33 Reiki sessions with patients who rated their well-being as a 10 before and after the session were eliminated from these data (felt excellent to start with), the average increase in the well-being scale improved to 2.1 points. These results were published in an article in *Reiki News Magazine* (Johnson and Fuerst, 2011). In this article, the authors conclude:

The pilot study data, with each patient serving as their own "control," showing pain decreasing 15–22%, anxiety 27–32%, and well-being improving 19–21%, is impressive

Table 14.1 Reported metrics from St. Charles Cancer Center (Bend, OR): effects of Reiki treatment on pain, anxiety and well-being in cancer patients			
Data gathered	Jan 7 to Sept 13, 2010		
Number of patients	79		
Number of sessions	312		
Pain Scale	**Average Change**	**Range**	**"Corrected" Average**
0=no pain 10=severe pain	1.53	0 to 8	2.26
Anxiety Scale	**Average Change**	**Range**	**"Corrected" Average**
10=feel great 0=feel miserable	2.7	0 to 9	3.2
Well-Being Scale	**Average Change**	**Range**	**"Corrected" Average**
10=feel great 0=feel miserable	1.9	10 to 0	2.1

(From: Johnson R, Fuerst R. Reiki at St. Charles Cancer Center. *Reiki News Magazine*, Spring 2011, 36–40. SCCC Reiki Session Data Table).

and encourages the pursuit of a study rigorous enough to be published in a medical journal. Reiki has enhanced the lives of staff, patients, and volunteers through the St. Charles Cancer Center Reiki program."

Reiki Training for Nurses, Caregivers, and Volunteers

According to Pamela Miles (Miles, 2017):

When full Reiki treatment is offered in hospital, it is generally by volunteers; hospital Reiki practitioners are rarely paid. Hospitals often rely on staff members who have become Reiki Masters. Some hospitals offer Reiki training to staff and some offer training to the community as well.

For this reason, this section will focus on the training of volunteers only.

The Brigham and Women's Hospital Reiki Volunteer Program

An excellent paper by Hahn et al. (2014) describes how a Reiki training program for volunteers was developed at Boston's Brigham and Women's Hospital (BWH):

Creating a healing and healthy environment for patients, families, and staff is an ongoing challenge. As part of our hospital's Integrative Care Program, a Reiki Volunteer Program has helped to foster a caring and healing environment, providing a means for patients, family, and staff to reduce pain and anxiety and improve their ability to relax and be present. Because direct care providers manage multiple and competing needs at any given time, they may not be available to provide Reiki when it is needed. This program demonstrates that a volunteer-based program can successfully support nurses in meeting patient, family, and staff demand for Reiki services.

Creating the program

- As a first step, the existing Hospital Reiki Policy was amended to include the use of trained volunteers in providing Reiki to patients, families, and staff.

- Each volunteer was interviewed by the Integrative Care Program director to evaluate whether they could adapt to the hospital environment, withstand the emotional strain caused from experiencing the pain and suffering of patients, and make a minimal one-year, 2-hours-per-week commitment to the program.

- Funding was provided by the vice president for nursing to hire a part-time coordinator for the Reiki Volunteer Program (RVP). Working with the Integrative Care Program director and a nurse educator, she created the structure, processes, and educational materials required to get the program up and running. A Reiki Volunteer Handbook was created, as well as a brochure to be used by staff in speaking with patients about Reiki.

Volunteer and Staff Preparation

- Each volunteer underwent a standard hospital orientation, followed by training in Reiki levels one and two classes taught by a Reiki Master.

- Each volunteer was taught by the RVP coordinator, in an empty patient room, how to create a treatment environment (using music, therapeutic suggestion, and breathing techniques) and was given the opportunity to practice Reiki on other volunteers.

- The volunteer was then introduced to the nurse manager and staff (who had been trained how to consent a patient, document results, and work with the Reiki volunteer), and the process for obtaining names of patients and staff interested in having sessions was discussed.

- Successful completion of volunteer training required the coordinator to be present for the first three patient sessions provided by the volunteer and to evaluate their performance before Reiki sessions could be given independently.

Chapter **14**

The competency tool used to evaluate the volunteers is shown in Table 14.2.

Consent of Patient

It is very important when giving Reiki treatments in hospitals to make sure the patient understands what Reiki is and to only provide a Reiki treatment if the patient has requested one. It is the responsibility of the Reiki team to explain Reiki to the patient before giving the treatment. This usually works best by the Reiki practitioner first taking a few minutes to introduce themselves and get to know the patient, and then explain the work they do. In most hospitals, a patient must sign a consent form and sometimes the attending physician or nurse must also give permission for a patient to receive Reiki. When giving Reiki to minors, or to those without the mental capacity to decide for themselves, the Code of Ethics and Practice for Professional Reiki Practitioners (created by The Reiki Council, UK), states that the written consent of a parent, guardian or relevant medical practitioner must be obtained. However, the wishes of the person must override any consent of a third party if they do not wish to receive Reiki. If a patient is unconscious, some Reiki practitioners use their inner guidance to determine whether or not the higher self of the patient is willing to receive Reiki. It is also advisable to obtain consent from a friend or relative, if available.

Condition of Patient

Reiki can do no harm. For that reason, Reiki is usually available to any patient who requests it in hospitals with Reiki programs. Conditions treated with Reiki include cancer, pain, chronic conditions, postoperative surgery, and childbirth.

The California Pacific Medical Center is one of the largest hospitals in northern California. Its Health and Healing Clinic provides care for both acute and chronic illness using a wide range of complementary therapies, including Reiki. The clinic is currently staffed by two physicians, Dr. Mike Cantwell and Dr. Amy Saltzman. Dr. Cantwell, a pediatrician specializing in infectious diseases, is also a Reiki Master. Dr. Cantwell states:

I have found Reiki to be useful in the treatment of acute illnesses such as musculoskeletal injury/pain, headache, acute infections, and asthma. Reiki is also useful for patients with chronic illnesses, especially those associated with chronic pain.

Number, Frequency, and Duration of Sessions

As described in Chapter 13, there are no hard data on the optimal number of Reiki sessions, length of sessions, and frequency of sessions necessary to alleviate symptoms of different diseases and issues. For that reason, it is often necessary to "play it by ear", observing the responses and listening to the comments of the patient during and after each session. In a hospital, it is generally wise to limit sessions to 20–30 minutes, so that other medical and service staff can have easy access to the patient in order to fulfil their obligations. Dr. Cantwell, from the California Pacific Medical Center, provides between one and three sessions, after which he assigns the patient to a Reiki level two internist who continues to provide Reiki sessions outside the clinic. Patients who continue to respond well to the Reiki treatments are referred for Reiki training so they can continue Reiki self-treatments on a continuing basis.

Role of Relatives and Friends

Sometimes the patients' relatives and friends like to act as caregivers, especially if the patient has a serious or chronic condition. In the Department of Anesthesiology and Pain Medicine, Seattle Children's Hospital, Seattle, Washington, USA, a pilot program was developed to train caregivers of hospitalized pediatric patients to give Reiki (Kundu et al., 2013). Seventeen out of 18 families agreed to participate. Caregivers indicated more confidence about using Reiki therapy for their children if they had received two or more training sessions and if they themselves had experienced Reiki therapy. Most families (65%) attended three Reiki training sessions and reported that Reiki benefited their child by improving the child's comfort (76%), helping the child relax (88%), and relieving pain (41%). Following this training, 10 caregivers (59%) reported that they regularly used Reiki with their children. Six of these 10 were directly observed providing therapy for their children, by the Rei-

Table 14.2 Table showing competency tool for assessing volunteers trained to provide Reiki to inpatients at the Brigham and Women's Hospital (BWH), Boston, MA, USA.

Competency Tool: Providing Reiki to patients on inpatient units	Meets: Y/N
1 Volunteer is able to locate list of patients, families and staff requesting Reiki	
2 Explains Reiki in simple, understandable language	

3   Creates a calm, quiet treatment environment
    • Places "do not disturb, Reiki session in progress" on patient door
    • Chooses and plays calming music with patient permission
    • Acts and speaks in calm & hospitable manner	

4   Adheres to the BWH Reiki Protocol
    • Utilizes therapeutic suggestion that invites patient to envision a peaceful place that is relevant for that person
    • Teaches the patient breathing techniques as described in protocol
    • Keeps hands above shoulders and below groin
    • Sessions are no more than 30 minutes in length	

5   Maintains patient safety as demonstrated by:
    Before entering room:
    • Uses "Purell" on hands
    • Checks signs on/near door indicating precautions, and follows instructions on sign (e.g. don gloves, gown, mask)
    Before leaving room:
    • Bed is placed in low position
    • Upper side rails are in upright position	

6 At completion of Reiki session, informs nurse of outcome (e.g. sleeping, more relaxed, etc.)	

7   Completes and submits the Reiki follow- up sheet indicating:
    • Date, location of session
    • Whether Reiki provided to patient, family or staff member
    • Reason Reiki given and outcome	

(From: Hahn J, Reilly PM, Buchanan TM. Development of a hospital reiki training program: training volunteers to provide reiki to patients, families, and staff in the acute care setting. *Dimensions of Critical Care Nursing* 2014; 33(1): 15–21. Figure: Reiki volunteer competency evaluation tool).

ki Master. The majority of caregivers (10/17) expressed an interest in further participation in Reiki training, including a specific request for an advanced level Reiki training by one. All caregivers found that participating in Reiki training helped them become active participants in their child's care. This small study suggests that having friends and relatives learn Reiki positively impacts the patients and their families.

Implementation Strategies for Reiki Programs

Plan: The first step is to form an executive planning team. This is easier if there is already a Complementary and Integrative Medicine program. Ideally, the team should include:

- Clinical nurse specialist for integrative medicine

- Integrative medicine coordinator

Chapter 14

- Volunteer program coordinator

- Physician with Reiki training

- Reiki Master trainer

- Several clinical nurse practitioners with Reiki training

Volunteers are vital to Reiki programs and it is essential to develop an effective screening process that includes a background check, verification of immunizations, and a review of hospital policies and requirements of a volunteer.

The next step is to develop a service description containing program details for review and approval by the volunteer coordinators, the executive planning team, and hospital leadership. The service description should cover requirements for training, requirements to become a volunteer, and details for oversight of the program. Fliers that describe Reiki should be developed to give to staff and patients. A flier is also needed to explain how to become a volunteer.

Design: The executive planning committee develops an educational module for nursing staff, as shown below, for presentation at team meetings.

Educational content on Reiki therapy for nurses:

- Definition of Reiki

- When Reiki might be useful for a nursing unit's patient population

- How to request Reiki for a specific patient

- Role of the Reiki volunteer

- Nursing role for documenting, in an electronic health record, the patient's response to treatment

Communication to physician practice committees about Reiki therapy:

- Definition of Reiki therapy

- Potential benefits for patients

- Other prestigious hospitals and clinics that offer Reiki treatments

- Proposed process to bring Reiki therapy to patients at point of care

A diagram summarizing the components of building a Reiki volunteer program is shown in Figure 14.1.

Payment of Reiki Practitioners

Since most Reiki practitioners who participate in hospital Reiki programs are volunteers, they do not receive any payment. However, as hospital Reiki programs become more widespread, it might be prudent, and fair to offer some incentive in order to recruit enough practitioners. According to a recent study (Montross-Thomas et al., 2017), hospital patients are willing to pay cash for services such as Reiki treatment. Many Reiki practitioners are perfectly happy to volunteer their services to the sick for free, but there is no reason that Reiki practitioners should not be paid, just as masseuses, for example, are paid for their services. As stated by William Rand, Director of the International Center for Reiki Training, in his piece "Developing your Reiki Practice" (reiki.org/reikipractice/practicehomepage.html):

They are not paying for the Reiki energy which is free but for your time and the effort you have put forth to learn Reiki. When people receive a treatment for free they often feel indebted to the practitioner and guilty feelings can develop. This creates an imbalance that can get in the way of continued treatments.

Tools for Talking About Reiki

Articles from several Reiki programs, at hospitals such as Tucson Medical Center, Tucson, Arizona, and Portsmouth Regional Hospital, Portsmouth, New Hampshire, indicate that they have found it best not to use the word "Reiki" with patients at first, but to talk about healing energy. They explain that healing energy exists in the body but is deplet-

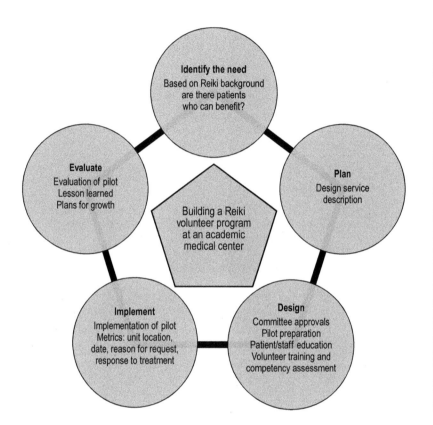

Identify the need
Based on Reiki background
are there patients
who can benefit?

Plan
Design service
description

Evaluate
Evaluation of pilot
Lesson learned
Plans for growth

Building a Reiki
volunteer program
at an academic
medical center

Implement
Implementation of pilot
Metrics: unit location,
date, reason for request,
response to treatment

Design
Committee approvals
Pilot preparation
Patient/staff education
Volunteer training and
competency assessment

Figure 14.1
Flow diagram showing steps for building a Reiki and Healing Touch volunteer program at an academic medical center.
(From: Anderson DM, Loth AR, Stuart-Mullen LG, Thomley BS, Cutshall SM. Building a Reiki and Healing Touch volunteer program at an academic medical center. *Advances in Integrative Medicine* 2017; 4: 74–79. Figure 2.)

ed when a person is unwell, and they describe their work as helping to increase the patient's healing energy supply. After that, they explain more about the technique and say that it is called Reiki. Reiki is better accepted by conventional doctors and hospitals if it is explained in conventional terms, such as a technique that reduces stress and promotes relaxation and healing, rather than in metaphysical terms. The action of Reiki can be described as enhancing the body's natural ability to heal itself.

Resources for Starting a Hospital-Based Reiki Program

The resources below include:

- Guidelines for setting up Reiki programs in hospitals

- Descriptions of Reiki training programs for hospital workers

- Patient responses to a successful hospital-based Reiki program

- An example of a Reiki fact sheet for hospital patients

- Lists of existing hospital-based Reiki programs worldwide

A good start for developing a hospital-based Reiki program is to read the article by Vitale (2014) in which she lays out the requisite components of a business plan that will appeal to healthcare organizations. The main factors to be considered are as follows:

1. An executive summary about the Reiki program.

2. Reiki program description, that is, program type – volunteer or paid – and initial target audience.

3. Vision/mission statement congruent with the organization's vision/mission/philosophy of care.

4. Background information that supports the decision to start a Reiki program (include emerging research data from the workshop delivered in understandable terms).

5. Reiki program objectives.

6. Reiki practitioner educational requirements, that is, evidence of Reiki training level.

7. Program management requirements (resources needed).

8. Capital/financial requirements to implement and sustain a Reiki program.

9. Marketing strategies.

10. Potential outcomes, that is, benefits of a Reiki program and potential risks.

11. Future expansion of Reiki services.

Two other excellent guides to developing Reiki programs in hospitals are: "Development of a hospital Reiki training program: training volunteers to provide Reiki to patients, families, and staff in the acute care setting" (Hahn et al., 2014), and "Building a Reiki and Healing Touch volunteer program at an academic medical center" (Anderson et al., 2017).

A PowerPoint presentation created by Anne Vitale, PhD, APN, AHN-BC and Elise Brownell, PhD as part of their work for the Center for Reiki Research, that provides guidelines for setting up a hospital Reiki program, is available at: http://www.rcpaconference.org/wp-content/uploads/2016/09/W51_Garver_-Reiki-In-Hospitals.pdf.

Two papers that describe programs to train caregivers and nurses in Reiki practice are: "Reiki training for caregivers of hospitalized pediatric patients: A pilot program", by Kundu et al. (2013) and "Reiki: a supportive therapy in nursing practice and self-care for nurses", by Gallob (2003).

An article describing patient responses to the successful Hartford Hospital Reiki program is available at: https://hartfordhospital.org/services/integrative-medicine/departments-services/reiki-therapy.

The Reiki Fact Sheet provided to patients by The Leonard P. Zakim Center for Integrative Therapies and Healthy Living, Dana Faber Cancer Institute, Boston, MA, explains what Reiki is, its benefits, and what happens during a Reiki session (below).

Existing Hospital-Based Reiki Programs

Details about hospital-based Reiki programs in the USA are provided on the website of The International Center for Reiki Training:

www.reiki.org/reikinews/reiki_in_hospitals.html

This website includes a list of 76 hospital, medical clinic, and hospice programs where Reiki is offered as a standard part of care. The information in the hospital list has been provided by individuals who are part of the Reiki program listed. A detailed description of each program including organization, number of practitioners, and contact person(s) is provided. The basic facts of each program have been verified and approved by the hospital before they are listed.

A list of hospitals and other healthcare establishments in the USA, Australia, Germany, Switzerland, and New Zealand where Reiki is used to treat their patients, and in some cases, treat the families and carers of their patients is provided by the following link:

www.olistiq.com/full-list-of-reiki-in-hospital/4585659483

Some of the hospitals and hospices in the Republic of Ireland where Reiki is available are listed on the website of Reiki Federation Ireland. This list is shown in the box below.

Some of the National Health Service (NHS) hospitals and other UK healthcare institutions that offer Reiki to patients and/or staff are available, with permission of Amber Kelly, at:

http://c4362503.myzen.co.uk/wp-content/uploads/2014/02/NHS-energy-healing.pdf

Box 14.1A

Integrative Therapy Fact Sheet: Reiki

What is Reiki?

Reiki is an ancient, hands-on energy healing therapy. The Japanese word *Reiki* describes a system for tapping into universal life force, sometimes referred to as *Chi* or *qi*, the energy that creates and sustains all life. Reiki can be used before cancer treatment, during treatment, and after treatment.

How Can Reiki Help Me?

Reiki is non-invasive and is known to be safe. It facilitates a deep state of relaxation, and can be used to manage stress, and promote well-being and comfort.

The use of Reiki as an integrative therapy in hospitals is increasing. Research and clinical experience show that it may help with treatment symptoms such as pain, anxiety and depression, fatigue, insomnia, and nausea.

Reiki should not be used to replace medical care or to postpone seeing a healthcare provider about a health problem. You are encouraged to tell your healthcare provider about any and all therapies you are using outside of your conventional care.

Reiki at the Zakim Center

The Reiki Practitioners at the Zakim Center are licensed massage therapists, who specialize in working with people with cancer. Reiki sessions are 45 minutes long and include a check-in with your therapist. Your first visit may require a bit more time to allow you and your practitioner to discuss:

- your medical history, treatment, laboratory results, and any pertinent information that will help your therapist provide you with a safe and effective session;
- any adjustments that may be needed to make you comfortable during your session;
- benefits of Reiki for your condition and symptoms;
- what your goals are for this session and/or ongoing sessions; and
- any questions that you might have before starting the Reiki session.

The Reiki session is generally done with hands on the body through one's clothing, but can also be done with hands off the body. When using Reiki with other touch modalities (such as massage), you can choose to receive it on exposed skin. Whether seated in a chair or receiving Reiki on a table, your comfort and safety is our first concern, and you are encouraged to discuss your comfort needs with the Reiki Practitioner.

(From: The Leonard P Zakim Center for Integrative Therapies and Healthy Living, Dana-Faber Cancer Institute. www.dana-farber.org).

Box 14.1B

At the end of the Reiki session, you will be encouraged to get up slowly, and your practitioner will give you privacy if you need to dress. Afterwards, your Reiki Practitioner will check in with you and see how you are doing, and will discuss:

- any questions you may have;
- observations, expectations, and recommendations; and
- resources that are available and may be appropriate for you.

(Continued)

Box 14.1B *(continued)*

To schedule a Reiki Appointment at the Zakim Center

To schedule a Reiki appointment, please call **617-632-3006**. Reiki services are available to Dana-Farber Patients only.

Cost of Reiki

We do not accept insurance for Reiki appointments. However, you may request a detailed receipt to submit to your insurance company for reimbursement if Reiki is a covered service. Adult patients pay $65 for each Reiki appointment. Reiki is complimentary to pediatric patients aged 21 and younger.

Thanks to the generosity of donors, financial assistance is available to those who qualify. For more information, please contact the Zakim Center office at **617-632-3322** or **Zakim_Center@dfci.harvard.edu**.

Additional information

National Center for Complementary and Integrative Health's "Reiki" Page

https://nccih.nih.gov/health/reiki-info

Reiki for Mind, Body, and Spirt Support of Cancer Patients

http://advancesjournal.com/pdfarticles/miles.pdf

To learn more about the Zakim Center's programs and services, please visit our website at **dana-farber.org/zakim**, e-mail **Zakim_Center@dfci.harvard.edu**, or call **617-632-3322**.

This document is for informational purpose only. The content is not intended as a substitute for professional medical advice, diagnosis, or treatment. Always seek the advice of your physician or other qualified health provider with any questions you may have regarding a medical condition.

(From: The Leonard P Zakim Center for Integrative Therapies and Healthy Living, Dana-Faber Cancer Institute. www.dana-farber.org).

Box 14.2

Where Reiki is provided in the Republic of Ireland

Reiki is used in many health settings. This is not a complete listing.

Reiki is used in the following Hospitals, Hospices and Nursing Homes:

- Cancer Information and Support Centre Limerick

Address: Mid-Western Regional Hospital, Dooradoyle, Limerick

- Cuisle Centre Portlaoise

Address: Block Road, Portlaoise, Co Laois

- Dochas Offaly Cancer Support
- Gort Cancer Support Centre

Address: The Hawthorn, Ennis Road, Gort, Co Galway

- Greystone Cancer Support Group

(Continued)

Address: La Touche Centre, Greystone, Co Wicklow

- Lios Aoibhinn Cancer Support Centre – Dublin

Address: St Vincents Hospital, Dublin

- Tuam Cancer Care Centre

Address: 30 Temple Jarlath Court, High Street, Tuam, Co Galway

- Sligo Cancer Support Centre

Address: 44 Wine Street, Sligo

Reiki has also been offered in Palliative Care in the following Hospitals and Hospices:

- Palliative Care: Glenaulin Nursing Home, Chapelizod.
- Palliative Care: Reiki for Staff of Palliative Care. Nurses, Physiotherapist, Administration Staff: Once a year in St Mary's Hospital. (Four years)
- Palliative Care: Reiki for Staff. St Josephs Hospital, Clonsilla, Dublin. (Once for afternoon)
- Palliative Care: Reiki for Staff in Hospice in Raheny, Dublin.
- Cancer Care: Irish Reiki Practitioner worked with Cancer Care in a Hospital in Sweden with a client.

Complementary Nurse is working in Palliative Care using a number of different therapies, Reiki included. We are a community based service which covers any location our patients are . . . . home, nursing home and hospital. Our team is multidisciplinary, made up of a consultant, doctors, clinical nurse specialists, physiotherapist, occupational therapist, social workers, dietician and nurse in complementary therapy.

Reiki is also used in St. Francis' Hospice Rehany, but not in Harold's Cross Hospice on an official basis. Reiki Practitioners have given Reiki to friends in Harold's Cross Hospice.

Reiki Practitioner when living in the UK offered Reiki to patients at a Marie Curie Hospice. Here, she gave Reiki to two male cancer patients so far, and later she would hope to be able to offer it in Hospices or in Cancer Support Groups.

Cancer Care: Four Reiki therapists work in Cancer Support Centre, Limerick.

(From: Reiki Federation Ireland. www.reikifederationireland.com/Where-Reiki-is-provided-in-Ireland.pdf).

References

Anderson DM, Loth AR, Stuart-Mullen LG, Thomley BS, Cutshall SM. Building a Reiki and Healing Touch volunteer program at an academic medical center. *Advances in Integrative Medicine* 2017; 4: 74–79.

Baldwin AL, Vitale A, Brownel E, Kryak E, Rand W. Effects of Reiki on pain, anxiety, and blood pressure in patients undergoing knee replacement surgery. *Holistic Nursing Practice* 2017; 31(2): 80–89.

Clark SC. An integral nursing education experience. Outcomes from a BSN Reiki course. *Reiki Holistic Nursing Practice* 2013; 27(1): 13–22.

Diaz-Rodríguez L, Arroyo-Morales M, Fernández-de-las-Peñas C, García-Lafuente F, García-Royo C, Tomás-Rojas I. Immediate effects of Reiki on heart rate variability, cortisol levels, and body temperature in healthcare professionals with burnout. *Biological Research for Nursing* 2011a; 13(4): 376–382.

Diaz-Rodriguez L, Arroyo-Morales M, Cantarero-Villanueva I, Férnandez-Lao C, Polley M, Fernández de-las-Peñas C. The application of Reiki in nurses diagnosed with Burnout Syndrome has beneficial effects on concentration of salivary IgA and blood pressure. *Revista Latino- Americana de Enfermagem* [online], 2011b; 19(5):1132–1138.

Gallob R. Reiki: a supportive therapy in nursing practice and self-care for nurses. *Journal of New York State Nurses Association* Spring/Summer 2003; 34(1): 9–13.

Hahn J, Reilly PM, Buchanan TM. Development of a hospital Reiki training program: training volunteers to provide Reiki to patients, families, and staff in the acute care setting. *Dimensions of Critical Care Nursing* 2014; 33(1): 15–21.

Johnson R, Fuerst R. Reiki at St. Charles Cancer Center. *Reiki News Magazine* Spring 2011; 36–40.

Kiecolt-Glaser JK, Page GG, Marucha PT, MacCallum RC, Glaser R. Psychological influences on surgical recovery: Perspectives from psychoneuroimmunology. *American Psychologist* 1998; 53: 1209–18.

Kundu A, Dolan-Oves R, Dimmers MA, Towle CB, Doorenbos AZ. Reiki training for caregivers of hospitalized pediatric patients: a pilot program. *Complementary Therapies in Clinical Practice* 2013; 19(1): 50–54.

Miles P. *Reiki in Hospitals: An Update,* April 15, 2017. Available at: reikiinmedicine.org/clinical-practice/reiki-in-hospitals-an-update.

Montross-Thomas LP, Meier E, Reynolds-Norolahi K, Raskin EE, Mills PJ, MacElhern L, Kallenberg G. Inpatients' preferences, beliefs and stated willingness to pay for complementary and alternative medicine treatments. *Journal of Alternative and Complementary Medicine* 2017; 23(4): 259–263.

Rosada RM, Rubik B, Mainguy B, Plummer J, Mehl-Madrona L. Reiki Reduces Burnout Among Community Mental Health Clinicians. *The Journal of Alternative and Complementary Medicine* 2015; 21(8): 489–495.

Ross C, Blau M, Sheridan K. Medicine with a side of mysticism: Top hospitals promote unproven therapies. *STAT News* March 7, 2017.

Vitale A. Nurses' lived experience of Reiki for self-care. *Holistic Nursing Practice* 2009; 23(3): 129–145.

Vitale A. Initiating a Reiki or CAM program in a healthcare organization – developing a business plan. *Holistic Nursing Practice* 2014; 28(6): 376–380.

Walburn J, Vedhara K, Hankins M, Rixon L, Weinman J. Psychological stress and wound healing in humans: a systematic review and meta-analysis. *Journal of Psychosomatic Research* 2009; 67(3): 253–271.

Zach H, Dirkx MF, Pasman JW, Bloem BR, Helmich RC. Cognitive Stress Reduces the Effect of Levodopa on Parkinson's Resting Tremor. *CNS Neuroscience & Therapeutics* 2017; 23(3): 209–215.

Chapter 15
Role of Basic Preclinical Research in Reiki

Scientific research is necessary for understanding and documenting how Reiki affects physiological and emotional well-being and also for determining a mechanism by which Reiki works. Although many Reiki practitioners do not think that they need this information to be effective healers, its lack is a handicap when it comes to Reiki's acceptance as an effective therapy in the medical field. That is because most clinicians are resistant to innovative principles outside the realm of established fact. So far, there is no tested scientific model for how Reiki works that fits our current understanding of chemical and physical principles, which increases resistance to Reiki by major decision-makers in public health.

Preclinical research on Reiki is essential for the following reasons:

- To define the characteristics of Reiki – under what conditions is it most effective?

- To provide physiological and psychological measures of Reiki's effects that quantify clinical outcomes. Here, animal studies should also be included to remove the effects of bias, expectation, prejudice, etc. from the data.

This chapter starts with a section about my personal experience of resistance to Reiki that was shown by scientists when I was ready to publish my first research paper on Reiki. It then leads in to the need for large scale clinical studies based on the requirements of the National Institutes of Health (NIH), the largest funder of biomedical and public health research in the world. The chapter ends with a list of physiological and psychological endpoints for use in future large scale research studies to determine the effectiveness of Reiki at improving all aspects of health.

Resistance to Reiki from Scientists: A Personal Experience

Although I had personally experienced real benefits of Reiki and was convinced that it promoted relaxation and pain relief, I soon discovered how resistant other scientists were to Reiki. This realization was highlighted when I was ready to submit my first manuscript describing the effects of Reiki on rats that had been stressed by their housing environment. After obtaining robust and reproducible quantitative results showing that Reiki reduced inflammation in rats, I was confident that the scientific world would be interested in this finding. The first journal I approached for publication was *Science*, the peer-reviewed academic journal of the American Association for the Advancement of Science and one of the world's top academic journals. Their website proclaims:

Publishing with us puts your best work in the company of the most cited and most discussed scientific research. It's the work that's read, covered, talked about and shared. Authors of papers that are not selected for in depth review are notified promptly, within about two weeks.

I was promptly notified of the rejection within two days. The next journal was *Nature*, an English multidisciplinary scientific journal ranked as the world's most-cited scientific journal. Once again, the editorial staff did not send the manuscript out for peer review. At this point I decided to contact the National Center for Complementary and Integrative Health (then the National Center for Complementary and Alternative Medicine), a part of NIH, who had funded the Reiki study, and ask their advice about where to submit my manuscript. They suggested *The British Medical Journal*. The personnel from *The British Medical Journal* were more polite in their rejection, informing me that although the study was interesting, it would not be of interest to their readers. I reluctantly decided to submit the paper to *The American Journal of Physiology* that had published 13 of my scientific papers in the past few years. I was reluctant because I knew that the readership of *The American Journal of Physiology* would be considerably smaller than that of the other, more prestigious journals I had tried. Although this time the manuscript was sent out for peer review, it was rejected following review. Both reviewers commented: "interesting but you have not demonstrated a physiological mechanism for its effect". This response surprised me. After all, the first clinical study on the active component of aspirin, salicylic acid, was published in 1763 (Stone, "An Account of the Success of the Bark of the Willow in the Cure of Agues") but its mechanism of action as an inflammatory agent was only discovered more than 200 years later, in 1971 by Robert Vane. So, why was the first study on the "success of Reiki in the cure of inflammation in rats" rejected on the basis that the mechanism had not yet been discovered? What was so different about Reiki compared to aspirin that made its effects on the body not worth reporting?

That was when I realized that my only option was to submit the paper to a journal specializing in complementary medicine; the disadvantage being that I would be preaching to the converted. This time the manuscript was accepted, with barely any revision required, by *The Journal of Complementary and Alternative Medicine* in 2006, for which I am grateful. By the end of 2006, there were 18 published peer-reviewed scientific studies on Reiki, 11 (61%) of which appeared in journals focusing on complementary and integrative medicine. Currently, there are 77 published peer-reviewed research studies on Reiki, and 32 (41%) appear in journals associated with complementary and integrative medicine. Most of the remaining papers appear in nursing journals, so it is still very difficult to break out of the restricted enclave of specialized journals that appeal to integrative healthcare practitioners rather than to a more general readership.

The Need for Large Scale Studies

Givers and receivers of Reiki experience first-hand, the benefits of Reiki for mind and body. However, people who are not familiar with Reiki may be doubtful that it can help them because it is not generally offered to patients by medical practitioners nor paid for by medical insurance. In order for Reiki to become an established, routine therapy that is widely available on request, its benefits must be evidence-based rather than just anecdotal. Although, as

demonstrated in this book, a body of supportive research evidence is emerging, it is still not adequate at this point to break through the threshold of acceptance by skeptical medical professionals.

The National Center for Complementary and Integrative Health (NCCIH) is the main institution in the USA that provides grant funds for medical research addressing complementary and alternative therapies such as Reiki, acupuncture, Chinese herbs, yoga, etc. At first glance, it would seem that NCCIH would be supportive of efforts to enhance the standing of Reiki in the public eye. However, on the contrary, NCCIH has a Reiki fact sheet available on its website (https://nccih.nih.gov/health/reiki-info) that states:

Reiki hasn't been clearly shown to be useful for any health-related purpose. [...] There's no scientific evidence supporting the existence of the energy field thought to play a role in Reiki.

This attitude is surprising considering that there are currently 77 peer-reviewed published papers on Reiki research, the vast majority of which show positive results. When NCCIH was asked in 2016 for evidence supporting its negative statements about Reiki, an NCCIH official replied that the comments were based on a lack of Reiki research studies that fit the following criteria:

- Must be published within the last five years

- The study size must be large

- The study must be a randomized clinical trial, etc.

"Published Within the Last Five Years"

Although there are currently 26 peer-reviewed research articles on Reiki published within the last five years, 2015–2019 (see www.centerforreikiresearch.org), all except three are "pilot studies". A pilot study is a small-scale preliminary study conducted in order to evaluate feasibility, time, cost, adverse events, and effect size (statistical variability) in an attempt to predict an appropriate sample size and improve upon the study design prior to performance of a full-scale research project (Hulley, 2007). Pilot experiments are frequently carried out before large scale research in an attempt to avoid time and money being wasted on an inadequately designed project.

"The Study Size Must be Large"

The term "large" is rather vague. A website (clinicaltrials. gov) that lists NCCIH-funded clinical trials reveals that there are currently seven completed clinical trials involving Reiki. Clinical trials are designed with large numbers of subjects to remove the bias that could occur on a study with small subject sampling. This helps to rule out the effects of random samples or outliers in the experimental results. The numbers of participants enrolled in the seven completed Reiki clinical trials listed on clinicaltrials.gov are: 26, 30, 79, 100, 146, 207, and 257. The numbers 26 and 30 are definitely not large, so based on the other numbers, "large" appears to be about 100–300 participants. The exact number will depend on the number of experimental groups in the protocol. The greater the number of groups in the experimental design, the more participants will be required to account for statistical variation between people in the measured parameters. Large studies obviously require far more funding than pilot studies.

"The Study Must be a Randomized Clinical Trial"

By including the word "randomized" the NCCIH is implying that there will be at least two groups in the study, one of which will be a "control" group, and the participants will be allocated to each group at random. Control is a vital element of a well-designed experiment because there needs to be a way to rule out the effects of extraneous variables other than the ones being studied. The control group usually receives a placebo or no treatment at all. In a double-blind, controlled clinical trial, neither the patient nor the researcher knows who is receiving the real treatment, and who the placebo.

A placebo is a substance or treatment with no active therapeutic effect (Oxford University Press). A placebo may be given to a person in order to deceive the recipient into thinking that it is an active treatment. In medical research, a placebo can be made to resemble an active therapy so that it functions as a control, in that it prevents the recipient and others from knowing (with their consent), whether the treatment is active or inactive. Consequently, there will be no added expectation of efficacy that can influence results. In randomized controlled trials, the participants are allocated by chance alone to receive the placebo or experimental intervention, or no treatment. If the assignment is not randomized, and people choose which group they are in, then there may be significant differences between the groups that will affect the results. For example, if one group in a hypothetical experiment to test effects of exercise on blood pressure were asked to walk half a mile and a second group three miles, then the second group would almost certainly attract people who were younger and fitter than those in the first group and this would affect the results.

Controlled experiments with Reiki are complicated by the possibility that sham Reiki, in which a person untrained in Reiki pretends to give the patient Reiki using the same hand positions as a Reiki practitioner, may also have a therapeutic effect. For example, previous studies showed that simple touch may reduce patients' self-reported anxiety (Weze et al., 2004; Henricson et al., 2008; Lindgren et al., 2013). Touch alone may also reduce self-reported pain (Baldwin et al., 2013), but pain relief induced by touch has not been shown to last very long (Fishman et al., 1995; Baldwin et al., 2013; 2017). In addition, there is currently no published evidence that simple touch (not including healing touch or therapeutic touch, or studies involving touching between friends and relatives), reduces physiological measures related to stress (such as elevated blood pressure or cortisol concentrations). Thus, although sham Reiki has some therapeutic benefits, Reiki appears to

Chapter 15

be more effective than sham Reiki based on current pilot studies (Dressen and Singg, 1998; Witte and Dundes, 2001; Shore, 2004; Mackay et al., 2004; Diaz-Rodríguez et al., 2011; Sagkal and Ganduzoglu, 2016; Baldwin et al., 2006; 2008; 2013; 2017).

Scientific Status of Reiki Based on NCCIH Criteria

There are three large scale Reiki clinical research studies that have been published within the last five years:

- **Kurebayashi et al., 2016.** This study was performed on 122 cancer survivors who were divided into three treatment groups: massage with rest, massage with Reiki, and standard of care (SOC). The combination of massage and Reiki was somewhat better than massage alone at reducing pain, and both were better than SOC.

- **Charkhandeh et al., 2016.** This study was performed on 188 adolescents who were divided into three treatment groups: cognitive behavioral therapy (CBT), Reiki, and SOC. Four hours of Reiki treatment was just as effective as 36 hours of CBT at reducing depression, and both were better than SOC.

- **Chirico et al., 2017.** This study was performed on 110 cancer patients who were divided into two treatment groups: Reiki and SOC. Anxiety was significantly decreased in the patients who received Reiki, whereas anxiety was either increased or stayed the same in patients in the control group. Of the patients in the Reiki group, the calming benefit of Reiki was enhanced in those who also had good self-coping skills.

These three large scale clinical studies do support the use of Reiki for reducing pain, depression and anxiety, but it is obvious that more such studies are needed, and this may explain the negative viewpoint of NCCIH regarding the effectiveness of Reiki.

Scientific Status of Reiki is Based Largely on Results of Pilot Studies

There are currently 77 peer-reviewed research articles published on Reiki (1989–2019). Seventeen trials included Reiki and SOC groups, 11 included Reiki and sham Reiki groups, 10 included Reiki, sham Reiki and SOC groups (plus another two studies on animals) and six included groups receiving Reiki, sham Reiki, or some other modality. Of the higher quality studies, those comparing Reiki to at least sham Reiki or SOC largely support the hypothesis that Reiki may help in reducing pain, burnout, and, in some cases, anxiety and depression, and in increasing relaxation and well-being. For this reason, it is worthwhile extending the more promising pilot studies to develop further large scale randomized controlled clinical trials. Only through successful, scientifically robust, large scale clinical trials is there a chance that the decision makers at the top scientific and medical institutions may eventually be convinced to support the widespread use of Reiki in hospitals, clinics, and hospices.

It should be noted that presently there are three additional large scale clinical trials, funded by NCCIH, that are recruiting participants. This means that although the attitude of NCCIH officers as reflected by their Reiki Fact Sheet seems bleak, they are definitely still open to giving Reiki a chance.

Physiological and Psychological Measures for Monitoring Reiki's Effects

In preparation for development of further high quality, large scale clinical trials on Reiki, here is a short description of the physiological and psychological measures that are routinely used to evaluate new therapies in the clinic. Only by utilizing these tried and tested outcome parameters that are accepted by all scientists in the medical field, will the quality of future Reiki research reach a level that merits serious consideration.

Physiological Measures

Experiments have indicated that Reiki improves relaxation and decreases anxiety. These responses are mediated through the autonomic nervous system (ANS) and hypothalamus–pituitary–adrenal (HPA) axis. The ANS is the part of the nervous system that regulates the organs, including the heart, as well as glands, and the smooth muscle of blood vessels and airways. It has two components: sympathetic and parasympathetic. The sympathetic nerves increase body arousal when stimulated, resulting in increased heart rate, blood pressure, dilation of the airways and dilation of the pupils. The parasympathetic nerves calm down the body, slowing the heart, reducing blood pressure, and promoting salivation and digestion of food. This response is commonly known as "rest and digest". Physiological measures for assessing the ANS are listed as follows:

- Heart rate

- Heart rate variability (the degree to which heart rate varies with time)

- Blood pressure (systolic and diastolic)

- Respiration rate

- Skin conductance (the ease with which an electric current can pass between two electrodes placed on the skin when a potential difference, or voltage, is applied). Skin conductance increases with sweating and is related to arousal of the sympathetic nervous system.

When a person becomes calmer, or less aroused, their heart rate, respiration rate, blood pressure, and skin conductance all decrease. Their heart rate variability (HRV) increases, indicating that in a relaxed state, their heart is able to rapidly adapt to second-by-second changes in the body's need for oxygen and other nutrients. A high HRV means that the sympathetic and parasympathetic nerves are working alternately to increase and decrease cardiac output as dictated by the body's needs. It is rather like driving in traffic; sometimes your foot is on the accelerator, and sometimes on the brake. Sometimes heart rate is going up and sometimes down and that is why the variability (HRV) is high. When a person becomes stressed, one of the components (usually sympathetic) becomes dominant, so that heart rate, respiration rate, and blood pressure all increase. The foot is mostly on the accelerator. Heart rate variability is low because the parasympathetic nerves never get a chance to bring the heart rate down. Experiments conducted so far in which participants have been given one or more Reiki sessions, have largely produced a relaxation response as judged by the reactions of the ANS.

The HPA axis is also stimulated by stress, and one well-known response is the release of the stress hormone, cortisol. One function of cortisol is to help the body metabolize carbohydrates to provide energy, which is obviously vital in times of stress. However, too much cortisol in the bloodstream too much of the time has many deleterious effects, such as suppressing the immune response, increasing body fat stores, elevating blood sugar (sometimes leading to type 2 diabetes), depleting skeletal muscles, causing osteoporosis, increasing cholesterol deposits in the artery (coronary artery disease) and damaging neurons in the hippocampus, leading to memory loss. Data are scarce on the effects of Reiki on concentrations of cortisol in the saliva and blood and more experiments need to be conducted. If Reiki produces a calming effect, we would expect to see decreases in cortisol concentrations.

Other physiological measures that have been used to test the effects of Reiki as a healing modality are:

- Neutrophil and white blood cell counts (to demonstrate effectiveness of the immune response)

- Skin blood flow in the fingertips. Blood flow in the skin of the fingertips of Reiki Masters markedly increased when they performed Reiki on themselves, indicating dilation of the finger blood vessels, and consistent with the feeling of heat in the hands that is commonly observed by givers and receivers of Reiki (Baldwin and Schwartz, 2012).

- Skin temperature

- Blood hemoglobin and hematocrit

- Range of motion (ROM) of arm elevation in the scapular plane (in participants already diagnosed with limited ROM due to shoulder injuries, arthritis, etc.). In this study, a single session of Reiki was just as effective as a single session of physical therapy in significantly improving ROM (Baldwin et al., 2013).

- Theta brainwaves as assessed from electroencephalogram. Theta brainwaves occur most often in sleep but are also dominant in deep meditation.

- Microvascular permeability in rats. Microvascular permeability refers to the degree to which substances can pass through the walls of tiny blood vessels from the blood to surrounding tissue. In this case, microvascular permeability was abnormally enhanced due to an inflammatory response, and Reiki significantly reduced the microvascular permeability (Baldwin and Schwartz, 2006).

Psychological Measures

In the opinion of the author, psychological measures are not as convincing as physiological measures because they are not objective, as they rely on self-report. However, they are useful because they do add a more personal dimension to the scientific evaluation of Reiki's effects on human beings.

- Self-Reported Pain level (VAS)

- Trace State Anxiety Inventory

- State-Trait Anxiety Inventory

- State Anxiety Scale

- Spielberger State Anxiety Inventory

- Vasconcelo's Stress Symptom List

- Perceived Stress Scale

- Beck Depression Inventory

- CES Depression Scale

- Maslach Burnout Inventory

- Annotated Mini Mental State Examination

- Well-Being Questionnaire

Where Do We Go From Here?

Reiki research has now reached a point at which sufficient promising pilot data have been obtained to support the funding of the large scale clinical trials that are needed to provide scientific validation for offering Reiki routinely in hospitals, hospices, and clinics. If the results of further large scale studies are positive, there is a chance that Reiki will become employed more routinely as an adjunct to allopathic medicine. Reiki would best be used in this way to reduce stress and anxiety, to relieve pain and inflammation and to improve physiological and psychological well-being. According to William Lee Rand ("Reiki and the Future", *Reiki News Articles*, The International Center for Reiki Training, 2019):

The current attitude is so positive for Reiki and other alternative practices in the US that this trend will certainly grow. I predict that in a short time, Reiki will be offered at most hospitals across the US. In addition, health insurance programs are now looking at Reiki as a possible insurance benefit. As soon as a few add it, the competitive nature of the health insurance industry will cause all of them to include Reiki. Then health insurance will pay for Reiki treatments. The need for Reiki practitioners will grow quickly and Reiki will have become established as a normal part of healthcare in the US. This will happen easily within the next 10 years!

References

Baldwin AL, Schwartz GE. Personal interaction with a Reiki practitioner decreases noise-induced microvascular damage in an animal model. *The Journal of Alternative and Complementary Medicine* 2006; 12(1): 15–22.

Baldwin AL, Wagers C, Schwartz GE. Reiki improves heart rate homeostasis in laboratory rats. *The Journal of Alternative and Complementary Medicine* 2008; 14(4): 417–422.

Baldwin AL, Schwartz GE. Physiological changes in energy healers during self-practice. *Complementary Therapies in Medicine* 2012; 20: 299–305.

Baldwin AL, Fullmer K, Schwartz GE. Comparison of physical therapy with energy healing for improving range of motion in subjects with restricted shoulder mobility. *Journal of Evidence-Based Complementary and Alternative Medicine* 2013; 2013: 329731.

Baldwin AL, Vitale A, Brownell E, Rand W. Effects of Reiki on pain, anxiety and blood pressure in knee replacement patients. *Holistic Nursing Practice* 2017; 31(2): 80–89.

Charkhandeh M, Talib, MA, Hunt CJ. The clinical evidence of cognitive behavior therapy and an alternative medicine approach in reducing symptoms of depression in adolescents. *Psychiatry Research* 2016; 239: 325–330.

Chirico, A, D'Aiuto G, Penon A, Mallia L, De Laurentiis M, Lucidi F, Botti G, Giordano A. Self-efficacy for coping with cancer enhances the effect of Reiki treatments during the pre-surgery phase of breast cancer patients. *Anticancer Research* 2017; 37(7): 3657–3665.

Diaz-Rodríguez L, Arroyo-Morales M, Fernández-de-las-Peñas C, García-Lafuente F, García-Royo C, Tomás-Rojas I. Immediate effects of Reiki on heart rate variability, cortisol levels, and body temperature in healthcare professionals with burnout. *Biological Research for Nursing* 2011; 13: 376–382.

Dressen LJ, Singg S. Effects of Reiki on pain and selected affective and personality variables of chronically ill patients. *Subtle Energies & Energy Medicine* 1998; 9(1): 53–82.

Fishman E, Turkheimer E, DeGood DE. Touch relieves stress and pain. *Journal of Behavioral Medicine* 1995; 18(1): 69–79.

Henricson M, Ersson A, Maata S, Segesten K, Bergland AL. The outcome of tactile touch on stress parameters in intensive care: a randomized controlled trial. *Complementary Therapies in Clinical Practice* 2008; 14(4): 244–254.

Hulley SB. *Designing Clinical Research.* Lippincott Williams & Wilkins, 2007, pp.168–169.

Kurebayashi, LFS, Turrini, RNT, Souza, TPB, Takiguchi, RS, Kuba, G, Nagumo, MT. Massage and Reiki used to reduce stress and anxiety: randomized clinical trial. 2016; *Revista Latino-Americana de Enfermagem* 24: e2834.

Lindgren L, Lehtipalo S, Winso O, Karlsson M, Wiklund U, Brulin C. Touch massage: a pilot study of a complex intervention. *Nursing in Critical Care* 2013; 18(6): 269–277.

Mackay N, Hansen S, McFarlane O. Autonomic nervous system changes during Reiki treatment: a preliminary study. *The Journal of Alternative and Complementary Medicine* 2004; 10(6): 1077–1081.

Sagkal MT, Ganduzoglu N. Effects of Reiki on pain and vital signs when applied to the incision area of the body after Cesarean section surgery: a single-blinded, randomized, double-controlled study. *Holistic Nursing Practice* 2016; 30(6): 368–378.

Shore AG. Long-term effects of energetic healing on symptoms of psychological depression and self-perceived stress. *Alternative Therapies in Health and Medicine* 2004; 10(3): 42–48.

Stone E. An Account of the Success of the Bark of the Willow in the Cure of Agues. In a Letter to the Right Honourable George Earl of Macclesfield, President of R. S. from the Rev. Mr. Edmund Stone, of Chipping-Norton in Oxfordshire. *Philosophical Transactions (1683-1775)*, 1763; 53: 195–200.

Weze C, Leathard HL, Grange J, Tiplady P, Stevens G. Evaluation of healing by gentle touch in 33 clients with cancer. *European Journal of Oncology Nursing* 2004; 8(1): 40–49.

Witte D, Dundes L. Harnessing life energy or wishful thinking? Reiki, placebo Reiki, meditation and music. *Alternative and Complementary Therapies* 2001; 7(5): 304–309.

INDEX

Index *continued*